Encyclopedia of Neuroimaging: Cognitive Neuroscience

Volume I

Encyclopedia of Neuroimaging: Cognitive Neuroscience
Volume I

Edited by **Miles Scott**

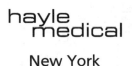

New York

Published by Hayle Medical,
30 West, 37th Street, Suite 612,
New York, NY 10018, USA
www.haylemedical.com

Encyclopedia of Neuroimaging: Cognitive Neuroscience
Volume I
Edited by Miles Scott

International Standard Book Number: 978-1-63241-182-2 (Hardback)

Contents

Preface

Every book is a source of knowledge and this one is no exception. The idea that led to the conceptualization of this book was the fact that the world is advancing rapidly; which makes it crucial to document the progress in every field. I am aware that a lot of data is already available, yet, there is a lot more to learn. Hence, I accepted the responsibility of editing this book and contributing my knowledge to the community.

The cognitive neurosciences of neuroimaging are described in this all-inclusive book. The rate of technological advancement is stimulating increasingly comprehensive lines of enquiry in cognitive neuroscience, which displays no sign of slowing down in the distant future. However, it is unlikely that even the most powerful advocates of the cognitive neuroscience approach would maintain that developments in cognitive theory have kept in step with techniques-based advancements. There are numerous reasons for the failure of neuroimaging studies to satisfactorily resolve a number of most significant theoretical debates in the literature. For example, a crucial proportion of published functional magnetic resonance imaging (fMRI) studies are not well explained in cognitive theory, and this depicts a step away from the conventional approach in experimental psychology of systematically and technically building on (or chipping away at) present theoretical models using authentic methodologies. Unless, the experimental analysis design is set up within a vividly outlined theoretical framework, any inferences that are drawn are unlikely to be accepted as anything other than analytical. The book includes excellent research chapters on images of the cognitive brain across age and culture, functional and structural magnetic resonance, neuroimaging and outcome assessments, and cognitive and psychological functions of sleep.

While editing this book, I had multiple visions for it. Then I finally narrowed down to make every chapter a sole standing text explaining a particular topic, so that they can be used independently. However, the umbrella subject sinews them into a common theme. This makes the book a unique platform of knowledge.

I would like to give the major credit of this book to the experts from every corner of the world, who took the time to share their expertise with us. Also, I owe the completion of this book to the never-ending support of my family, who supported me throughout the project.

Editor

1

Cytoarchitectonics of the Human Cerebral Cortex: The 1926 Presentation by Georg N. Koskinas (1885–1975) to the Athens Medical Society

Lazaros C. Triarhou
University of Macedonia, Thessaloniki
Greece

1. Introduction

The Greek neurologist-psychiatrist Georg N. Koskinas (1885–1975) is better known for his collaboration with Constantin von Economo (1876–1931) on the cytoarchitectonic study of the human cerebral cortex (von Economo & Koskinas, 1925, 2008). Koskinas seems to have been one of those classically unrecognised and unrewarded figures of science (Jones, 2008, 2010). Such an injustice has been remedied in part in recent years (Triarhou, 2005, 2006). The

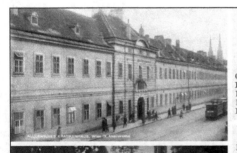
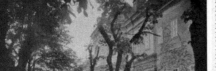

Mitgliederverzeichnis
des Vereines für Psychiatrie und Neurologie in Wien
(Stand: Juli 1926)

Ehrenmitglieder

CAJAL, RAMON Y (Madrid).   MARIE, PIERRE (Paris).
DERCUM, FRANCIS (Philadelphia).   MINGAZZINI, GIOVANNI (Rom).
HEAD, HENRY (London).   NONNE, MAX (Hamburg).
KRAEPELIN, EMIL (München).   STARR, ALLEN (New-York).
LAEHR, MAX (Wernigerode).   WILSON, S. KINNIER (London).

Ordentliche Mitglieder

KALMUS, ERNST, Ob.-Bez.-Arzt, Prag, Podskalerstr. 335.
KARPLUS, JOHANN PAUL, Prof., Wien I, Oppolzerstraße 6.
KATTINGER, OTTO, Dr., Gräfenberg b. Freiwaldau, Sanatorium.
KAUDERS, OTTO, Assistent, Wien IX, Lazarettgasse 14.
KLEBELSBERG, ERNST, Dr., Hall in Tirol, Landes-Heilanstalt.
KLUGE, EDWIN, Direktor, Tobelbad bei Graz.
KNÖPFELMACHER, WILHELM, Prof., Wien IX, Günthergasse 3.
KOGERER, HEINRICH, Assistent, Wien IX, Schwarzspanierstraße 9.
KOHN, ALFRED, Dr., Inzersdorf bei Wien, Sanatorium.
KOLBEN, SIEGFRIED, Hofrat, Wien XIX, Döblinger Hauptstraße 71.
KORNER, FRIEDRICH, Dr., Wien I, Rathausstraße 20.
KOSKINAS, GEORG, Dr., Wien VIII, Alserstraße 43.
KOVACS, FRIEDRICH, Prof., Hofrat, Wien I, Spiegelgasse 3.
KURE, SHUZO, Prof., Tokio, Psych. Klinik.
KURZ-GOLDENSTEIN, Primarius, Niederhart b. Linz, Irrenanstalt.

Fig. 1. The Vienna General Hospital on the left, where Koskinas worked between 1916 and 1927 under the supervision of Julius Wagner von Jauregg (1857–1940) and Ernst Sträussler (1872–1959) (author's archive). The 1926 roster of the Vienna Society for Psychiatry and Neurology on the right, showing Koskinas as a regular member (Hartmann et al., 1926)

year 2010 has marked the 125th birthday anniversary of Koskinas (1 December 1885) and the centennial of his graduation from the University of Athens (M.D., 1910).

As soon as the Atlas and Textbook of Cytoarchitectonics were published in 1925, Koskinas briefly returned to Greece and donated a set to the Athens Medical Society. On that occasion, he delivered a keynote address, which summarises the main points of his research with von Economo. That address (Koskinas, 1926) forms the main focus of this paper. There are only two other presentations known to have been made by Koskinas: one with von Economo at the Society for Psychiatry and Neurology in Vienna in February 1923 (von Economo & Koskinas, 1923), presenting an initial summary of cytoarchitectonic findings on the granularity of sensory cortical areas especially in layers II and IV; and the other with Sträussler at the 88th Meeting of the German Natural Scientists and Physicians in Innsbruck in September 1924 (Sträussler & Koskinas, 1925), reporting histopathological findings on the experimental malaria treatment of patients with general paralysis from neurosyphilis.

2. The 1926 presentation by Koskinas

The following is an exact English translation of the *Proceedings* of the Athens Medical Society, Session of Saturday, 23 January 1926, rendered from the original Greek text (Koskinas, 1926) by the author of the present chapter.

2.1 Introductory comment by Constantin Mermingas, presiding

"I am in the gratifying position of announcing an exceptional donation, made to the Society by the colleague Dr. G. Koskinas, sojourning in Athens; having temporarily come from Vienna, he brought with him a copy, as voluminous as you see, but also as valuable, of the truly monumental compilation, produced by the two Hellenic scientists in Vienna, C. Economo and G. Koskinas, who is among us today. It involves the book—text volume and atlas—*Cytoarchitektonik der Hirnrinde des erwachsenen Menschen*, about the value of which we had learnt from reviews published in foreign journals, but also convinced directly. Dr. Koskinas deserves our warm thanks, as well as our gratitude, for being willing to deliver a synopsis of that original scientific research and achievement."

2.2 Main lecture by Georg N. Koskinas, keynote speaker

"Thanks to the ardour of the honourable President of the Society, Professor Dr. Mermingas, who is meritoriously making every attempt to highlight the Society as a centre of noble emulation in scientific research and the promotion of science and at the encouragement of whom I have the honour of being a guest at the Society today. Enchanted by that, I owe acknowledgments because you are offering me the opportunity to briefly occupy you in person about the work published by Professor von Economo and myself in German, and deposited to the chair of the Society, "The Cytoarchitectonics of the Human Cerebral Cortex" *(Die Cytoarchitektonik der Hirnrinde des erwachsenen Menschen)*. An attempt on my behalf to analyse that work requires much time and many auxiliary media which, simply hither passing through, I lack. That is why I wish to confine myself, such that I very briefly cover the following simply and to the extent possible.

Cytoarchitectonics of the Human Cerebral Cortex: The 1926 Presentation by Georg N. Koskinas (1885–1975) to the Athens Medical Society

3

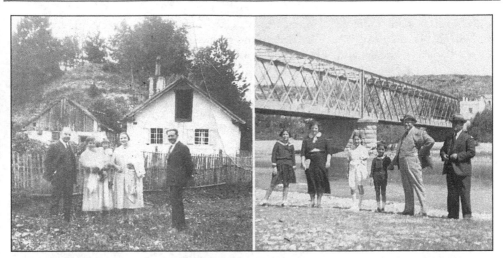

Fig. 2. Previously unpublished photographs of Koskinas and family members. The left photograph, taken in Vienna around 1926, shows Koskinas (first from the right) with his wife Stefanie, their daughter, his sister Paraskevi and her husband. The right photograph shows Koskinas (second from the right) in the Peloponnese in the 1940s — the bridge of the Eurotas River appears in the background — with his wife and daughter (left), and the children of his sister Irene and their father (photos courtesy of Rena Kostopoulou)

2.2.1 Incentives and aim
The incomplete and largely imperfect knowledge of the histological structure of the brain constituted the main reason that led us to its detailed architectonic research, and its ultimate goal was the localisation, to the extent possible, of the various cerebral functions and the pathological changes in mental disorders, as well as the interpretation of numerous problems, such as individual mental attributes, i.e. the talent in mathematics, music, rhetoric, etc.

2.2.2 Methods
At the outset of our studies we came across various obstacles and difficulties deriving on one hand from the very structure of the brain and on the other from the deficiency of the hitherto available research means. That is why we were obliged to modify numerous of the known means, to incise absolutely new paths, taking advantage of any possible means towards a precise, reliable and indelible rendition of nature. We modelled an entire system of new methods of brain research from the autopsy to the definitive photographic documentation of the preparations. Thus, we were able to not only solve many of the problems, but also, and above all, to provide to anyone interested various topics for investigation, as well as the manner for exploring them.

Allow me to mention some of the employed research means.

Sectioning method. Instead of the hitherto used method of sectioning the whole brain serially perpendicular to its fronto-occipital axis (Fig. 5), whereby gyri are rarely sectioned perpendicularly, we effected the sections always perpendicular to the surface of each gyrus and in directions corresponding to their convoluted pattern (Fig. 6). We arrived at that act by the idea that, in order to compare various parts of the brain cytoarchitectonically, sections must be oriented perpendicularly to the surface of the gyri, insofar as only then is provided precisely the breadth of both the overall cerebral cortex and of each cortical layer.

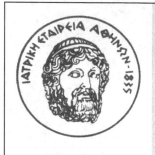

Ἰστολογία καὶ φυσιολογία τοῦ ἐγκεφάλου. Κατὰ τὴν συνεδρίαν τῆς 23ης Ἰανουαρίου 1926 ὁ Γ. Κοσκινᾶς ἐδώρησε τῇ Ἑταιρείᾳ ἐν ἀντίτυπον τοῦ συγγράμματος «Ἡ κυτταροαρχιτεκτονικὴ τοῦ φλοιοῦ τοῦ ἐγκεφάλου τοῦ ἀνθρώπου», ἐν συνεργασίᾳ μετὰ τοῦ Οἰκονόμου, ἐν Βιέννῃ δημοσιευθέντος, καὶ ἀνέπτυξεν ἀκολούθως τὴν ἀφετηρίαν καὶ τὸν σκοπὸν τοῦ ἔργου, τὸν τρόπον τῆς ἐρεύνης, τὰ ἐπιτευχθέντα καὶ προσδοκώμενα ἀποτελέσματα. Κατὰ τὴν συνεδρίαν τῆς 12ης Ἀπριλίου 1930 ὁ M. Minkowski, Καθηγητὴς τῆς Νευρολογίας ἐν τῷ Πανεπιστημίῳ τῆς Ζυρίχης διαλέγεται τὸ θέμα «ὀφθαλμὸς καὶ ἐγκέφαλος» προσκομίσας τῇ Ἑταιρείᾳ τὰ πορίσματα τῶν ἐρευνῶν του ἀπὸ φυλοοντογονικῆς, ἀνατομικῆς, φυσιολογικῆς ἅμα δὲ καὶ κλινικῆς ἀπόψεως.

ΣΥΝΕΔΡΙΑ 23ΗΣ ΙΑΝΟΥΑΡΙΟΥ 1926
ΠΡΟΕΔΡΕΙΑ Κ. ΜΕΡΜΗΓΚΑ

Γίνονται (παμψηφεὶ) δεκτοὶ ὡς τακτικοὶ ἑταῖροι οἱ Κοι Α. Θρου βάλας, Α. Κατσαρός, Κ. Μαχαίρας, Α. Φραγκούλης καὶ ἡ Δις Σ. Λεμπέση.

1) Πρόεδρος: Εὑρίσκομαι εἰς τὴν εὐάρεστον θέσιν ὅπως ἀναγγείλω ἐξαιρετικὴν δωρεάν, γενομένην πρὸς τὴν Ἑταιρείαν ἐκ μέρους τοῦ παρεπιδημοῦντος ἐν Ἀθήναις συναδέλφου Κου Γ. Κοσκινᾶ, ὅστις, ἐλθὼν προσκαίρως ἐκ Βιέννης, ἐκόμισε μεθ' ἑαυτοῦ ἵνα δωρήσῃ πρὸς τὴν Ἑταιρείαν ἡμῶν ἓν ἀντίτυπον, τοσοῦτον ὀγκῶδες ὡς βλέπετε, ἀλλὰ καὶ τοσοῦτον πολύτιμον, τῆς ὄντως μνημειώδους συγγραφῆς, ἣν παρήγαγον δύο Ἕλληνες ἐπιστήμονες ἐν Βιέννῃ, ὁ Κ. Οἰκονόμος καὶ ὁ μεταξὺ ἡμῶν σήμερον εὑρισκόμενος Γ. Κοσκινᾶς. Πρόκειται περὶ τοῦ συγγράμματος, βιβλίου καὶ ἄτλαντος, «Cytoarchitektonik der Hirn-

Fig. 3. The *Proceedings* of the Athens Medical Society for the Session of 23 January 1926

Staining method. The staining of the preparations was perfected by us such that a uniform tone was achieved not only of a single section, but of all the countless series of sections into which each brain was cut for study. And that was absolutely mandatory, on one hand in order to define the gradual differences of the histological elements of the neighbouring areas of the cerebral cortex, and on the other hand to achieve a consistent photographic representation.

Specimen depiction method. The hitherto occasional histological investigations of the brain depicted things schematically and therefore subjectively. Instead of such a schematic depiction, aiming at a precise representation of the preparations with all the relationships of the countless and polymorphous cells, we used photography. Photographic documentation constitutes the most truthful testimony of the exact depiction of nature, providing truly objective images of things as they bear in natural form, size and arrangement (Fig. 7). But to succeed in the photographic method it became necessary to turn to the study of branches foreign to medicine, such as advanced optics and photochemistry. We took advantage of both of these as much as we could. Lenses, light beams, filters, photographic plates and finally the photographic paper itself were all adopted towards the accomplishment of the intended goal of the most perfect, i.e. the photographic, depiction.

Cytoarchitectonics of the Human Cerebral Cortex: The 1926 Presentation by Georg N. Koskinas (1885–1975) to the Athens Medical Society

5

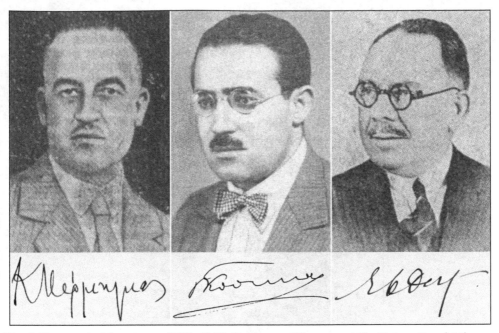

Fig. 4. Constantin Mermingas (1874–1942), Professor of Surgery at the University of Athens and President of the Athens Medical Society (left), Georg N. Koskinas (1885–1975) in the centre, and Spyridon Dontas (1878–1958), Professor of Physiology and Pharmacology at the University of Athens and President of the Academy of Athens (right). © 1957 *Helios Encyclopaedical Lexicon* (signatures from the author's archive)

2.2.3 Accomplished and anticipated results

Through our work an extremely precise and detailed description was achieved of the normal histological structure of the cerebral cortex as it is depicted in the photographic plates and explained in the text. Our photographic plates in the atlas, as such, constitute an ageless, imprescriptible opus, the basis and the control of any future research on the cerebral cortex. Whatever in such research is in agreement with the plates, must be considered as normal, and whatever diverges constitutes a pathological condition. From that precise knowledge of the architectonic structure of the cerebral cortex, which we achieved, it is allowable to anticipate the solution of numerous and different questions and issues of utmost importance; from their endless number I suffice in mentioning e.g. the following.

a. *The problem of problems, i.e. the problem of the psyche.* When, as anatomists and physiologists, we speak of the psyche, we do not refer to it as a metaphysical being that finds itself a priori outside any anatomical and physiological weight, but as a moral, mental, active and historical personality which interacts with others and influences ourselves.

b. *The problem of individual mental attributes, i.e. intellectual talents,* such as rhetoric, music, mathematics, delinquency and the variations in the mental development of human phyla on the earth. By comparing e.g. the centres of music in individuals who genetically present a total lack of music perception to individuals who possess an evolved musical talent we may exactly pinpoint differences in such music centres.

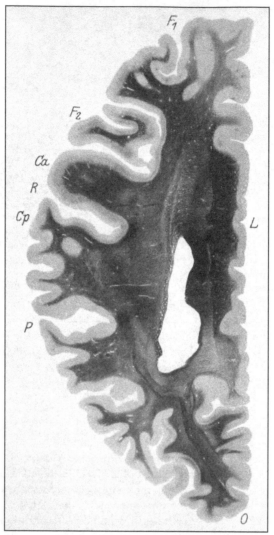

Fig. 5. Horizontal section through the left human cerebral hemisphere, depicting the sizeable regional differences in cortical thickness and the random orientation of the gyri (Koskinas, 2009). Weigert method. F_1 and F_2, superior and middle frontal gyrus; Ca, precentral gyrus; R, central sulcus; Cp, postcentral gyrus, P, parietal lobe; O, occipital lobe; L, limbic gyrus

c. *The problem of pathological lesions in numerous mental disorders* both primarily and secondarily encountered in the brain.

d. *The problem of the localisation of various centres.* The various localisations of sensation, movement, stereognosis, speech, etc., which thus far were mostly defined without an exact histological control, from now on, admittedly, can be readily and precisely defined on the basis of the cerebral cortical areas that we have designated, which from a total number of 52 known thus far we brought to 107 (Fig. 8–10). The solution of this

Cytoarchitectonics of the Human Cerebral Cortex: The 1926 Presentation by Georg N. Koskinas (1885–1975) to the Athens Medical Society

7

problem also possesses utmost sense, insofar as in that way diagnosis can be readily effected, foci can be defined with precision and brain surgery can be enhanced.

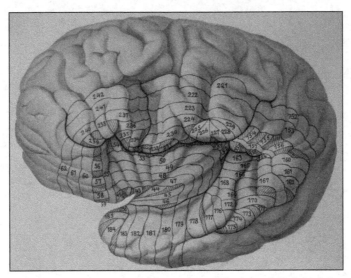

Fig. 6. Indication on the convex cerebral facies around the lateral (Sylvian) fissure of the von Economo & Koskinas (1925, 2008) method for dissecting each hemisphere into an average of 280 4mm-thick blocks perpendicular to the course of each gyrus for cytoarchitectonic study; hatched areas indicate the "cancelled" tissue

Sirs, in the phylogenetic line of living beings, nature, at times acting slowly and at times saltatorily, but always continually, produces new complex and viable animal forms. The same resourceful force that has given over the eons wings to the eagle to fly, has indirectly bestowed humans, by understanding their mind, with the capacity to construct wings themselves in order to defeat the law of gravity and to conquer the air. Nonetheless, the mind has its organic locus, its seat, its altar in the cerebral cortex. That is why one would be justified in saying that the anatomical and the physiological exploration of that noblest of organs deserves the utmost attention of science. The mind which explores and tends to subjugate everything, which tames everything and cannot be tamed, has to fall."

2.3 Response by Spyridon Dontas, annotator

"The work of Drs. Economo and Koskinas is monumental and constitutes a milestone of science, opening up new pathways towards the understanding of the brain from an anatomical, physiological and pathological viewpoint. It further forms the first comprehensive reference on the architecture of the adult human brain. And because the most precise of known methods was used, the optical, and through it a reproduction of the structure of the brain was achieved, in the natural, I reckon that this work will persevere as an everlasting possession of science. I further wish that Drs. Economo and Koskinas continue and complement their work, studying the remaining parts of the nervous system as well, to the great benefit of science."

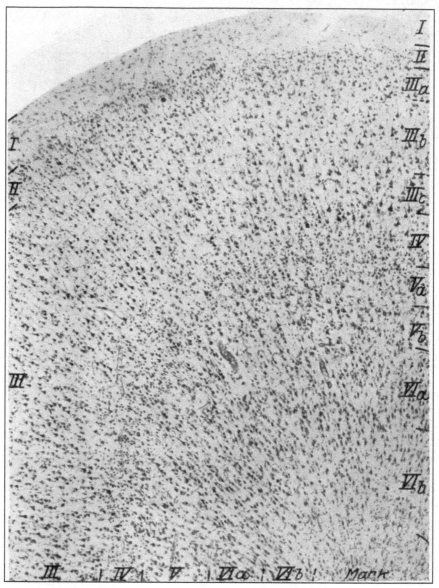

Fig. 7. Section of the dome of a gyrus from the frontal lobe of a human cerebral hemisphere, showing the normal six-layered (hexalaminar) cortex. The white matter (*Mark* in German), which is devoid of nerve cells, is seen on the lower-right hand corner. The six superimposed cortical cell layers are denoted in Latin numbers (I–VI). Photographed with a Carl Zeiss 2.0 cm Planar, a special objective lens with a considerably larger field than could be obtained with common microscopy objectives, especially valuable for large area objects under comparatively large magnifications and an evenly illuminated image free from marginal distortion. Planar micro-lenses are used without an eyepiece. ×50 (von Economo, 2009)

Cytoarchitectonics of the Human Cerebral Cortex: The 1926 Presentation by Georg N. Koskinas (1885–1975) to the Athens Medical Society

9

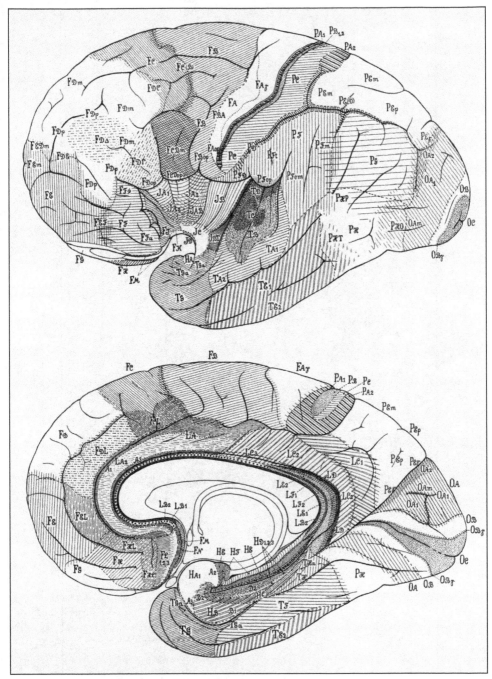

Fig. 8. The cytoarchitectonic map of von Economo and Koskinas, depicting their 107 cortical modification areas on the convex and median hemispheric facies of the human cerebrum

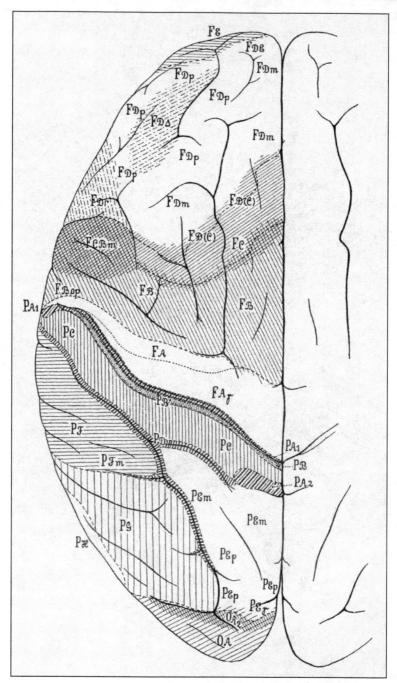

Fig. 9. The cytoarchitectonic map of von Economo and Koskinas, depicting their 107 cortical modification areas on the dorsal hemispheric surface of the human cerebrum

Cytoarchitectonics of the Human Cerebral Cortex: The 1926 Presentation by Georg N. Koskinas (1885–1975) to the Athens Medical Society

11

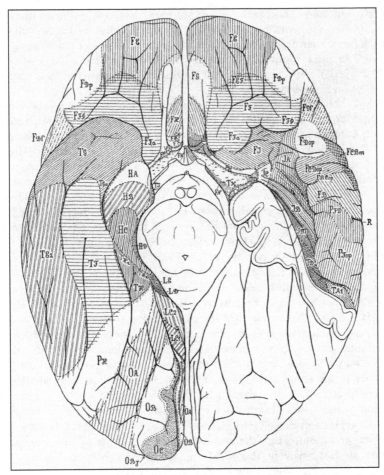

Fig. 10. The cytoarchitectonic map of von Economo and Koskinas, depicting their 107 cortical modification areas on the ventral hemispheric surface of the human cerebrum

3. Conclusion

Besides a histological mapping criterion, variations in cellular structure (cytoarchitecture) of the mammalian cerebral cortex reflect regional functional specificities linked to individual cell properties and intercellular connections. With the current interest in functional brain imaging, maps of the human cerebral cortex based on the classical cytoarchitectonic studies of Korbinian Brodmann (1868–1918) in Berlin are still in wide use (Brodmann, 1909; Garey, 2006; Olry, 2010; Olry & Haines, 2010; Zilles & Amunts, 2010). The Brodmann number system comprises 44 human cortical areas subdivided into 4 postcentral, 2 precentral, 8 frontal, 4 parietal, 3 occipital, 10 temporal, 6 cingulate, 3 retrosplenial, and 4 hippocampal. Following in the footsteps of the Viennese psychiatrist and neuroanatomist Theodor Meynert (1833–1892), who is considered to be the founder of the cytoarchitectonics of the cerebral cortex (Meynert, 1872), von Economo and Koskinas, also working at the University of Vienna (Triarhou, 2005, 2006), took cytoarchitectonics to a new zenith almost two decades after Brodmann's groundwork by defining 5 "supercategories" of fundamental structural types of cortex (agranular, frontal, parietal, polar, and granulous or *koniocortex*), subdivided into 54 *ground*, 76 *variant* and 107 cytoarchitectonic *modification* areas (von Economo & Koskinas, 1925, 2008), plus more than 60 additional intermediate *transition* areas (von Economo, 2009; von Economo & Horn, 1930).

Topographically, the 107 Economo-Koskinas modification areas are subdivided into 35 frontal, 13 superior limbic, 6 insular, 18 parietal, 7 occipital, 14 temporal, and 14 inferior limbic or hippocampal. Moreover, the frontal lobe is subdivided into prerolandic, anterior (prefrontal), and orbital (orbitomedial) regions; the superior limbic lobe into anterior, posterior and retrosplenial regions; the parietal lobe into postcentral (anterior parietal), superior, inferior and basal regions; and the temporal lobe into supratemporal, proper, fusiform and temporopolar regions (von Economo, 2009; von Economo & Koskinas, 2008).

The detailed cytoarchitectonic criteria of von Economo & Koskinas (1925, 2008) confer a clear advantage over Brodmann's scheme; their work represents a gigantic intellectual and technical effort (van Bogaert & Théodoridès, 1979), an attempt to bring the existing knowledge into a more orderly pattern (Zülch, 1975), and the only subdivision to be later acknowledged by von Bonin (1950) and by Bailey & von Bonin (1951). It is meaningful that basic and clinical neuroscientists adopt the Economo-Koskinas system of cytoarchitectonic areas over the commonly used Brodmann areas (see also discussion by Smith, 2010a, 2010b).

Brodmann (1909; Garey, 2006) described the comparative anatomy and cytoarchitecture of the cerebral cortex in numerous mammalian orders, from the hedgehog—with its unusually large archipallium—up to non-human primate and human brains; he introduced terms such as *homogenetic* and *heterogenetic formations* to denote two different basic cortical patterns, which, respectively, are either derived from the basic six-layer type or do not demostrate the six-layer stage. Brodmann was intrigued by the phylogenetic increase in the number of cytoarchitectonic cortical areas in primates, and was astute in pointing out the phenomenon of phylogenetic regression as well (Striedter, 2005). Vogt & Vogt (1919) laid the foundations of fiber pathway architecture; they defined the structural features of allocortex, proisocortex, and isocortex, and extensively discussed the differences between paleo-, archi-, and neocortical regions (Vogt & Vogt, 1919; Vogt, 1927; Zilles, 2006).

Combining cyto- and myeloarchitectonics, Sanides (1962, 1964) placed emphasis on the transition regions *(Gradationen)* that accompany the "streams" of neocortical regions coming from paleo- and archicortical sources (Pandya & Sanides, 1973). [Vogt & Vogt (1919) had already spoken of "areal gradations".] The idea of a "koniocortex core" and "prokoniocortex belt areas" in the temporal operculum (Pandya & Sanides, 1973) was modified by Kaas & Hackett (1998, 2000), who speak of histologically and functionally distinct "core", "belt" and "parabelt" subdivisions in the monkey auditory cortex, with specified connections.

There are three major advantages in using the system of cytoarchitectonic areas defined by von Economo and Koskinas as opposed to the maps defined by Brodmann (von Economo, 2009; Triarhou, 2007a, 2007b):

3.1 Timing of publication

Brodmann published his monograph in 1909. Von Economo began work on cytoarchitectonics in 1912, with Koskinas joining in 1919; their *Textband* and *Atlas* were published in 1925, almost two decades after Brodmann, and comprised 150 new discoveries

Cytoarchitectonics of the Human Cerebral Cortex: The 1926 Presentation by Georg N. Koskinas (1885–1975)
to the Athens Medical Society

13

(Koskinas, 1931, 2009), including the description of the large, spindle-shaped bipolar cells in the inferior ganglionic layer (Vb) of the dome of the transverse insular gyrus, currently referred to as "von Economo neurons" (Watson et al., 2006) — although a more accurate term would be "von Economo-Koskinas neurons". Ngowyang (1932) appears to be the first author to refer to fusiform neurons as "von Economo cells".

3.2 Defined cytoarchitectonic fields
Brodmann defined 44 cortical areas in the human brain. Von Economo and Koskinas defined 107 areas (von Economo, 2009; von Economo & Koskinas, 2008), plus another more than 60 *transition* areas (von Economo, 2009), thus providing a greater "resolution" over the Brodmann areas for the human cerebral hemispheres by a factor of four. Brodmann correlations can be found in the *Atlas* (von Economo & Koskinas, 2008) and in a related review (Triarhou, 2007b).

3.3 Extrapolated versus real surface designations
Brodmann maps are commonly used to either designate cytoarchitectonic areas as such, or as a "shorthand system" to designate some region on the cerebral *surface* (DeMyer, 1988). Macroscopic extrapolation of Brodmann projection maps are effected on the atlas of Talairach & Tournoux (1988), rather than being based on real microscopic cytoarchitectonics. Such a specification of Brodmann areas is inappropriate and may lead to erroneous results in delineating specific cortical regions, which may in turn lead to erroneous hypotheses concerning the involvement of particular brain systems in normal and pathological situations (Uylings et al., 2005). On the other hand, the unique sectioning method of von Economo and Koskinas, whereby each gyrus is dissected into blocks *always perpendicular to the gyral surface*, be it dome, wall or sulcus floor, essentially offers a "mechanical" solution to the generalized mapmaker's problem of flattening nonconvex polyhedral surfaces (Schwartz et al., 1989), one of the commonest problems at the epicentre of cortical research.

Furthermore, microscopically defined borders usually differ from gross anatomical landmarks, cytoarchitectonics reflecting the inner organisation of cortical areas and their morphofunctional correlates (Zilles, 2006). Despite the integration of multifactorial descriptors such as chemoarchitecture, angioarchitecture, neurotransmitter, receptor and gene expression patterns, as well as white matter tracts, it is clear that the knowledge of the classical anatomy remains fundamental (Toga & Thompson, 2007). The structure of cortical layers incorporates, and reflects, the form of their constitutive cells and their functional connections; the underpinnings of neuronal connectivity at the microscopic level are paramount to interpreting any clues afforded by neuroimaging pertinent to cognition.

4. Acknowledgment

I thank the Aristotelian University Central Library for providing a copy of the *Proceedings*, as well as Ms. Rena Kostopoulou and Dr. Vassilis Kostopoulos for providing archival material of the Koskinas family.

5. References

Bailey, P. & von Bonin, G. (1951). *The Isocortex of Man*, University of Illinois Press, Urbana, IL, U.S.A.

Brodmann, K. (1909). *Vergleichende Lokalisationslehre der Großhirnrinde*, J.A. Barth, Leipzig, Germany

DeMyer, W. (1988). *Neuroanatomy*, Harwal Publishing Company, ISBN 0-683-06236-0, Malvern, PA, U.S.A.

Garey, L.J. (2006). *Brodmann's Localisation in the Cerebral Cortex*, Springer Science, ISBN 978-0-387-26917-7, New York, U.S.A.

Hartmann, F.; Mayer, C.; Pötzl, O.; Wagner-Jauregg, J.; Pollak, E. & Raimann, E. (1926). Mitgliederverzeichnis des Vereines für Psychiatrie und Neurologie in Wien (Stand: Juli 1926). *Jahrbücher für Psychiatrie und Neurologie*, Vol. 45, pp. 80–84

Jones, E.G. (2008). Cortical maps and modern phrenology. *Brain*, Vol. 131, No. 8, (August 2008), pp. 2227–2233, ISSN 0006-8950

Jones, E.G. (2010). Cellular structure of the human cerebral cortex. Brain, vol. 133, No. 3, (March 2010), pp. 945–946, ISSN 0006-8950

Kaas, J.H. & Hackett, T.A. (1998). Subdivisions of auditory cortex and levels of processing in primates. *Audiology and Neuro-Otology*, Vol. 3, No. 2–3, (March-June 1998), pp. 73–85, ISSN 1420-3030

Kaas, J.H. & Hackett, T.A. (2000). Subdivisions of auditory cortex and processing streams in primates. *Proceedings of the National Academy of Sciences of USA*, Vol. 97, No. 22, (24 October 2000), pp. 11793–11799, ISSN 0027-8424

Koskinas, G.N. (1926). Cytoarchitectonics of the human cerebral cortex [in Greek]. *Proceedings of the Athens Medical Society*, Vol. 92, pp. 44–48

Koskinas, G.N. (1931). *Scientific Works Published in German – Their Analyses and Principal Assessments by Eminent Scientists* [in Greek], Pyrsus, Athens, Greece

Koskinas, G.N. (2009). An outline of cytoarchitectonics of the adult human cerebral cortex, In: *Cellular Structure of the Human Cerebral Cortex*, C. von Economo (translated and edited by L. C. Triarhou), pp. 194–226, S. Karger, ISBN 978-3-8055-9061-7, Basel, Switzerland

Meynert, T. (1872). *Der Bau der Gross-Hirnrinde und Seine Örtlichen Verschiedenheiten, Nebst Einem Pathologisch-Anatomischen Corollarium*, J.H. Heuser, Neuwied, Germany

Ngowyang, G. (1932) Beschreibung einer Art von Spezialzellen in der Inselrinde zugleich Bemerkungen über die v. Economoschen Spezialzellen. *Journal für Psychologie und Neurologie*, Vol. 44, pp. 671–674

Olry, R. (2010). Korbinian Brodmann (1868–1918). *Journal of Neurology*, Vol. 257, No. 12, (December 2010), pp. 2112–2113, ISSN 0340-5354

Olry, R. & Haines, D.E. (2010) Korbinian Brodmann: The Victor Hugo of cytoarchitectonic brain maps. *Journal of the History of the Neurosciences*, Vol. 19, No. 2, (May 2005), pp. 195–198, ISSN 0964-704X

Pandya, D.N. & Sanides, F. (1973). Architectonic parcellation of the temporal operculum in rhesus monkey and its projection pattern. *Zeitschrift für Anatomie und Entwicklungs-Geschischte*, Vol. 139, No. 2, (20 March 1973), pp. 127–161, ISSN 0044-2232

Sanides, F. (1962) *Die Architektonik des Menschlichen Stirnhirns*, Springer-Verlag, Berlin-Göttingen-Heidelberg, Germany

Sanides, F. (1964) The cyto-myeloarchitecture of the human frontal lobe and its relation to phylogenetic differentiation of the cerebral cortex. *Journal für Hirnforschung*, Vol. 47, pp. 269–282, ISSN 0944-8160

Cytoarchitectonics of the Human Cerebral Cortex: The 1926 Presentation by Georg N. Koskinas (1885–1975)
to the Athens Medical Society

15

Schwartz, E.L., Shaw, A. & Wolfson, E. (1989) A numerical solution to the generalized mapmaker's problem: Flattening nonconvex polyhedral surfaces. *IEEE Transactions on Pattern Analysis and Machine Intelligence*, Vol. 11, No. 9, (September 1989), pp. 1005–1008, ISSN 0162-8828

Smith, C.U.M. (2010a). Does history repeat itself? Cortical columns: 1. Introduction. *Cortex*, Vol. 46, No. 3, (March 2010), pp. 279–280, ISSN 0010-9452

Smith, C.U.M. (2010b). Does history repeat itself? Cortical columns: 4. Déjà vu? *Cortex*, Vol. 46, No. 8, (September 2010), pp. 947–948, ISSN 0010-9452

Sträussler, E. & Koskinas, G.N. (1925). Untersuchungen zwecks Feststellung des Einflusses der Malariabehandlung auf den histologischen Prozeß der progressiven Paralyse. *Zentralblatt für die Gesamte Neurologie und Psychiatrie*, Vol. 39, pp. 471–480

Striedter, G.F. (2005) *Principles of Brain Evolution*, Sinauer Associates, ISBN 0-87893-820-6, Sunderland, MA, U.S.A.

Talairach, J. & Tournoux, P. (1988). *Co-planar Stereotaxic Atlas of the Human Brain. 3-Dimensional Proportional System: An Approach to Cerebral Imaging* (translated by M. Rayport), G. Thieme Verlag, ISBN 3-13-711701-1, Stuttgart, Germany

Toga, A.W. & Thompson, P.M. (2007). What is where and why it is important. *NeuroImage*, Vol. 37, No. 4, (1 October 2007), pp. 1045–1049, ISSN 1053-8119

Triarhou, L.C. (2005). Georg N. Koskinas (1885–1975) and his scientific contributions to the normal and pathological anatomy of the human brain. *Brain Reseach Bulletin*, Vol. 68, No. 3, (30 December 2005), pp. 121–139, ISSN 0361-9230

Triarhou, L.C. (2006). Georg N. Koskinas (1885–1975). *Journal of Neurology*, Vol. 253, No. 10, (October 2006), pp. 1377–1378, ISSN 0340-5354

Triarhou, L.C. (2007a). The Economo-Koskinas Atlas revisited: Cytoarchitectonics and functional context. *Stereotactic and Functional Neurosurgery*, Vol. 85, No. 5, (August 2007), pp. 195–203, ISSN 1011-6125

Triarhou, L.C. (2007b). A proposed number system for the 107 cortical areas of Economo and Koskinas, and Brodmann area correlations. *Stereotactic and Functional Neurosurgery*, vol. 85, No. 5, (August 2007), pp. 204–215, ISSN 1011-6125

Uylings, H.B.M.; Rajkowska, G.; Sanz-Arigita, E.; Amunts, K. & Zilles, K. (2005). Consequences of large interindividual variability for human brain atlases: Converging macroscopical imaging and microscopical neuroanatomy. *Anatomy and Embryology*, Vol. 210, No. 5–6, (December 2005), pp. 423–431, ISSN 0340-2061

van Bogaert, L. & Théodoridès, J. (1979). Constantin von Economo: The Man and the Scientist, Verlag der Österreichischen Akademie der Wissenschaften, ISBN 3-7001-0284-4, Vienna, Austria

Vogt, C. & Vogt, O. (1919). Allgemeinere Ergebnisse unserer Hirnforschung. *Journal für Psychologie und Neurologie*, Vol. 25, pp. 279–461

Vogt, O. (1927). Architektonik der menschlichen Hirnrinde. *Zentralblatt für die Gesamte Neurologie und Psychiatrie*, Vol. 45, pp. 510–512

von Bonin, G. (1950). *Essay on the Cerebral Cortex*, Charles C Thomas, Springfield, IL, U.S.A.

von Economo, C. (2009). *Cellular Structure of the Human Cerebral Cortex* (translated and edited by L. C. Triarhou), S. Karger, ISBN 978-3-8055-9061-7, Basel, Switzerland

von Economo, C. & Horn, L. (1930). Über Windungsrelief, Maße und Rindenarchitektonik der Supratemporalfläche, ihre individuellen und ihre Seitenunterschiede. *Zeitschrift für die Gesamte Neurologie und Psychiatrie*, Vol. 130, pp. 678–757 von Economo, C. & Koskinas, G.N. (1923). Die sensiblen Zonen des Großhirns. *Klinische Wochenschrift*, Vol. 2, No. 19, (7 May 1923), p. 905

von Economo, C. & Koskinas, G.N. (1925). *Die Cytoarchitektonik der Hirnrinde des Erwachsenen Menschen – Textband und Atlas mit 112 Mikrophotographischen Tafeln*, J. Springer, Vienna, Austria

von Economo, C. & Koskinas, G.N. (2008). *Atlas of Cytoarchitectonics of the Adult Human Cerebral Cortex* (translated, revised and edited by L. C. Triarhou), S. Karger, ISBN 978-3-8055-8289-6, Basel, Switzerland

Watson, K.K.; Jones, T.K. & Allman, J.M. (2006). Dendritic architecture of the von Economo neurons. *Neuroscience*, Vol. 141, No. 3, (1 September 2006), pp. 1107–1112, ISSN 0306-4522

Zilles, K. (2006). Architektonik und funktionelle Neuroanatomie der Hirnrinde des Menschen, In: *Neurobiologie Psychischer Störungen*, H. Förstl, M. Hautzinger & G. Roth (eds.), pp. 75–140, Springer Medizin, ISBN 978-3-540-25694-6, Heidelberg-Berlin, Germany

Zilles, K. & Amunts, K. (2010). Centenary of Brodmann's map—Conception and fate. *Nature Reviews Neuroscience*, Vol. 11, No. 2, (February 2010), pp. 139–145, ISSN 1471-003X

Zülch, K.J. (1975). Critical remarks on "Lokalisationslehre", In: *Cerebral Localization*, K.J. Zülch, O. Creutzfeldt & G.C. Galbraith (eds.), pp. 3–16, Springer-Verlag, ISBN 0-387-07379-5, Berlin-Heidelberg, Germany

Neuroimaging of Single Cases: Benefits and Pitfalls

James Danckert[1] and Seyed M. Mirsattarri[2]
[1]Dept of Psychology, University of Waterloo
[2]Depts of CNS, Med Biophys, Med Imaging, & Psychology,
University of Western Ontario
Canada

1. Introduction

Single case studies of neurological patients has a long and storied history (Zillmer & Spiers, 2001). First used as a teaching tool (Haas, 2001), the method of thoroughly exploring the cognitive and motor functions of a unique individual patient has led to extraordinary advances in our understanding of structure-function relationships in the human brain. Single cases have led to important advances in many fields, including pioneering work on language (Broca, 1861; see also Ryalls & Lecours, 1996) and visual perception (Poppelreuter, 1917/1990; see also Humphreys & Riddoch, 1996) to more recent work on memory systems (Scoville & Milner, 1957; Milner & Penfield, 1955-1956; see Milner, 2005 for a recent review) where one patient (HM) has arguably done more to advance that field than any other single case study in history. Prior to the advent of x-rays and eventually computerised axial tomography (CT scans), the method of studying single cases was the only way to determine the location of a patient's pathology. The advent of CT scans in the 1970's obviated, to some degree, the need for detailed neuropsychological testing, at least as it was needed to determine the *location* of pathology (Banich, 2004; Lezak, et al., 2004; Kolb & Wishaw, 2009). A few decades later and the advent of functional MRI (fMRI) provides an even more powerful tool for examining the nature of structure-function relationships in humans and in non-human primates (Ogawa et al., 1992; Ford et al., 2009). Indeed, the rapid rise of fMRI studies (Fox, 1997; Raichle, 1994) has outstripped the pace of single case studies in the past few decades (Figure 1).

By 2005 the proportion of neuroimaging abstracts accepted for presentation at the Cognitive Neuroscience Society meeting was around 35% compared to only 15% for patient studies (which included group and single case methods; Chatterjee, 2005[1]).

There are a range of reasons behind the rise of functional neuroimaging studies including the ease and relatively low cost with which these studies can be carried out (Chatterjee, 2005). Although per hour imaging costs seem high to most, the cost of patient research is undoubtedly far higher both in time committed and real costs related to screening and following patients over longer periods of time (Chatterjee, 2005). In addition, each method

---

[1] A search of the 2011 CNS program using "fMRI", "neuroimaging" and "patients" separately showed that neuroimaging references were almost double those of references to patients.

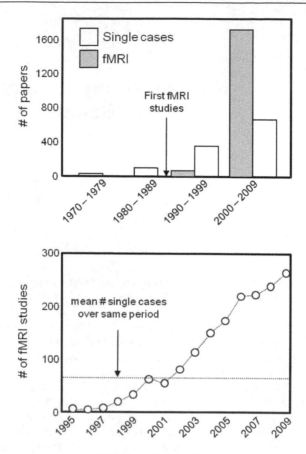

Fig. 1. Proportion of single case and fMRI studies in the past few decades. Upper panel shows the results of two Pubmed searches, the first using the term 'memory' (open bars) and the second using the conjunction search terms 'memory AND fMRI'. The first search included the following constraints: case studies published in English, dating from 1970 onwards (under the 'limits' tab of Pubmed the following criteria were selected: 'English', 'Humans', 'Case Studies', 'dates from 1970.01.01 to 2010.01.01'). The resulting abstracts were inspected to ensure that only single case studies of neurological patients were included. The second search term included the same constraints with the exception that the constraint 'case studies' was removed from the search term. Again, all abstracts were inspected to ensure that only fMRI studies examining memory processes were included.

provides distinct information. By design, human functional neuroimaging studies are necessarily correlational and as such can not address which brain regions are *necessary* for a given function but highlight only those regions or networks that are *sufficient* (Chatterjee, 2005; Friston & Price, 2003). In fact, given that the vast majority of fMRI studies present only group averaged data, it is feasible that much of what we see represents 'cognitively degenerate' neural systems - that is, typical imaging findings may highlight only one of several regions or networks each capable of subserving the same cognitive function (Friston

& Price, 2003). On the other hand, case studies of neurological patients, while capable of demonstrating which brain regions are necessary for a given function, encounter a range of distinct problems (Rorden & Karnath, 2004). Human lesions tend to be large and highly variable and in turn lead to heterogeneous behavioural symptoms. Furthermore, it is not possible to determine the effects of disconnection – the consequences not only of damage to a particular brain region but of removing that 'node' from the network of regions it once participated in (e.g., Bartolomeo, et al., 2007).

Perhaps the best way to compensate for the shortcoming of single case and neuroimaging methods is to combine the two (Friston & Price, 2003; Price et al., 2006, 1999; Chatterjee, 2005). Unfortunately, both methods demonstrate a strong within citation bias (although the bias is stronger in neuroimaging work; Chatterjee, 2005). There have been elegant studies using fMRI in groups of patients to address a wide variety of behaviours from motor control in Parkinson's disease (e.g., Nandhagopal et al., 2008), to strategy selection in social games in psychopathy (Rilling et al., 2007; see also Hoff et al., 2009 for a single case study of psychopathy) and recovery of function in neglect patients – a common disorder typically arising from right hemisphere strokes (Corbetta et al., 2005). Far fewer studies have made use of fMRI to examine single case studies. In this chapter we will first discuss some of the challenges to using fMRI as another tool for exploring single cases before giving some examples of how such an approach could be used to advance our understanding of structure-function relationships in humans.

2. Design issues relevant to single case studies in fMRI

Several technical aspects related to collecting the Blood Oxygenated Level Dependent (BOLD) response that forms the basis of fMRI data pose problems for single case studies. First, the shape of the haemodynamic response function (HRF) may vary from one experimental session to another (Aguirre et al., 1998). Within a given subject the shape of the HRF tends to be robust particularly within a single scanning session (Aguirre et al., 1998). More variability is evident within individuals when scanning runs span multiple sessions. This may be related to hardware issues in the scanner itself with some variability in measures of magnetic susceptibility from one session or day to the next (Huettel et al., 2004). Noise may also be introduced from the subject themselves with differing levels of alertness being an important factor in testing neurological patients (Lerdal et al., 2009; see also Tyvaert et al., 2008 for a study of the effects of alertness on BOLD signals). Even factors such as levels of caffeine influence the BOLD signal (Chen & Parrish, 2009). The variability of the HRF and subsequent BOLD measures when testing over multiple sessions is particularly problematic for single case designs as it constrains the number of tasks, and repetition of those tasks, one can expect to complete in a given session. Commonly, fMRI designs require multiple repetitions of the same task within a single session to achieve the appropriate statistical power to demonstrate a robust change in the BOLD signal (Huettel et al., 2004; Monti, 2011). While the same can be said of behavioural studies of single cases, such studies can often extend over days or weeks with an opportunity to replicate findings within the patient and to examine an extensive range of behaviours (e.g., Danckert et al., 2002; Branch-Coslett & Lie, 2008). Issues of fatigue in this instance can be addressed by testing the patient at the same time of day in each instance or collecting a control task as an index of fluctuations in alertness (e.g., a basic information processing task such as the Trails A test would suffice for this purpose; e.g., Gaudino et al., 1995). In contrast, collecting fMRI data across a range of cognitive functions within one scanning session can be time prohibitive, especially in instances where repetition of each domain specific task is ideal to achieve the appropriate statistical power (Huettel et al., 2004). These limitations can in part be overcome through the choice of tasks to be implemented and the design chosen (i.e., block design vs. the various forms of event-related designs). In general, block designs lead to larger percent signal changes than do event-related designs (Bandettini & Cox, 2000) due to a loss of signal-to-noise ratio for the latter. Tasks exploring basic sensory or motor functions also tend to lead to larger BOLD signal changes than do tasks exploring more complex cognitive functions (Huettel et al., 2004).

A second issue in fMRI scanning impacting upon single case studies using this methodology relates to susceptibility artefacts (Huettel et al., 2004). Susceptibility artefacts can be readily distinguished from true BOLD signal and other artefacts such as motion, using a range of statistical techniques including independent components analysis (e.g., DeMartino et al., 2008). With abnormally developed or injured brains, however, these issues could be compounded. In particular, if one is interested in examining hemispheric differences in activation, it is important to determine that susceptibility artefacts do not impact the damaged and undamaged hemispheres differentially (e.g., Danckert et al., 2007). This can be overcome statistically by contrasting activation for similar regions across each hemisphere (Adcock et al., 2003; Danckert et al., 2007; Shulman et al., 2010). In this instance, however, it is crucial to first determine what one might expect in the healthy brain. For example, basic sensory processes may be expected to lead to symmetrical activations across the two hemispheres (e.g., motion processing and object perception; Dukelow et al., 2001; Kourtzi & Kanwisher, 2000), whereas more complex cognitive processes may be expected to lead to asymmetric activations (e.g., language processing; Price, 2000, 2010). Language functions represent a pertinent case as many individuals may be expected to have bilateral activations during language tasks (Fernandes et al., 2006; Fernandes & Smith, 2000) or even shifted language dominance to the right hemisphere (e.g., Peng & Wang, 2011; Wong et al., 2009). In this instance, fMRI with a single case suffers from the same methodological issues that behavioural studies do – without a baseline measure of performance in some cognitive domains it is difficult if not impossible to determine what has *changed* for the patient. This is particularly problematic for patients suffering from traumatic brain injury (TBI), especially at the mild end of the spectrum, in which subtle changes to executive functions, social functioning and personality are difficult to quantify (e.g., Vaishnavi et al., 2009).

Another issue to consider concerns the nature of damaged or abnormal tissue in neurological patients. More to the point, given that BOLD fMRI depends on changes in oxygenation at the level of capillaries (Huettel et al., 2004; Price et al., 1999), it is possible that damaged or abnormal tissue will also demonstrate abnormal, or at the very least altered, vascularization (Beck & Plate, 2009). Cerebral angiograms are not useful in this circumstance as only gross vascular morphology can be imaged (e.g., obvious abnormalities such as arterioveinous malformations can be detected but the consequences of such malformations for the capillary bed are more complex). This is particularly problematic when faced with null results, an issue we will explore in more detail below. Briefly, any absence of activation could, among other things, be explained due to abnormal vascularization related to the pathology in question. This could be related to abnormally developed tissue (e.g., heterotopias; Guerrini & Barba, 2010) or changes to vascularization due to insults such as stroke (Beck & Plate, 2009). Statistical approaches can in part address this issue (i.e., lowering statistical thresholds should show some level of activity even in abnormal tissue) and comparisons with similar patients and healthy controls can also partly address these concerns (e.g., Danckert et al., 2007; Danckert & Culham, 2010). These approaches however, never fully remove the concerns surrounding null results and can be seen only as increasing the degree of confidence regarding alternate reasons for an absence of activation. This issue will be revisited with the examples to be discussed in more detail below.

One final vital issue when utilising neuroimaging techniques with neurological patients concerns task design. As already suggested, it is often best to make use of tasks that lead to well documented, robust activation patterns (e.g., tasks known to activate primary sensory and motor cortices). Given that each patient presents with a unique behavioural deficit, however, it is not always possible to stick with the robust, simple tasks. In that sense, task choice and design necessarily feeds off neuropsychological testing – in other words single case methodology. While the temptation may be to choose tasks that fully highlight the patient's particular deficits, this may not be the ideal approach (Price & Friston, 1999). If the patient is completely incapable of performing a given task, interpretation of any neural activity (should any even exist) is limited. Instead, those tasks that the patient can perform either to the same level as healthy controls or to some suboptimal level, should be preferred. In the first instance, when a patient performs to an equivalent level of controls, it is possible to explore the extent to which the same networks are invoked (e.g.,. Yucel et al., 2002). In many instances, patients will utilise alternate neural networks to achieve the same level of behavioural performance as controls (this may be especially important when investigating disorders such as schizophrenia). The difficulty with this kind of finding comes from interpreting the abnormal neural responses as either *causing* the behavioural syndrome or deficit in question or arising as a *consequence* of the syndrome/deficit (note: in this case the task used may show no deficit per se but tap into a component process known to be impaired in the patient; Price & Friston, 2006). Essentially this arises from the fact that neuroimaging data are correlational in nature and do not allow for conclusions related to the cause of changed patterns of activation. In the second instance, in which the patient performs a task at suboptimal levels, it is possible to correlate performance with the BOLD signal directly (i.e., activations related to correct vs. error trials; Price & Friston, 2006) or to address which parts of the normal neural network are necessary for the task at hand (e.g., Steeves et al., 2004). For example, Steeves and colleagues (2004) examined object processing in a visual form agnosic patient who performed at above chance levels, but well below that of healthy individuals, when asked to recognise visual representations of objects. In their study they were able to examine more precisely which components of object recognition, including colour diagnostics, form outlines and greyscaled images, were most impaired in their patient thereby enabling a more detailed exploration of the variety of processes involved in object perception (Steeves et al., 2004). In instances such as these, however, there remains the possibility that abnormal neural activation patterns arise due to either a loss of function from the damaged region or as a consequence of the fact that the damaged region is disconnected from a broader network (see Price & Friston, 2006 for a detailed review of these and related issues in single case neuroimaging).

Task choice and design are ultimately dictated by the nature of the question being asked. In many instances (including the first two patients to be discussed below) the questions asked are primarily patient focused - that is, the studies represent an attempt to determine the degree of recovery or reorganisation of function in a given patient. In this instance tasks with well-described patterns of activation in the healthy population are essential. In other instances, the patient serves as a means to understanding normal cognitive processes by virtue of either the demonstrated behavioural deficits or alterations in neural functioning needed attain normal performance (Price & Friston, 2006). Here one can utilise behavioural performance in conjunction with imaging data (e.g., correlate BOLD with correct vs. incorrect trials) to examine changes in neural function.

In summary, single cases of unique neurological patients provides an opportunity to examine structure-function relationships, with a particular focus on which brain regions may be necessary for a given behaviour. Functional MRI provides another tool that can be used with single cases to examine a broad range of issues. In utilising fMRI with single cases it is important to consider the nature of the pathology for the particular patient, expectations regarding activation in the healthy brain (i.e., is there a demonstrated pattern of activity in healthy individuals related to the task at hand?) and the limitations of the paradigms to be employed (e.g., block designs focussing on well-documented structure-function relationships vs. event-related designs focussing on more complex behaviours). Some of these issues will be explored further below relative to particular examples of fMRI used with single cases.

3. Potential uses of fMRI in single case studies

Below we examine three distinct uses of fMRI in single case studies to illustrate some of the benefits and potential pitfalls of combining the two methodologies. These examples are by no means exhaustive, but represent a disparate range of approaches to combining fMRI and single case studies.

3.1 Examining the consequences of unusual neuropathologies

We recently examined a range of cognitive functions in two patients with epileptic disorders arising from distinct etiologies (Danckert et al., 2004; 2007). The aims for these studies were varied and so posed distinct challenges. Our first case involved a patient with a large left hemisphere porencaphalic cyst (Figure 2). The remaining left frontal tissue was also the site of seizure onset for the patient and fMRI was employed in the first instance to determine whether or not that residual tissue supported cognitive and motor functions. In this sense then, fMRI becomes an additional tool for the clinician that has the potential to aid in treatment decisions. In fact, fMRI serves another important clinical function in epilepsy research as it has recently begun to surpass traditional methods of determining language lateralisation in epilepsy patients (i.e., the WADA; Abou-Khalil & Schlaggar, 2002; Jones et al., 2011; Woermann et al., 2003). A secondary aim in this case, was to use fMRI to determine the extent to which normal structure-function relationships had been distorted in this patient. In other words, to what extent had his pathology led to a reorganisation of function? Our approach in this instance was to examine basic motor and somatosensory functions and language functions that would all be expected to activate left frontal regions (i.e., when using the right hand for the motor and somatosensory tasks; Toma & Nakai, 2002; Price, 2000). The motor and somatosensory tasks have the added benefit of being robust, simple tasks with predictable activation patterns expected in the unaffected hemisphere, thereby enabling comparisons between the intact and affected cortex. Results showed that the remaining tissue in the left frontal region of this patient did in fact support a range of cognitive and motor functions (Figure 2). Importantly, this indicated that tissue that was demonstrated to be the focus of seizure activity was also capable of supporting normal functioning.

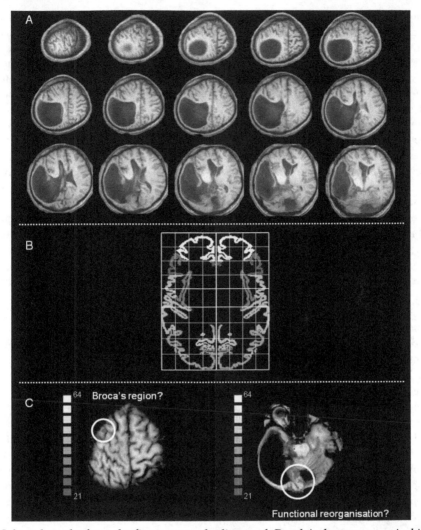

Fig. 2. Selected results from the first case study discussed. Panel A shows anatomical images showing that the patient's skull had been deformed by his porencephalic cyst making it difficult to align the patient's images to a standardised space (indicated in the Panel B using the Talairach template from BrainVoyager software). Panel C shows two data points from this patient. To the left is activity during a silent word naming task in which a left frontal region was activated. Given the distortions evident in the patient's brain and skull it is impossible to know whether this region represents Broca's area. Similarly, the data to the right shows activity in a remaining portion of occipital cortex during silent word naming. This region would not normally be activated in this task (and the undamaged hemisphere showed no occipital activity) and the patient was hemianopic suggesting that the remaining occipital cortex was unlikely to support visual functioning. Nevertheless, caution should be employed when interpreting data of this sort in terms of functional reorganisation. Data adapted from Danckert et al., 2004.

Challenges arising from the case described above that are pertinent to studies of this kind included alignment of the patient's structural scan to a standardised space and a lack of exhaustive testing, especially for unusual activations. As can be seen in Figure 2, the patient's skull had been deformed by the cyst making it difficult to find the landmarks normally used to align structural scans to a normalised space (e.g., Talairach & Tournoux, 1988; see Price & Friston, 2006 for further discussion of this issue). In instances such as this estimates of missing or distorted landmarks are required. This is relatively trivial given that the patient's data will stand alone (i.e., there is no 'group average' to worry about). Where it does pose a problem is in localising activations one would normally expect to see. For example, we found a region of frontal cortex that was active for silent word production that may have been analogous to Broca's region (Danckert et al., 2004). However, given the obvious distortion in gross morphology and without appropriate landmarks, this kind of association was at best speculative.

Perhaps more difficult to address was the fact that it was simply not possible to perform the full range of tasks we would have liked to have collected on this patient. This is likely a problem for all single case studies using fMRI for all of the reasons noted above. For our patient, silent word naming activated a small region of remaining occipital cortex. Given that the patient was hemianopic, any activation in this region is difficult to interpret without further testing. For example, visual perceptual tasks (e.g., object recognition protocols; even retinotopy; Kourtzi & Kanwisher, 2000; Sereno et al., 1995; Tootell et al., 1995) may have been informative regarding the role this remaining region of occipital cortex played in the patient's behaviour (e.g., would the patient have shown residual functions akin to blindsight, or would visual imagery evoke activity in this region even though it receives no afferent input?). Unfortunately, we had been guided in the first instance by other aspects of his presentation (e.g., some mild apraxia) and the fact that his seizures originated not in the sliver of remaining occipital tissue, but in the frontal cortex. This merely serves to highlight some of the restrictions one encounters when addressing unusual single cases in fMRI. Perhaps more important to highlight is the fact that this work was able to demonstrate that a range of functions were subserved by the compromised left hemisphere which in turn guided treatment decisions to some extent. That is, surgery to remove the remaining left frontal tissue had been considered a treatment option, with the fMRI demonstrating just how devastating this approach would have been for the patient's daily functioning.

In our second case, we examined a patient with heterotopic tissue in the anterior temporal cortex (Danckert et al., 2007). In contrast to our first patient, this patient's pathology was not the site of the origin of his seizures, which was more posterior in normally differentiated tissue. Here we wanted to know whether the heterotopic tissue supported any normal cognitive functioning. In addition, what if any, were the consequences to expected structure-function relationships in the tissue where seizures originated? Here we were able to take advantage of imaging results in healthy individuals to examine laterality effects in our patient. Using tasks that would normally activate brain regions identified as the origin of his seizures or tasks that would activate neighbouring regions (i.e., object recognition and motion processing tasks) we were able to demonstrate that our patient had asymmetrical activations where symmetrical activation patterns would have been expected (Figure 3). Taken together with results from our first case, this highlights an important finding in epilepsy research such that tissue that supports epileptic activity is also likely to support normal function. In the current case we were able to demonstrate an asymmetry of processing such that the epileptic hemisphere showed less activity than the unaffected hemisphere (Figure 3).

The challenges in this case were more substantial than in our first case for several reasons. First, we were unable to demonstrate activation in the heterotopic tissue for any of the tasks we used (Danckert et al., 2007). This raises the spectre of null results briefly mentioned above with the obvious caveat that an absence of evidence is not evidence of absence. This issue would be particularly important if fMRI results of this kind were to be used to guide surgery. Although there was no gross distortion of the patient's brain, the heterotopic tissue also raises concerns regarding abnormal vascularization (see D'Esposito, et al., 2003 for a review of this issue). Any such abnormalities may well have been the root cause of the failure to find significant activations. In addition, task choice may well determine whether or not activation is observed. Without the right task, one would not expect to see activation in a given region. Two approaches can be utilised to address these concerns although it should be noted that what is provided here is some degree of corroborating evidence and not certainty. First, data from healthy individuals using the same tasks/protocols used in the patient can demonstrate what would normally be expected with respect to a given brain region (note, we were unable to do this for all tasks in our case). If the same task that fails to activate a brain region in the patient nevertheless leads to robust and reliable (i.e., evident in all subjects) activity in healthy individuals, one can have more confidence that the patient's pathology has disrupted normal function.

A second approach to dealing with null results involves lowering the threshold for significant activation to determine whether changes in the BOLD response will be evident with less stringent statistical approaches (Figure 3; Danckert et al., 2007; Danckert & Culham, 2010). In our case, even at the lowest statistical thresholds there was no evidence of activity within the heterotopic tissue. Even instances where lowering the statistical threshold does show changes in BOLD signal that were not evident at more conventional thresholds can be informative (Danckert & Culham, 2010). Changes in BOLD signal seen at lower statistical thresholds that fail to modulate with task manipulations (i.e., no difference between BOLD in the task vs. baseline conditions) should be considered meaningless (Danckert & Culham, 2010).

In both cases described above, careful neuropsychological testing was also carried out to compliment the imaging findings. Where possible, such clinical and/or experimental testing is vital as it can cover more ground than imaging alone. In our first case, neuropsychological results (i.e., mild apraxia) directed us towards tasks that would examine basic and more complex (i.e., praxic) motor skills. Similarly, our second case exhibited some mild object naming deficits on neuropsychological testing that guided our choice of tasks (i.e., both language and object naming tasks were used; Danckert et al., 2007). Not only do neuropsychological findings of this kind help guide the choice of tasks for imaging, they can corroborate certain imaging findings. For example, our patient with heterotopic tissue showed asymmetric activation of the lateral occipital complex when naming objects, which could be interpreted in the context of both his pathology (i.e., LOC was proximal to the region of cortex deemed to be the origin of his seizures) and his neuropsychological profile (i.e., mild naming deficits).

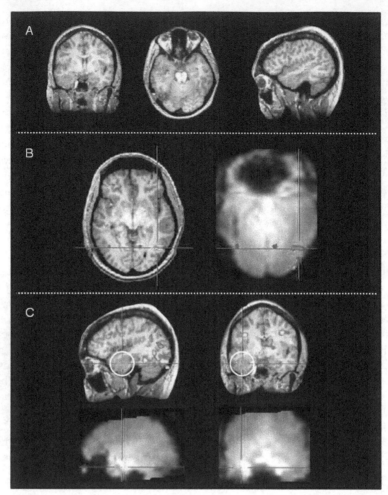

Fig. 3. Selected results from the second case study discussed. Panel A shows anatomical images highlighting the region of heterotopic tissue in the left anterior temporal cortex. Panel B shows activity in response to expanding and contracting concentric circles in area MT bilaterally. Both area and peak BOLD signal were weaker in the damaged hemisphere. Importantly, the raw fMRI data shows no drop-off in signal-to-noise ratio in the damaged hemisphere. Panel C shows activity (both raw and overlaid data) from an object naming task in which the statistical thresholds have been lowered to determine whether heterotopic tissue supported activity. This shows that a failure to detect activity in this region was not due to a lack of statistical power. Nevertheless, caution should be exercised in this instance as other explanations (e.g., abnormal vascularization) can not be ruled out. Data adapted from Danckert et al., 2007.

In both instances discussed above tasks were chosen that would lead to robust, predictable activations with a limited number of experimental runs to maximise the range of behaviours that could addressed within a single scanning session. This allowed us to explore issues of symmetry, reorganisation of function and the association between epileptiform activity and function across a reasonably large range of tasks. In other instances, the *range* of tasks to be explored is less relevant as specific hypotheses regarding particular functions allow the focus to be narrowed. For instance, recent investigations into memory functioning in an epilepsy patient who underwent resective surgery of anterior temporal cortex, focused only on specific component processes of memory – namely, familiarity vs. recollection, to determine the role played in each process by the region surgically removed (Bowles et al., 2007). Another instance in which the fMRI approach to single cases can be more narrowly focussed – that of blindsight – is discussed in more detail below.

3.2 Residual visual pathways in blindsight

Patients presenting with visual field defects, such as hemianopias, arising from lesions of primary occipital cortex (area V1) can nevertheless respond to blind field stimuli at better than chance levels (Pöppel et al., 1973; Weiskrantz et al., 1974). The term 'blindsight' was first coined by Weiskrantz and colleagues (1974) to refer to these residual visual abilities. Initial demonstrations of above chance responding to blind field stimuli showed that some patients were surprisingly accurate when reaching to, or making a saccade to target locations that had been briefly flashed in their 'blind' field (Weiskrantz et al., 1974; Zihl & Werth, 1984). Note, that the patients were "guessing" at these locations as they had no conscious experience of the targets themselves. Research on blindsight has demonstrated a myriad of residual abilities including motion discrimination, colour and form interference effects, wavelength discrimination and even semantic priming (Danckert et al., 1998; Magnussen & Mathiesen, 1989; Marcel, 1998; Morland et al., 1999; Stoerig & Cowey, 1989).

The demonstration of a broad range of residual abilities in blindsight patients indicates that secondary visual pathways carry information to extrastriate cortex in the absence of input from V1 (Cowey, 2004; Danckert & Goodale, 2000; Danckert & Rossetti, 2005; Stoerig & Cowey, 1997; Weiskrantz et al., 1974). The most prominent of these pathways spared following damage to V1 connects the superior colliculus directly to the pulvinar nucleus of the thalamus, which in turn has direct connections with extrastriate visual cortex (Cowey, 2004; Stoerig & Cowey, 1997; see Sincich et al., 2004 for demonstration of another pathway in the monkey from koniocellular layers of the LGN directly to motion-selective regions of extrastriate cortex).

One key issue in blindsight research involves demonstrating conclusively that the residual visual functions demonstrated are not in fact explained by factors not related to secondary visual pathways. Light scattering from blind to sighted portions of the retina (intraocular scatter) or from blind to sighted portions of the visual field (extraocular scatter) represent a major challenge to blindsight research (Campion et al., 1983). Masking off regions of the blind field and modifying the physical properties of the target stimuli can address these issues to some extent (King et al., 1996; Danckert et al., 2003; Danckert & Culham, 2010). A second challenge can be addressed through both anatomical and functional MRI. Some have suggested that blindsight does not rely on residual pathways bypassing V1, but instead reflects subthreshold activation in residual 'islands' of cortex within V1 (Campion et al., 1983; Fendrich et al., 1992; Gazzaniga et al., 1994). Anatomical scans in this case can conclusively address whether such islands even exist in a given patient. Functional scans have suggested that, in at least one blindsight patient, despite evidence of anatomical sparing of V1, there was no evidence that the spared region supported any functions (Stoerig et al., 1998). Although this work suffers from the absence of evidence argument discussed above, activation in the undamaged hemisphere can act as a 'control' site for the patient. In other words, if stimuli presented to the sighted field leads to robust activation in the undamaged hemisphere one can be reasonably confident that the task, equipment and statistics are not responsible for a lack of activation when the same stimuli are presented to the blind field (Stoerig et al., 1998). Furthermore, the fact that extrastriate regions *did* show activity in this patient goes a long way towards dismissing the hypothesis that residual visual capacities are in fact reliant on spared islands of cortex in V1.

Functional neuroimaging can also provide insights into the neural structures and potentially the pathways connecting those structures, that would support the range of blindsight phenomena observed. One of the more robust activation paradigms in fMRI makes use of simple flickering checkerboard stimuli to highlight retinotopic maps in striate and extrastriate cortex (e.g., Tootell et al., 1998). For example, various neuroimaging techniques, including fMRI, positron emission tomography (PET) and visual evoked potentials, have been used in the most extensively tested blindsight patient, GY, to demonstrate that, although V1 has been almost completely destroyed in this patient's left hemisphere, spared processing occurs in the visual motion complex, MT+/V5 (Barbur et al., 1993; ffytche et al., 1996; Zeki & ffytche, 1998; Bridge et al., 2008; Goebel, Muckli et al., 2001), in dorsal extrastriate cortex (Baseler et al., 1999; Goebel, et al., 2001), and even in the amygdala, colliculus and prefrontal cortex within the damaged hemisphere in response to blind field stimuli (Morris et al., 2001; Sahraie et al., 1997). Finally, diffusion tensor imaging has the potential to illuminate the white matter pathways that until recently were merely hypothesised to support the range of blindsight phenomena discussed (Leh et al., 2006).

We recently used fMRI to determine the veracity of an unusual case of responding to blind field stimuli (Danckert & Culham, 2010). Our patient had surgery to remove V1 as treatment for medication resistant epilepsy. The patient presented with unusual responses to blind field stimuli in that she consistently localised targets presented in the periphery of her blind field to locations closer to the midline of her field defect and vice versa (Figure 4).

We used fMRI to determine whether we would see residual activation in MT to blind field motion stimuli – a phenomenon evident in other blindsight patients (Magnussen & Mathiesen, 1989). We were also able to contrast our patient's performance with that of GY on similar tasks. Results showed there was no residual activation in the extrastriate cortex of the damaged hemisphere in response to blind field motion stimuli in our patient (Danckert & Culham, 2010). Again, this result suffers from the 'absence of evidence' argument. Here we were able to show reliable activity to blind field motion stimuli in GY's damaged hemisphere and were then able to show that this activity was evident in only one experimental run (Figure 4). That is, responses to blind field stimuli were reliable and robust in patient GY with only minimal exposure. The same could not be said of our patient who showed no reliable activity on any single experimental run even at lowered statistical thresholds (Figure 4). Just as in our case of heterotopic tissue discussed above (Figure 3), this kind of evidence provides additional support to the notion that the absence of activity is not simply due to a lack of statistical power. In contrast to that patient, lowering statistical thresholds in this case did show some level of signal in the voxels of the damaged hemisphere that would be expected to support blindsight motion processing (Figure 4). In this case, however, we were able to show that the 'activity' in these voxels did not show any reliable modulation with the experimental paradigm (Figure 4). Again, caution is still needed with respect to evidence of this kind as it does not rule out other potential explanations for the lack of activation.

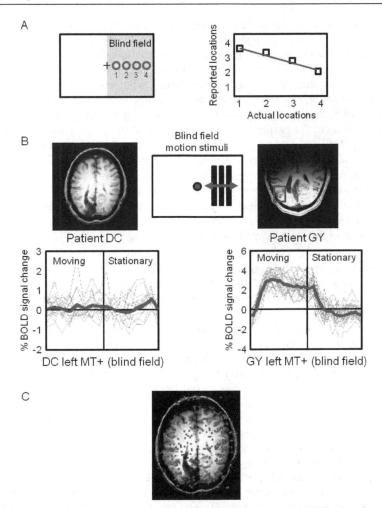

Fig. 4. Panel A shows behavioural data from a hemianopic patient (DC) who showed unusual residual behaviour. To the left is the stimulus setup in which targets could be flashed to either her sighted or blind fields (only blind field targets are shown). When asked to guess blind field target locations DC consistently mislocalised targets - that is, she consistently guessed that targets presented at location 1 in her blind field had instead appeared at location 4 and vice versa. Panel B shows fMRI data from DC and GY, a well tested blindsight patient, when motion stimuli were presented to their blind fields. For GY (to the right) blind field motion stimuli reliably activated MT bilaterally despite a lack of awareness of the stimuli (the red line below represents mean activation across a number of runs for the region highlighted on the anatomical scan show above). This response was evident even in single experimental runs (indicated by the grey lines in the event-related average). In contrast, DC showed no reliable activation to blind field motion stimuli. Panel C shows activity for DC when statistical thresholds were lowered which failed to show any reliable activation suggesting that statistical power was not responsible for the lack of activity to blind field stimuli. Data adapted from Danckert & Culham, 2010

The approaches to examining residual vision in hemianopic patients discussed above highlight many of the issues facing single case studies with fMRI. In most instances robust paradigms (e.g., retinotopy, motion processing) with known activation patterns localised to specific brain regions in the healthy brain (Sereno et al., 1995) were utilised. This enables the testing of specific and directed hypotheses concerning what one would expect to see in the patient. In contrast to the cases of epilepsy discussed above, these cases did not require an extensive range of behaviours to be tested (or accompanying neuropsychological profiling) and instead could focus on particular aspects of residual visual processing in more detail. Finally, utilising fMRI in single cases of residual vision (suspected or demonstrated) can inform not only the neural pathways necessary for supporting residual vision but also the neural signatures of conscious experience. For example, it is possible to contrast activations to stimuli that the patient does report some degree of awareness of with those instances in which they responded to stimuli without any conscious perceptual experience. The final use of fMRI in single cases to be discussed below – synaesthesia – has similar potential to inform our understanding of the neural correlates of consciousness.

3.3 Synaesthesia and the neural bases of consciousness

Synaesthesia represents an unusual perceptual phenomenon in which the subject perceives multiple percepts in response to a single sensory stimulus (Rich & Mattingley, 2002, Ward & Mattingley, 2006). Perhaps the most common synaesthetic experience is grapheme-colour associations in which a digit presented in black ink is perceived by the synaesthete to have an additional, consistent colour associated with it (e.g., 7 is always red; Rich & Mattingley, 2002, Ward & Mattingley, 2006; Ramachandran & Hubbard, 2001; Dixon et al., 2000). The study of this unusual phenomenon has the potential to offer new insights into two key issues in cognitive neuroscience: first, how are different perceptual characteristics bound to the same object? That is, colour-grapheme synaesthesia may represent an unusual form of binding in the absence of an external percept (Robertson, 2003). Second, given that synaesthetes experience conscious percepts in the absence of external stimuli, they present an interesting avenue for exploring the neural bases of consciousness and in particular, in discriminating between preconscious and conscious processes (i.e., a synaesthetic experience is by definition not preconscious; Gray 2003; Gray et al., 2006). Functional neuroimaging represents another tool through which these and other questions related to synaesthesia (e.g., is attention necessary for a synaesthetic experience?) can be addressed (Rich et al., 2005).

A key issue in synaesthesia research is the idiosyncratic nature of the individual's experience (see Hochel & Milán, 2008 and Ward & Mattingley, 2006 for review). The authenticity of the particular experience must first be verified through behavioural testing. In essence then, functional imaging approaches to synaesthesia largely *require* single case methodology. That is, given the idiosyncratic experiences of individual synaesthetes, any imaging study will need to tailor tasks to the individual's experience making group comparisons problematic (although see van Leeuwen et al., 2010). A key issue highlighted by fMRI in synaesthetes is the need for appropriate control tasks and participants. For example, Blakemore and colleagues (2005) tested a synaesthete who experienced touch sensations when observing others being touched. They first demonstrated that the synaesthete and controls showed similar patterns of activity for somatosensory stimuli of the self before examining the potential differences in activation when observing others being touched. In the latter case the intention was to determine whether the synaesthete would show differential activation to the observation of touch in the form of either *increased* activity in regions also shown to be active in controls or *additional* regions not normally activated. Results showed that the synaesthete demonstrated both kinds of activation patterns, with higher activation relative to controls in somatosensory cortex when observing others being touched and additional regions of activity in the anterior insular cortex bilaterally.

One problem with interpreting activations in synaesthetes (or indeed in neurological patients) not evident in controls is that it remains possible that statistical power or other analysis variables may have led to the failure to see those same regions in controls (Friston & Price, 2003). Essentially, additional activations seen in the synaesthete may be evidence of a cognitively degenerate system. That is, there may be more than one brain region or network capable of performing a given cognitive task with only a subset of those regions evident in the analysis of the control group (Friston & Price, 2003; Price & Friston, 2006). One approach to address this concern is to match the synaesthete (or patient, as in the blindsight example above) with a control subject with similar behavioural competencies or idiosyncracies (or similar deficits in the case of neurological patients). Elias and colleagues (2003) did this by contrasting a grapheme-colour synaesthete with a cross-stitch expert. Cross-stitching involves consistent, overlearned associations between colours and numbers. Both the synaesthete and the cross-stitch expert showed Stroop-like interference effects for incongruently coloured numbers (i.e., for the synaesthete this means presenting a number in a colour inconsistent with her perceptual experience, whereas for the cross-stitch expert this meant presenting a number is an incorrectly associated colour with respect to the standards used in cross-stitching). Despite similar behavioural effects, the synaesthete showed distinct neural activations (Elias et al., 2003). The power of this design is that the two individuals (who were also contrasted with a healthy control group) demonstrated comparable behaviours. Some would argue that this is an essential component of using fMRI to explore neurological cases (Price & Friston, 2006) although it is far more challenging to find tasks that patients and controls perform at a similar level. Regardless, the advantage is that with identical behavioural performance, differences in neural activation are less ambiguous. In the example discussed above, the cross-stitch expert represents an 'over-trained' normal control individual, whereas the synaesthete, by virtue of the distinct neural activations observed, clearly invokes different neural patterns to support her unique perceptual experience. Without such a control participant (and beyond the most commonly experienced form of synaesthesia it is hard to see how one would obtain such controls; Smilek et al., 2007) additional activations evident in synaesthesia are difficult to interpret.

As already mentioned in the other examples presented in this chapter, choosing tasks with well documented activation patterns in the healthy brain represents an important component of the approach to investigating the neural basis of synaesthesia. For example, retinotopic mapping demonstrates the borders of visual areas in the healthy brain including those regions most responsive to colour – areas V4 and V8 (Sereno, et al., 1995; Tootell, et al., 1998). Sperling and colleagues (2006) tested four grapheme-colour synaethetes using retinotopic mapping to first delineate areas V4/V8. Subsequent tests then presented graphemes that did and did not have associated syneasthetic colour experiences (idiosyncratic to the individual synaesthete) in regions corresponding to the retinotopically mapped V4/V8. For the synaesthetes, graphemes with associated colours led to higher activity in V4/V8 than did graphemes with no colour association (Sperling et al., 2006). In contrast, van Leeuwen and colleagues (2010) used another fMRI technique – MR adaptation, in which repeated presentation of a stimulus leads to reduced BOLD signal – to demonstrate that adaptation occurred not in colour responsive cortex but in the left superior parietal lobule. This result was taken to suggest that synaesthetic experiences depend on feedback from higher cortical regions. Nevertheless, in both instances conclusions regarding the neural basis of syneasthetic experiences benefited from the use of robust paradigms with well documented activation patterns.

Perhaps the primary concern in fMRI with syneasthetes involves the interpretation of additional activations not seen in the healthy brain (Price & Friston, 2003). Closely matched controls, robust tasks with predictable activation patterns and closely matching BOLD signal with behaviour (e.g., dissociating BOLD signal to graphemes that do vs. do not lead to syneasthetic percepts) represent important considerations that can at least partly assist with interpretations of additional activations.

4. Conclusion

Neuroimaging techniques, including functional MRI, are necessarily correlational in nature. From neuroimaging then, we can make conclusions regarding which regions are *sufficient* for a particular function (Friston & Price, 2003; Price & Friston, 2006). In addition, activity may reflect one or many regions/systems capable of subserving the function under consideration (i.e., cognitive degeneracy; Friston & Price, 2003). In contrast, single case studies of neurological patients can demonstrate which brain regions are *necessary* for a given behaviour. The combination of the two methodologies has the potential to provide insights into brain-behaviour relationships that each technique alone can not address, with both clinical and basic science implications. Issues concerning changes to vascularisation as a consequence of neural insult or abnormal neural development, altered signal-to-noise ratios in those regions and consistency of the haemodynamic response function across sessions all represent challenges to implementing single case fMRI studies. In addition, task choice and design involve a number of important considerations: can the patient perform the task? Can performance be correlated with changes in BOLD signal (e.g., differences related to errors vs. correct trials, conscious vs. unconscious percepts, etc.)? Are there precedents in the healthy population (i.e., does the task lead to robust, reliable patterns of activation)? Contrasting activation with similar patients (e.g., Danckert & Culham, 2010) also represents an important strategy with the potential to bolster interpretations of either additional activations or a lack of activation. Nevertheless, the absence of activations in expected regions represents a significant challenge in applying fMRI to single case methods. One approach might be to conduct large scale normative fMRI studies or meta-analyses to provide robust expectations regarding patterns of activation for a range of behaviours that could then be applied to single case studies with either a basic or clinical focus (see Vigneau et al., 2006 for an example of this with respect to language tasks). Given appropriate consideration, the combination of fMRI and single case methodologies has the potential to lead to insights into a wide range of important issues in clinical and cognitive neuroscience.

5. References

Abou-Khalil, B., & Schlaggar, B.L. (2002). Is it time to replace the Wada test? *Neurology, 59,* 160–161.

Adcock, J.E., Wise, R.G., Oxbury, J.M., Oxbury, S.M., & Matthews, P.M. (2003). Quantitative fMRI assessment of the differences in lateralization of language-related brain activation in patients with temporal lobe epilepsy. *Neuroimage, 18,* 423–438.

Aguirre, G.K., Zarahn, E., & D'Esposito, M. (1998). The variability of human, BOLD hemodynamic responses. *Neuroimage, 8,* 360–369.

Bandettini, P.A., & Cox, R.W. (2000) Event-related fMRI contrast when using constant interstimulus interval: theory and experiment. *Magnetic Resonance Medicine, 43,* 540–548.

Banich, M.T. (2004). Cognitive Neuroscience and Neuropsychology, 2nd Edition. Houghton, Mifflin, Boston, USA.

Barbur, J.L., Watson, J.D.G., Frackowiak, R.S.J., & Zeki, S. (1993). Conscious visual perception without V1. *Brain, 116,* 1293–1302.

Bartolomeo, P., Thiebaut de Schotten, M., & Doricchi, F. (2007) Left unilateral neglect as a disconnection syndrome. *Cerebral Cortex, 17,* 2479–2490.

Baseler, H.A., Morland, A.B., & Wandell, B.A. (1999). Topographic organisation of human visual areas in the absence of input from primary cortex. *Journal of Neuroscience, 19,* 2619–2627.

Beck, H., & Plate, K.H. (2009) Angiogenesis after cerebral ischemia. *Acta Neuropathologica, 117,* 481–496.

Bittar, R.G., Ptito, M., Faubert, J., Dumoulin, S.O., & Ptito, A. (1999). Activation of the remaining hemisphere following stimulation of the blind hemifield in hemispherectomized subjects. *Neuroimage, 10,* 339–346.

Bowles, B., Crupi, C., Mirsattari, S.M., Pigott, S.E., Parrent, A.G., Pruessner, J.C., Yonelinas, A.P., & Köhler, S. (2007). Impaired familiarity with preserved recollection after anterior temporal-lobe resection that spares the hippocampus. *Proceedings of the National Academy of Science, U S A, 104,* 16382–16387.

Bridge, H., Thomas, O., Jbabdi, S., & Cowey, A. (2008). Changes in connectivity after visual cortical brain damage underlie altered visual function. *Brain, 131,* 1433–1444.

Broca, P. (1861). Nouvelle observation d'aphémie produite par une lésion de la moité postérieur des deuxiéme et troisiéme circonvolutions frontales. *Bulletins de la Société Anatomique de Paris, 36,* 398–407.

Campion, J., Latto, R., & Smith, Y.M. (1983). Is blindsight an effect of scattered light, spared cortex, and near-threshold vision? *The Behavioural and Brain Sciences, 6,* 423–486.

Chatterjee, A. (2005). A madness to the methods in cognitive neuroscience? *Journal of Cognitive Neuroscience, 17,* 847–849.

Chen, Y., & Parrish, T.B. (2009) Caffeine dose effect on activation-induced BOLD and CBF responses. *Neuroimage, 46,* 577–583.

Corbetta, M., Kincade, M.J., Lewis, C., Snyder, A.Z., & Sapir, A. (2005) Neural basis and recovery of spatial attention deficits in spatial neglect. *Nature Neuroscience, 8,* 1603–1610.

Coslett, H.B., & Lie, G. (2008) Simultanagnosia: when a rose is not red. *Journal of Cognitive Neuroscience, 20,* 36–48.

Cowey, A. (2004). The 30th Sir Frederick Bartlett lecture: Fact, artefact, and myth about blindsight. *The Quarterly Journal of Experimental Psychology, 57A,* 577–609.

Danckert, J., & Rossetti, Y. (2005). Blindsight in action: What can the different subtypes of blindsight tell us about the control of visually guided actions? *Neuroscience and Biobehavioural Reviews, 29,* 1035–1046.

Danckert, J., Revol, P., Pisella, L., Krolak-Salmon, P., Vighetto, A., Goodale, M.A., & Rossetti, Y. (2003). Measuring unconscious actions in action-blindsight: exploring the kinematics of pointing movements to targets in the blind field of two patients with cortical hemianopia. *Neuropsychologia, 41,* 1068–1081.

Danckert, J., & Goodale, M.A. (2000). Blindsight: A conscious route to unconscious vision. *Current Biology, 10,* R64–R67.

Danckert, J., Maruff, P., Kinsella, G., de Graff, S., & Currie, J. (1998). Investigating form and colour perception in blindsight using an interference task. *NeuroReport, 9,* 2919–2925.

Danckert, J., Ferber, S., Doherty, T., Steinmetz, H., Nicolle, D., & Goodale, M.A. (2002) Selective, non-lateralized impairment of motor imagery following right parietal damage. *Neurocase, 8,* 194–204.

Danckert, J., Mirsattari, S.M., Danckert, S., Wiebe, S., Blume, W.T., Carey, D., Menon, R., & Goodale, M.A. (2004) Spared somatomotor and cognitive functions in a patient with a large porencephalic cyst revealed by fMRI. *Neuropsychologia, 42,* 405–418.

Danckert, J., Mirsattari, S.M., Bihari, F., Danckert, S., Allman, A-A., Janzen, L. (2007) Functional MRI characteristics of a focal region of cortical malformation not associated with seizure onset. *Epilepsy & Behaviour, 10,* 615–625.

Danckert, J., & Culham, J.C. (2010) Reflections on blindsight: neuroimaging and behavioural explorations clarify a case of reversed localisation in the blind field of a patient with hemianopia. *Canadian Journal of Experimental Psychology, 64,* 86–101.

De Martino, F., Valente, G., Staeren, N., Ashburner, J., Goebel, R., & Formisano, E. (2008). Combining multivariate voxel selection and support vector machines for mapping and classification of fMRI spatial patterns. *Neuroimage, 43,* 44–58.

D'Esposito, M., Deouell, L.Y., & Gazzaley, A. (2003). Alterations in the BOLD fMRI signal with ageing and disease: A challenge for neuroimaging. *Nature Reviews Neuroscience, 4,* 863–872.

Dixon, M.J., Smilek, D., Cudahy, C., & Merikle, P.M. (2000). Five plus two equals yellow. *Nature, 406,* 365.

Dukelow, S.P., DeSouza, J.F., Culham, J.C., van den Berg, A.V., Menon, R.S., & Vilis, T. (2001) Distinguishing subregions of the human MT+ complex using visual fields and pursuit eye movements. *Journal of Neurophysiology, 86,* 1991–2000.

Fendrich, R., Wessinger, C.M., & Gazzaniga, M.S. (1992). Residual vision in a scotoma: Implications for blindsight. *Science, 258,* 1489–1491.

Fernandes, M.A., Smith, M.L., Logan, W., Crawley, A., & McAndrews, M.P. (2006) Comparing language lateralization determined by dichotic listening and fMRI activation in frontal and temporal lobes in children with epilepsy. *Brain and Language, 96,* 106–114.

Fernandes, M.A., & Smith, M.L. (2000) Comparing the Fused Dichotic Words Test and the Intracarotid Amobarbital Procedure in children with epilepsy. *Neuropsychologia, 38,* 1216–1228.

ffytche, D.H., Guy, C.N., & Zeki, S. (1996). Motion specific responses from a blind hemifield. *Brain, 199,* 1971–1982.

Ford, K.A., Gati, J.S., Menon, R.S.,& Everling, S. (2009) BOLD fMRI activation for anti-saccades in nonhuman primates. *Neuroimage, 45,* 470–476.

Fox, P.T. (1997). The growth of human brain mapping. *Human Brain Mapping, 5,* 1–2.

Friston, K.J., & Price, C.J. (2003) Degeneracy and redundancy in cognitive anatomy. *Trends in Cognitive Science, 7,* 151–152.

Gaudino, E.A., Geisler, M.W., & Squires, N.K. (1995) Construct validity in the Trail Making Test: What makes Part B harder? *Journal of Clinical and Experimental Neuropsychology, 17*, 529–535.

Gazzaniga, M.S., Fendrich, R., & Wessinger, C.M. (1994). Blindsight reconsidered. *Current Directions in Psychological Science, 3*, 93–96.

Goebel, R., Muckli, L., Zanella, F.E., Singer, W., & Stoerig, P. (2001). Sustained extrastriate cortical activation without visual awareness revealed by fMRI studies of hemianopic patients. *Vision Research, 41*, 1459–1474.

Gray, J.A. (2003). How are qualia coupled to functions? *Trends in Cognitive Sciences, 7*, 192–194.

Gray, J.A., Parslow, D.M., Brammer, M.J., Chopping, S., Vythelingum, G.N., & ffytche, D.H. (2006). Evidence against functionalism from neuroimaging of the alien colour effect in synaesthesia. *Cortex, 42*, 309–318.

Guerrini, R., & Barba, C. (2010) Malformations of cortical development and aberrant cortical networks: epileptogenesis and functional organization. *Journal of Clinical Neurophysiology, 27*, 372–379.

Haas, L.F. (2001) Jean Martin Charcot (1825-93) and Jean Baptiste Charcot (1867-1936). *Journal of Neurology, Neurosurgery & Psychiatry, 71*, 524.

Hochel, M. & Milán, E.G. (2008). Synaesthesia: The existing state of affairs. *Cognitive Neuropsychology, 25*, 93–117.

Huettel, S.A., Song, A.W., & McCarthy, G. (2004). Functional Magnetic Resonance Imaging. Sinauer Associates, Massachusetts, USA.

Humphreys, G.W., & Riddoch, M.J. (1996). Poppelreuter's case of Merk: The analysis of visual disturbances following a gunshot wound to the brain. In C. Code, C-W. Wallesch, Y. Joanette & A. Roch Lecours (Eds.) Classic Cases in Neuropsychology. Psychology Press, Erlbaum, East Sussex, UK.

Jones, S.E., Mahmoud, S.Y., & Phillips, M.D. (2011). A practical clinical method to quantify language lateralization in fMRI using whole-brain analysis. *Neuroimage, 54*, 2937–2949.

King, S.M., Azzopardi, P., Cowey, A., Oxbury, J., & Oxbury, S. (1996). The role of light scatter in the residual visual sensitivity of patients with complete cerebral hemispherectomy. *Vision Neuroscience, 13*, 1-13.

Kolb, B., & Wishaw, I.Q. (2009). Fundamentals of Human Neuropsychology, 6th Edition. Worth Publishers, USA.

Kourtzi, Z., & Kanwisher, N. (2000) Cortical regions involved in perceiving object shape. *Journal of Neuroscience, 20*, 3310–3318.

Leh, S.E., Johansen-Berg, H., & Ptito, A. (2006). Unconscious vision: new insights into the neuronal correlate of blindsight using diffusion tractography. *Brain, 129*, 1822–1832.

Lerdal, A., Bakken, L.N., Kouwenhoven, S.E., Pedersen, G., Kirkevold, M., Finset, A., & Kim, H.S. (2009)

Poststroke fatigue--a review. *Journal of Pain Symptom Management, 38*, 928–949.

Lezak, M.D., Howieson, D.B., & Loring, D.W. (2004). Neuropsychological Assessment, 4th Edition. Oxford, New York.

Magnussen, S., & Mathiesen, T. (1989). Detection of moving and stationary gratings in the absence of striate cortex. *Neuropsychologia, 27*, 725–728.

Marcel, A.J. (1998). Blindsight and shape perception: Deficit of visual consciousness or of visual function? *Brain, 121,* 1565-1588.

Milner, B. (2005) The medial temporal-lobe amnesic syndrome. *Psychiatry Clin North America,* 28, 599-611.

Milner, B., & Penfield, W. (1955-1956) The effect of hippocampal lesions on recent memory. *Transactions of the American Neurological Association, (80th Meeting),* 42-48.

Monti, M.M. (2011). Statistical Analysis of fMRI Time-Series: A Critical Review of the GLM Approach. *Frontiers in Human Neuroscience, 5,* 28.

Morland, A.B., Jones, S.R., Finlay, A.L., Deyzac, E., Le, S., & Kemp, S. (1999). Visual perception of motion, luminance and colour in a human hemianope. *Brain, 122,* 1183-1196.

Morris, J.S., de Gelder, B., Weiskrantz, L., & Dolan, R.J. (2001). Differential extrageniculostrate and amygdala responses to presentation of emotional faces in a cortically blind field. *Brain, 124,* 1241-1252.

Nandhagopal, R., McKeown, M.J., & Stoessl, A.J. (2008) Functional imaging in Parkinson disease. *Neurology, 70,* 1478-1488.

Ogawa, S., Tank, D.W., Menon, R., Ellermann, J.M., Kim, S.G., Merkle, H., & Ugurbil, K. (1992) Intrinsic signal changes accompanying sensory stimulation: functional brain mapping with magnetic resonance imaging. *Proceedings of the National Academy of Sciences, U S A, 89,* 5951-5955.

Peng, G., & Wang, W.S. (in press) Hemisphere lateralization is influenced by bilingual status and composition of words. *Neuropsychologia.*

Pöppel, E., Held, R., & Frost, D. (1973). Residual visual function after brain wounds involving the central visual pathways in man. *Nature, 243,* 295-296.

Poppelreuter, W. (1917/1990). Disturbances of lower and higher visual capacities caused by occipital damage. (J. Zihl with L. Weiskrantz, Tanslation). Clarendon Press, Oxford, UK.

Price, C.J. (2010) The anatomy of language: a review of 100 fMRI studies published in 2009. *Annals of the New York Academy of Science, 1191,* 62-88.

Price, C.J. (2000) The anatomy of language: contributions from functional neuroimaging. *Journal of Anatomy, 197,* 335-359.

Price, C.J., & Friston, K.J. (1999) Scanning patients with tasks they can perform. *Human Brain Mapping,8,* 102-108.

Price, C.J., Crinion, J., & Friston, K.J. (2006) Design and analysis of fMRI studies with neurologically impaired patients. *Journal of Magnetic Resonance Imaging, 23,* 816-826.

Ptito, M., Johannsen, P., Faubert, J., & Gjedde, A. (1999). Activation of human extrageniculostriate pathways after damage to area V1. *Neuroimage, 9,* 97-107.

Raichle, M.E. (1994) Images of the mind: studies with modern imaging techniques. *Annual Reviews in Psychology, 45,* 333-356.

Ramachandran, V.S., & Hubbard, E.M. (2001). Psychophysical investigations into the neural basis of synaesthesia. *Proceedings of Biological Sciences, 268,* 979-983.

Rich, A.N., Bradshaw, J.L., & Mattingley, J.B. (2005). A systematic, largescale study of synaesthesia: Implications for the role of early experience in lexical-colour associations. *Cognition, 98,* 53-84.

Rich, A.N., & Mattingley, J.B. (2002). Anomalous perception in synaesthesia: a cognitive neuroscience perspective. *Nature Reviews Neuroscience, 3,* 43-52.

Rilling, J.K., Glenn, A.L., Jairam, M.R., Pagnoni, G., Goldsmith, D.R., Elfenbein, H.A., & Lilienfeld, S.O. (2007) Neural correlates of social cooperation and non-cooperation as a function of psychopathy. *Biological Psychiatry, 61*, 1260–1271.

Robertson, L.C. (2003). Binding, spatial attention and perceptual awareness. *Nature Reviews Neuroscience, 4*, 93–102.

Rorden, C., & Karnath, H-O. (2004) Using human brain lesions to infer function: a relic from a past era in the fMRI age? *Nature Reviews Neuroscience, 5*, 813–819.

Ryalls, J., & Lecours, A.R. (1996). Broca's first two cases: from bumps on the head to cortical convolutions. In C. Code, C-W. Wallesch, Y. Joanette & A. Roch Lecours (Eds.) Classic Cases in Neuropsychology. Psychology Press, Erlbaum, East Sussex, UK.

Sahraie, A., Weiskrantz, L., Barbur, J.L., Simmons, A., Williams, S.C.R., & Brammer, M.J. (1997). Pattern of neuronal activity associated with conscious and unconscious processing of visual signals. *Proceedings of the National Academy of Sciences, USA, 94*, 9406–9411.

Scoville, W.B., & Milner, B. (1957). Loss of recent memory after bilateral hippocampal lesions. *Journal of Neurology, Neurosurgery, & Psychiatry, 20*, 11–21.

Sereno, M.I., Dale, A.M., Reppas, J.B., Kwong, K.K., Belliveau, J.W., Brady, T.J., Rosen, B.R., & Tootell, R.B. (1995) Borders of multiple visual areas in humans revealed by functional magnetic resonance imaging. *Science, 268*, 889–893.

Shulman, G.L., Pope, D.L.W., Astafiev, S.V., McAvoy, M.P., Snyder, A.Z., & Corbetta, M. (2010). Right hemisphere dominance during spatial selective attention and target detection occurs outside the dorsal frontoparietal network. *The Journal of Neuroscience, 30*, 3640–3651.

Sincich, L.C., Park, K.F., Wohlgemuth, M.J., & Horton, J.C. (2004). Bypassing V1: a direct geniculate input to area MT. *Nature Neuroscience, 7*, 1123–1128.

Smilek, D., Malcolmson, K.A., Carriere, J.S., Eller, M., Kwan, D., & Reynolds. M. (2007). When "3" is a jerk and "E" is a king: personifying inanimate objects in synesthesia. *Journal of Cognitive Neuroscience, 19*, 981–992.

Steeves, J.K., Humphrey, G.K., Culham, J.C., Menon, R.S., Milner, A.D., & Goodale, M.A. (2004). Behavioral and neuroimaging evidence for a contribution of color and texture information to scene classification in a patient with visual form agnosia. *Journal of Cognitive Neuroscience, 16*, 955–965.

Stoerig, P., & Cowey, A. (1989). Wavelength sensitivity in blindsight. *Nature, 342*, 916–918.

Stoerig, P., & Cowey, A. (1997). Blindsight in man and monkey. *Brain, 120*, 535–559.

Stoerig, P., Kleinschmidt, A., & Frahm, J. (1998). No visual responses in denervated V1: high-resolution functional magnetic resonance imaging of a blindsight patient. *Neuroreport, 9*, 21–25.

Toma, K., & Nakai, T. (2002) Functional MRI in human motor control studies and clinical applications. *Magnetic Resonance Medical Science, 1*, 109–120.

Tootell, R.B., Hadjikhani, N., Mendola, J.D., Marrett, S., & Dale, A.M. (1998). From retinotopy to recognition: fMRI in visual cortex. *Trends in Cognitive Science, 2*, 174–183.

Tootell, R.B., Reppas, J.B., Kwong, K.K., Malach, R., Born, R.T., Brady, T.J., Rosen, B.R., & Belliveau, J.W. (1995) Functional analysis of human MT and related visual cortical areas using magnetic resonance imaging. *Journal of Neuroscience, 15*, 3215–3230.

Tyvaert, L., Levan, P., Grova, C., Dubeau, F., & Gotman, J. (2008). Effects of fluctuating physiological rhythms during prolonged EEG-fMRI studies. *Clinical Neurophysiology, 119,* 2762–2774.

Vaishnavi, S., Rao, V., & Fann, J.R. (2009) Neuropsychiatric problems after traumatic brain injury: unraveling the silent epidemic. *Psychosomatics, 50,* 198–205.

van Leeuwen, T.M., Petersson, K.M., & Hagoort, P. (2010). Synaesthetic colour in the brain: Beyond colour areas. A functional magnetic resonance imaging study of synaesthetes and matched controls. *PLoS One, 5,* 1–12.

Vigneau, M., Beaucousin, V., Hervé, P.Y., Duffau, H., Crivello, F., Houdé, O., Mazoyer, B., & Tzourio-Mazoyer, N. (2006). Meta-analyzing left hemisphere language areas: phonology, semantics, and sentence processing. *Neuroimage, 30,* 1414–1432.

Ward, J., & Mattingley, J.B. (2006). Synaesthesia: an overview of contemporary findings and controversies. *Cortex, 42,* 129–136.

Weiskrantz, L., Warrington, E.K., Sanders, M.D., & Marshall, J. (1974). Visual capacity in the hemianopic field following a restricted occipital ablation. *Brain, 97,* 709–728.

Woermann, F.G., Jokeit, H., Luerding, R., Freitag, H., Schulz, R., Guertler, S., Okujava, M., Wolf, P., Tuxhorn, I., & Ebner, A. (2003). Language lateralisation by Wada test and fMRI in 100 patients with epilepsy. *Neurology, 61,*699–701.

Wong, S.W.H., Jong, L., Bandur, D., Bihari, F., Yen, Y.F., Takahashi, A.M., Lee, D.H., Steven, D.A., Parrent, A.G., Pigott, S.E., & Mirsattari, S.M. (2009). Cortical reorganization in temporal lobe epilepsy patients following anterior temporal lobectomy. *Neurology, 73,* 518–525.

Yücel, M., Pantelis, C., Stuart, G.W., Wood, S.J., Maruff, P., Velakoulis, D., Pipingas, A., Crowe, S.F., Tochon-Danguy, H.J., & Egan, G.F. (2002). Anterior cingulate activation during Stroop task performance: a PET to MRI coregistration study of individual patients with schizophrenia. *American Journal of Psychiatry, 159,* 251–254.

Zeki, S., & ffytche, D.H. (1998). The Riddoch syndrome: insights into the neurobiology of conscious vision. *Brain, 121,* 25–45.

Zihl, J., & Werth, R. (1984). Contributions to the study of "blindsight" – I. Can stray light account for saccadic localisation in patients with postgeniculate field defects? *Neuropsychologia, 22,* 1–11.

Zilmer, E.A., & Spiers, M.V. (2001). Principles of Neuropsychology. Wadsworth, Belmont, USA.

3

Functional and Structural Magnetic Resonance Imaging of Human Language: A Review

Manuel Martín-Loeches and Pilar Casado

Center UCM-ISCIII for Human Evolution and Behavior, UCM-ISCIII, Madrid
Spain

1. Introduction

In this review we outline the range of functional processes involved in language comprehension and their anatomical underpinnings, including recent data on neural connectivity specifically wired for language, using magnetic resonance imaging (MRI) as main tool. A review of this type certainly implies such a large number of references that, for the sake of concision, we have selected the most outstanding and representative studies and reviews. Our interests in identifying possible cues for the evolutionary origins of language partially guided this selection; this review is actually intended as a contribution to better understand human language.

To start with, a description of language and its components appears necessary. In this regard, we will follow the proposal by Ray Jackendoff (2002), who provides one of the most comprehensive and valuable current accounts from the linguistics. Jackendoff proposes at least three structural layers in language, all of them working simultaneously in the processing of every utterance. These layers consist of a *phonological structure*, a *syntactic structure*, and a *semantic/conceptual structure*. Additionally, a number of processes -or subprocesses- coexist within each of these three structures, all of them again working simultaneously.

The phonological structure, which roughly refers to the "sounds" of language, is probably the most complex one, containing the largest number of subprocesses. The auditory-verbal nature of human language may not be alien to this complexity. The phonological structure is actually subdivided into a *prosodic* one -referring to the different intonations along the course of a general envelope covering an entire utterance- and more partial processes referring to *syllabic, segmental,* and *morpho-phonological* structures. These latter three structures refer to what most people would call "phonology" as such, and roughly cover the sounds of single syllables, larger word segments, and complete words, respectively.

Syntax refers to the structure of a sentence; that is, the way in which the different words or morphemes constituting a sentence are organized -most often hierarchically-, determining their mutual relationships and dependencies. The hierarchical structure achieved by syntax establishes what the main information is and its relationships with other, secondary items of information; that is, the concrete state of affairs described in an utterance in which the meaning of individual words and morphemes combine. This structure appears "desemantized", i.e., it can be entirely independent of the individual meanings of its constituents, as in the classical example by Chomsky: "*Colorless green ideas sleep furiously*".

The semantic/conceptual structure of a linguistic utterance is probably the most central one. Indeed, the main aim of processing any linguistic message, regardless of its syntactic structure and transmission modality, is the realization of this semantic structure. This basically consists on the "meaning" of any whole sentence, that is, what it specifically means, or the idea in the mind of the speaker that she wants to elicit in the mind of the hearer. Although this information largely relies on syntax and phonology, the semantic/conceptual structure is completely independent of them –the same idea can actually be transmitted using the two other structures in many ways-. Although single words or morphemes in isolation convey semantic/conceptual information, the combination of these individual meanings by means of syntax, which in turn is achieved by means of phonology, gives place to a different, very specific meaning or semantic structure describing a concrete and detailed situation. It is not clear, however, to which extent the semantic/conceptual structure belongs to language as such, or whether it is a general process, common to other input options such as the non-linguistic interactions between the individual and her environment. In this regard, several authors still distinguish between semantic aspects specific of language and general semantic aspects common to any domain, and this distinction is particularly applicable at the level of the meaning of single words or morphemes. However, the distinction between semantics for language and general semantics appears difficult to embrace from the neural perspective, as we will see. Whatever the case, the semantic structure taps into reality, "*space* structure", i.e., the events in the real world a linguistic message refers to.

Semantics also applies to a layer not explicitly highlighted in Jackendoff's proposal but playing a significant role in language comprehension: the *discourse* level. This level refers to the situation in which two or more sentences are comprehended together, i.e., it is the semantic analysis beyond sentences. Indeed, many of the phenomena involved at this level are even less language-specific than those at the other layers or structures. In a discourse, although the hearer is attempting to get the whole comprehension of a longer message, the final picture does not depend for the most part on what is actually heard or read but, rather, on inferences and logical relationships between the ideas transmitted linguistically. These relationships are indeed extra information added by the hearer and based on her previous knowledge of the world. Although this might not be "language" as such, language would be useless if this level is not achieved.

All the processes described so far, i.e., the phonological, prosodic, syntactic, semantic, and discourse structures, may participate in sequential order –actually following this same order - or occur largely in parallel -mostly before the first 250 ms after stimulus onset (Pulvermüller et al., 2009b)-. In the literature, these two opposing views still remain. Whatever the case, the high degree of specialization and efficiency of the human brain for speech processing at all these levels is granted by most authors.

The fact that language can be transmitted using other than the auditory/verbal modality, as in the sign languages of deaf people, or, more frequently, in written form, also deserves some consideration. Consequently, a few lines in this review will be devoted to written language. Overall, most authors would agree that the linguistic machinery in the brain is largely common to any modality, with notable exceptions appearing only when specific peripheral mechanisms are engaged during the emission or decoding of a given message.

2. The sounds of language

Phonology has been less extensively studied using neuroimaging techniques than any other aspect of language. The perspective that phonology may not be as crucial in defining human language when compared to non-human forms of communication as other aspects of language, such as semantics or, particularly, syntax (Hauser et al., 2002), has probably biased the interests of the authors apart from this structure. However, human language is primarily an auditory-verbal process which, in turn, implies cerebral specializations at this level. On one hand, phonological aspects seem to be processed into specialized brain areas located within and around primary auditory ones (Brodmann Areas -BA- 41/42, Heschl's gyrus). In this regard, there is evidence of the use of extensive regions within the superior temporal gyrus largely specialized for these functions. These regions are mostly bilateral, though some degree of left-lateralization also emerges. Accordingly, a very first step in the processing of phonological information seems to be localized very dorsally in the temporal lobe, in Heschl's gyrus, where phonology would be already distinguished from non-linguistic sounds (Price, 2000). Thereafter, an antero-lateral functional gradient starting in Heschl's gyrus and progressing toward the temporal pole seems involved in further integrating heard sounds, identifying and distinguishing concrete phonological sounds such as familiar vowels against single formants (Leff et al., 2009). Additional data complete this picture by adding more ventral -middle temporal gyrus- and posterior areas of the left temporal lobe as involved as well in these functions (Specht et al., 2009).

An additional specialization for auditory language processing refers to whole words. This is known as "word-form" analysis, which means that, rather than the processing of single phonemes or longer auditory segments, what is processed and identified at this level is the overall specific sound of an entire word; a holistic analysis. There seem to be specialized cortical regions for the integration of phonological sounds into these larger and unitary sound chains, these regions corresponding to auditory association areas in the left hemisphere. A possible candidate for this process seems to be Wernicke's area. Its location next to primary auditory areas would favor such specialization. Wernicke's area is normally located in the posterior part of BA 22 within the superior temporal gyrus and sulcus (Wise et al., 2001). There are other alternatives for the location of Wernicke's area, however. Some of them spread the posterior part of BA 22 to also cover parts of BA 39 and 40 in the parietal lobe (Mesulam, 1998), whereas others locate Wernicke's area at the unimodal auditory association areas in the superior temporal gyrus just anterior to the primary auditory cortex (Démonet et al., 1992) -then covering portions that have been already mentioned here as participating in lower-level phonological analyses-. Indeed, irrespective of whether these more anterior regions can be considered or not as belonging to Wernicke's area, they have actually been claimed as the precise location for the "auditory word form area" (Cohen et al., 2004). Interestingly, however, it has been also claimed that there are no such specific cortical sites devoted to auditory word-form processing (Price et al., 2003; these authors also claim against a "visual word-form area" -see below-).

In any event, the systemic nature of the brain becomes already patent even at these very primary stages of language comprehension. In other words, the perception of speech sounds would not be limited to the temporal auditory and surrounding cortical areas, but is also significantly involving frontal cortical regions and subcortical nuclei normally implied in production (i.e., motor) processes. Accordingly, in addition to the superior temporal cortex, the most posterior portions of the left inferior frontal regions -comprising parts of Broca's area-, the left basal ganglia, and even the (right) cerebellum, seem to play a crucial role in identifying the phonemes and sounds used during speech processing (Bozic et al., 2010). Although specific roles for these neural circuits have still to be elucidated, their involvement has been proposed as a mechanism to better process speech sounds regardless of large variability in the input, a way to internally produce those sounds as if the hearer herself were the emitter (Lieberman, 2000). Kotz and Schwartze (2010) stress that these regions, particularly the basal ganglia and the cerebellum, process timing variables crucial for speech. Overal, this is an example of the conjoint action of perceptual and motor brain systems in cognitive processing, as supported by direct evidences as the mirror neurons (Rizzolatti & Craighero, 2004).

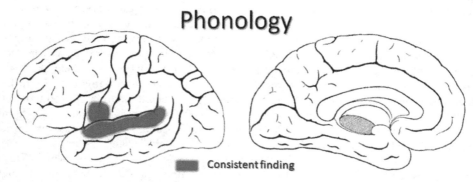

Fig. 1. Approximate locations of the phonological system

If, overall, phonology has been scarcely studied by means of MRI, the case is still worse specifically for prosody, even if this type of auditory information may be as relevant as to determining the syntactic structure of a linguistic message (Snedeker, 2008). There is evidence of the involvement of right fronto-lateral cortical areas (fronto-opercular portions in the right inferior frontal gyrus) and the right superior temporal regions in main analyses of prosody, as has been found when comparing normal speech and pseudo-speech (i.e., speech with normal prosodic intonations but devoid of known words) with degraded speech (e.g., Meyer et al., 2004). Even though, the role of the counterparts regions in the left hemisphere for the processing of prosodic information cannot be obliterated. A common circuit for language, music, and song perception comprising mid and superior temporal gyri as well as inferior and middle frontal gyri, all bilaterally, has been described (Schön et al., 2010). It is true, nonetheless, that the main implication of either hemisphere appears a function of the phonological vs. melodical nature of the input material (corresponding to left vs. right side, respectively).

3. The pictures of language

As mentioned, language can also be visual (as well as gestural), even if this is not originally the "natural" modality for human language. The human brain exhibits a high degree of flexibility and adaptability, yielding high levels of efficacy in tasks to which it is most probably not genetically prepared; reading is an outstanding example in this regard. For a long time, the place in the brain for the "visual word-from area" has been the target of strong debates, even its existence has been put into doubt (Price et al., 2003). The angular gyrus was originally proposed as playing this role by the very first (historical) neurolinguistic models, and indeed it has appeared as such occasionally in recent functional MRI (fMRI) studies (e.g., Bookheimer et al., 1995). However, the fact that this activation is not consistent, while this region seems better characterized as semantic, has encouraged researchers to look elsewhere. A number of studies locate this functional region into Wernicke's area. But this activation is common to both visual and auditory words (Price et al., 2003) and, indeed, the most plausible functional characterization of Wernicke's area as auditory associative is difficult to conform to a visual word-form area. Some portions of the occipito-temporal cortex appear as better candidates for this function. Specifically, the most outstanding in this regard is located within the fusiform gyrus and surrounding areas -such as the lingual gyrus- in the basal temporal cortex (Dehaene et al., 2002). Interestingly, these areas would be genetically prepared for the processing of faces and objects, these functions emerging as a result of natural selection. However, by virtue of education, a portion of these regions could turn into specifically devoted to the processing of letters and visual word-forms (Dehaene, 2009).

4. The structure of language

Common to any input modality there are processes involved in understanding linguistic messages that appear of the highest interest. Syntactic processes may be among the most outstanding of these factors. As outlined above, syntax permits to determine the hierarchical structure of a sentence composed by a sequence of words (word-forms and their meanings). Studies in this regard have usually approached brain areas involved in syntactic processing using either of two procedures. On the one hand, the comparison between syntactically incorrect and correct material would enhance the activity of brain areas specialized in detecting grammatical errors. As an example, the activation during a sentence like "the cake was eat" is compared with its corresponding correct version. On the other hand, comparing grammatically complex sentences with simpler sentences would imply activations in areas particularly handling the complexity of syntactic structures and, hence, areas presumably involved in the hierarchical organization of the sentences. Complexity is usually increased either by embedding material within (e.g.) a main clause, rendering what is called a "recursive" structure, or by changing canonical order (usually, SVO: subject-verb-object) to a non-canonical one, as in the case of passive sentences. Examples of these situations imply comparing "the child that my mother saw was small" or "the cake is being eaten by the children", respectively, with their corresponding simpler versions (i.e., "my mother saw a child; the child was small", and "the children are eating a cake"). The case of complexity poses a problem on whether it is actually syntax what is being measured or, instead, working or short-term memory activations necessary to hold information active until the corresponding structural assignments are completed. However, it is also possible to accept that the brain areas specifically involved in working memory for syntactic structures in fact pertain to syntax processing properly, as it can be assumed that working memory for syntax implies the transient activation of circuits actually devoted to syntactic processing (e.g., Fuster, 1999; MacDonald & Christiansen, 2002).

Overall, both types of approaches to the study of human syntax have been comparable, yielding largely similar results. As one of the most consistent findings, the left inferior frontal gyrus (IFG), emerges as a central place involved in syntactic errors detection, grammatical complexity processing, and verbal working memory (e.g., Bornkessel-

Schlesewsky et al., 2009; Friederici et al., 2006; Friederici et al., 2009; Koelsch et al., 2009; Meltzer et al., 2010; Newman et al., 2009; Raettig et al., 2010; Rogalsky et al., 2008). Accordingly, the left IFG can be viewed as a main hub in the brain networks supporting syntax.

Nonetheless, IFG is a relatively extensive area, whereas syntactic rules and processes comprise a number of apparently different operations. In this regard, it seems that there are differential demands within specific portions of the left IFG as a function of the task in course. It is difficult, however, to condense the results from the different studies due to systematic inconsistencies in the criteria employed to describe their main results. In terms of Brodmann's cytoarchitectonic areas, IFG occupies, approximately -and starting from a more posterior position next to the precentral sulcus towards a more anterior one, in the left hemisphere- the most inferior portion of BA6, the whole of BA 44, the inferior half of BA 45, and BA 47 (Gray, 1918/2000; Brodmann, 1909/1994). At the same time, the IFG can be anatomically subdivided, following the same spatial sequential order as before, into the *pars opercularis*, the *pars triangularis* and the *pars orbitalis* (Gray, 1998/2000). Whereas both the anatomical and the cytoarchitectonic divisions do not match largely, some studies adopt one system but not the other, and vice versa. Several studies refine their findings by focusing on Broca's area, which certainly pertains to the left IFG. However, this is not solving the problem since there are also historical inconsistencies about what exactly are the boundaries of Broca's area. In this regard, Broca's area corresponds to BA 44 for a number of authors; for several others, BA 44, 45, and 47 should be included; for a number of other authors, the areas involved are just BA 44 and 45 (e.g., Uylings et al., 1999). Finally, in an attempt to refine anatomical exactitude when describing main results, several studies use Talairach or MNI 3D coordinates (Price, 2010). This highly precise system nonetheless obliterates the fact that fMRI is not as precise as to use these millimetrical coordinates, particularly considering the number of processing stages needed for normalization and statistical processing of the data. In addition, results in 3D coordinates usually refer to the centroid of an activated region regardless of its total size or whether its limits overlap with or surpass the anatomical or cytoarchitectonical subdivisions. In the following, we will try to minimize as far as possible these current limitations when describing the main results reported in the literature, carefully inspecting and contrasting the data reported by the different authors.

According to some reports, the most ventral part of the *pars opercularis*, roughly -but not solely- coinciding with BA 44, appears involved in verbal (syntactical) working memory (Friederici et al., 2006; Price, 2010; Rogalsky et al., 2008). In line with this might also be interpreted different results for this area as those by Bornkessel-Schlesewsky et al. (2009) for the processing of word-order variations in sentences, or Christensen (2010) and Rodd et al. (2010) for garden-path and ambiguous sentences -in which the structure must be reanalyzed and reconstructed, or several candidate structures must be kept active during sentence processing-. This ventral part of the *pars opercularis* has further been subdivided into two depending on whether the portions belong to BA 44 or to BA 6; the former would be involved in phrase structure grammar, the latter in finite state grammar (Friedrici et al., 2006). The first type of grammar refers to the use of embedded sentences, therefore demanding more working memory than the latter, simpler (linear) structures with no nesting. Detecting grammatical errors also tap on BA 44 (e.g., Heim et al., 2010), a result consistent with a role of this area in syntactic working memory to the extent that the detection of errors also increases processing demands. Overall, all these data are in line with a syntactic working memory interpretation as a main role of BA 44 (or the anterior ventral *pars opercularis*). However, if we approach working memory in the sense mentioned above – i.e., that it consists of the transient activation of circuits devoted to accomplish specific operations- then BA 44 might be better seen as containing core circuits for syntactic processing determining the hierarchical syntactic structure of a sentence. This would harmonize with the variety of different syntactic operations that have been seen to tap on this area, as outlined above. In sum, BA 44 seems a central place for syntax in the brain.

The dorsal portion of the *pars opercularis* (overlapping with the most superior part of BA 44 and a portion of BA 9) appears also involved in the processing of syntactic complexity, even when working memory is factored out (Makuuchi et al., 2009). In this regard, however, it has also been claimed that this cortical region is involved in hierarchical ordering of sequences of events regardless of whether they are linguistic or not, as it has been seen to sequence (e.g.) colored shapes or nonlinguistic visual symbols (Bahlmann et al., 2009; Tettamenti et al., 2009). Its language-specificity, therefore, appears challenged. As we will see below, this is also the case for most, if not all of the areas involved in language.

This is in fact the case of BA 44 or the ventral portion of the *pars opercularis* described earlier. Tactile imagery (Yoo et al., 2003), word and face encoding (Leube et al., 2001), object manipulation (Binkofki et al. 1999), smelling familiar odors (Ciumas et al., 2008), or music enjoyment (Koelsch et al., 2006), among several others, are tasks in which BA 44 has been seen importantly involved. Moreover, and within the frame of language, even the role of BA 44 as exclusive for syntax processing does not appear to be proved. In this regard, semantic and articulatory (phonological) processes have been seen to tap also on this area (see our previous section for phonology and the next one for semantics). Possibly, these data might be understood if we assume the proposal of a functional gradient along the whole left IFG, in which -using Brodmann's areas as reference, and from left to right- BA 47 and 45 would appear mainly involved in semantic unification, BA 45 and 44 in syntactic unification, and BA 44 and ventral BA 6 in phonological unification (Hagoort, 2007). Unification is, in the end, the main defining purpose of syntactic operations: unify or "put together", according to the hierarchical structure of the sentence, the different constituents of a sentence. As the posterior part of BA 44 has been seen involved in articulation/phonology and the anterior part in semantics, it might appear that BA 44 is relevant for both phonology and semantics; or, rather, for something in between, maybe what we properly call "syntax". It might also be the case –we are here certainly speculating- that what we call syntax is indeed an abstraction that actually relies on both phonology and semantics. As can be seen, studying language with fMRI gives rise to core questions on the very nature of human language.

In this regard, the role of BA 45, roughly coinciding with the *pars triangularis* of the IFG, might also appear ambiguous. As has been just-mentioned, it seems involved in analyzing the semantic structure of the sentence. Several studies comparing sentences containing semantic anomalies with their correct counterparts (Kuperberg et al., 2008), or sentences with and without semantic ambiguities (Davis et al., 2007), consistently report activations in BA 45. But this area also appears particularly involved in analyzing embedded structures (Shetreet et al., 2009), which can be considered as a more genuine syntactic process. In line with this, BA 45 has also been seen to support the syntactic constituent structure of the sentence, in a study in which syntactic and semantic structures were disentangled (Pallier et al., 2011). In this latter study, the activation of BA 45 in *pars triangularis* spread also to IFG *pars orbitalis*, therefore including BA 47. However, it is a consistent finding the role of BA 47 in semantic processing (e.g., Binder et al., 2009; see also our section below). In sum, and as an eclectic solution, it might be possible that the most posterior part of BA 45 is relatively more syntactic in nature, conforming a somehow unitary system together with part of BA 44; the anterior part, in turn, would be more semantic, working together with BA 47. Overall, the above-mentioned functional gradient within the left IFG might actually be more gradual than the labels currently available to describe it (i.e., semantic, syntactic, and articulatory/phonological), which might also explain why the ventral portion of BA 6, most consistently described as an articulatory/phonological area (it actually belongs to the premotor cortex) has also been seen occasionally involved in detecting syntactic errors or analyzing syntactically ambiguous sentences (Christensen, 2010; Friederici et al., 2006). The picture can be yet more complicated when considering that even language processing at the discourse level consistently recruits large portions of the IFG, as we will see below.

Additionally, a number of studies also support the involvement of other regions apart from the IFG in syntactic processing. One of the most consistent findings in this regard is the existence of a fronto-temporal network supporting syntactic processing. Whereas the frontal pole of this network implies the left IFG, especially in and around BA 44, the temporal portion is mainly comprising the left superior temporal gyrus (STG) and superior temporal sulcus (STS), most likely excluding primary auditory areas (i.e., BA 41 and 42), and roughly corresponding to BA 22 (Christensen, 2010; Rodd et al., 2010). Interestingly, these activations may plainly include Wernicke's area (Shetreet et al., 2009), which is mainly involved in the processing of language sounds (see our previous section in this regard). In several studies, large (anterior and posterior) portions of BA 22 appear relevant in syntactic processes (Friederici, 2002; Rodd et al., 2010). In other occasions, however, it is only a small portion of BA 22 what is involved, such as the posterior portion of the STS (Pallier et al., 2011). Upper portions of the middle temporal gyrus (MTG), comprising part of BA 21, have been also reported to participate in syntactic processing (Christensen, 2010; Friederici et al., 2006; Shetreet et al., 2009). Interestingly, although the main findings are located within the left hemisphere, occasional activations in corresponding areas of the right hemisphere are also reported. Several studies also report activations in the ventral portion of the supramarginal gyrus (SMG, part of BA 40), together with the *planum temporale*, a posterior portion of BA 22 (Raettig et al., 2010), although these regions appear more consistently as rather semantic, particularly the SMG (Binder et al, 2009).

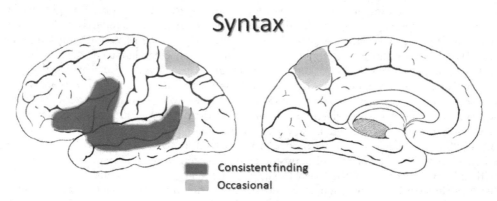

Fig. 2. Approximate locations of the syntactic system

Finally, still other brain regions have been seen also involved in syntactic processing, though less consistently. Among these, we can mention the precuneus (in the medial parietal lobe), small portions of BA 37 (next to BA 22), superior parietal cortex (BA 7), as well as the lentiform and the caudate nuclei (e.g., Chistensen, 2010; Friederici et al., 2006; Shetreet el al., 2009).

5. The meaning of language (I)

Linguistic messages normally tell something about the world and its components (objects, persons, places, and so forth). As such, a linguistic message includes words (word-forms with their individual semantic contents or meanings) that are combined, usually through syntax, rendering a concrete description of their relationships intended to mirror a real situation or an idea. Within the brain, indeed, extensive regions of the cerebral cortex appear devoted to semantic information processing. This seemingly provides a clue on the relationships between language and other cognitive processes. But it also poses some doubts on the boundaries between what can be labeled as "linguistic" and "non-linguistic". It is also the case that "semantic" might appear as a rather vague and imprecise term, covering a large number of otherwise different processes or operations. In fact, terms as "pragmatic", "conceptual", as well as several others, often appear next to "semantic" as equivalent or corresponding to a somehow unitary system.

Actually, the meaning of words, one of the main features that the term semantic can refer to, can be just about anything in the world. In other words, human languages have words –and, then, meanings- for absolutely all (or almost all) things known so far in the world, be they real, imagined, or with a large amount of ambiguity and abstraction (e.g., Pinker, 2007). In this regard, some authors even think that the so-called "syntactic words" (i.e., complements, determiners, suffixes, and so many words or particles with a specific syntactic function) have also a meaning to be considered as plainly pertaining to the same semantic system of the brain as any other type of content word, such as nouns or verbs. In this line, it could be the case that syntactic regions reviewed above might be part of the "semantic" system, but only the part preferentially dealing with abstract structural hierarchical relationships between a number of items, be they words or whatever. Indeed, it is a plausible scenario that syntax words emerged initially as any other, less functional words during the evolution of human language (Heine & Kuteva, 2007).

This said, it should not be surprising that semantic areas have been proposed to occupy most of the cerebral cortex. Providentially, Binder et al. (2009) have recently published an extensive review of functional neuroimaging studies of semantic processing, in which not only strict inclusion criteria were applied but also advanced statistical analyses for determining the probability of a given region as belonging to the semantic system. The studies included in that review used words as stimuli, so that we can be certain that the areas suggested as supporting the semantic system are indeed areas activated by language. This note is important because, as we will see, the areas constituting the semantic system are actually and for the most part classically considered as heteromodal association areas of the neocortex, located both in frontal and posterior regions. They are therefore common to a large amount of non-linguistic processes involved in either perception or action. Additionally, areas of the limbic system involved in emotional processing are also part of the semantic system.

According to the review by Binder et al. (2009), the semantic system in the brain can be subdivided into three main widespread locations. A first one includes large portions of the posterior multimodal and heteromodal cortex, namely the angular gyrus (AG, in BA 39), the

SMG, and the MTG, including part of the temporal pole (comprising small parts of BA 38 and 29). Also in the posterior parts of the brain other areas highly involved in semantics are basal temporal areas, particularly within the fusiform and parahippocampal gyri (comprising portions of BA 20 and 37; mainly high-order visual regions, as we saw for reading). A second location of the semantic system comprises portions of the heteromodal frontal cortex, namely the upper and –especially- medial portions of BA 8 and part of BA 9. Interestingly, BA 8 contains the supplementary motor area (SMA) and has been seen involved in a variety of tasks, including motor learning and imagery (Malouin et al., 2003; Matsumura et al., 2004), executive functions and planning (Kübler et al., 2006), and even speech motor programming (de Waele et al., 2001). On the other hand, BA 9 is also involved in executive functions (e.g. Kübler et al., 2006) and, as we will see below, in discourse processing. Another frontal heteromodal association area included in the second locus of the semantic system is BA 47 in the IFG, an area that was already mentioned in our previous section on syntactic processing, its most probable function being related to semantic/pragmatic unification. Finally, the third group of areas supporting the semantic system according to Binder et al. (2009) includes the posterior cingulate/precuneus region and the ventromedial prefrontal cortex. Whereas the former has been seen to be associated with emotional processing (Maddock, 1999), it has also been related to visuospatial memory and imagery (Burgess, 2008; Epstein et al., 2007), among several other functions, including – occasionally, as we saw- syntax. Indeed, the role of this area seems rather polyvalent; later on, we will see that it is implicated in the semantic analysis of whole sentences and longer language emissions (discourses). The ventromedial prefrontal cortex, roughly corresponding to BA 11 and other BAs (such as portions of the most ventral parts of BA 10, 24, 25, and 32), comprising the rostral part of the anterior-ventral cingulate, is linked to motivation, emotion, and decision making involving reward (e.g., Ernst et al., 2004), among several other functions such as olfaction (Royet et al., 1999).

It must be remarked that all the regions outlined so far in Binder et al. (2009) as constituting the semantic system are mainly and preferentially in the left hemisphere, in consonance with the fact that they were circuits activated by words. This in turn harmonizes with the left-lateralization of other linguistic functions, such as syntax and phonetics. Overall, it seems that the semantic system activated by words largely overlaps with the system used by our brain to understand and process, as well as to interact with, the external world. In fact, this is what language crucially conveys in the very end. We have seen that words can activate association areas involved in action planning, perception, and emotions, and certainly the meaning of words ultimately refers to any of these things, or to a combination of them. However, it is also possible that the view of the semantic system sketched by Binder et al. (2009) is to some extent a restrictive one. Indeed, interactions with the external (or internal) reality imply not only heteromodal association areas, but also more primary areas. Actually, the brain areas directly supporting body movements or first stages in the perceptual processing might also be part of our semantic system. This is the idea endorsed by Pulvermüler and colleages (e.g., Pulvermüler, 2010; Pulvermüller, & Fadiga, 2010). An overview of fMRI evidences in this regard by these authors (e.g., Boulenger et al., 2009), as well as by other groups (e.g., Martin & Chao, 2001; Tomasino et al., 2007) can be summarized as supporting that words referring to concepts in which movements or actions are crucial (e.g., tools, as well as many verbs), activate cortical areas specifically devoted to directly perform those movements or actions. When the words refer to arm movements (e.g., "catch"), leg movements (e.g., "run"), or face movements (as any facial expression, like "smile"), they activate corresponding areas for these actions within the primary motor cortex (BA 4), also largely respecting its somatotopic organization. The same is the case for words referring to specific stimulus features, or in which these features are crucial in their definition. Words such as "ellipse" or "red", or words belonging to semantic categories in which visual features prevail (like "animals"), activate visual areas specifically related to the processing of those perceptual features. Binder and colleagues, in their 2009 review, mention this type of findings, but consider them as secondary, less conspicuous and consistent than the other regions substantiating their proposal. It is possible, nonetheless, that the participation of these primary regions in the semantic system of the brain is less systematic namely because they refer to very specific actions or perceptions, so that only the linguistic material referring to these very concrete body features would activate them. This would not be the case, however, of the heteromodal and multimodal association areas, the main areas according to Binder et al. (2009) review, which by definition would be activated by any stimulus of any modality. This depiction is supported in Pulvermüller et al. (2009a).

By considering the semantic system as composed by both heteromodal and multimodal association areas as well as by primary or secondary areas of the perceptual and motor systems extends the size of the semantic system and is a very plausible scenario. Under this perspective, the semantic system would be substantiated by the cortical circuits involved in all of our interactions with the world; the semantic system would be equivalent to our whole "world knowledge" system. Part of this knowledge is concrete, but also part of it refers to abstractions and relations performed in the heteromodal and multimodal association areas. The involvement of limbic regions in the semantic system also fits with this line of reasoning, since emotions are also an important part of our world knowledge. Indeed, this depiction harmonizes well with recent theories of "embodied language" (e.g., de Vega et al., 2008), according to which language directly and straightforwardly makes use of the brain areas involved in performing or processing what is described in an utterance. Embodied language theories contrast with traditional proposals for a more "abstract" code created by language (or from which language emerges, in case of production) that can in turn be converted into the mental representation of specific perceptions and actions. Both views could complement each other, however, if both abstract and "body" codes working simultaneously and in cooperation are accepted. The former would be related to heteromodal and multimodal association areas, the latter to more primary or secondary areas. Indeed, not all that can be uttered can be visualized or executed externally. We can also add that there is a noticeable overlap between the most abstract and heteromodal portions of the semantic system -i.e., the proposed by Binder et al. (2009)- and part of the so-called "human default system", a rather bilateral network of activations in the human brain appearing when the subject is involved in mental tasks other than those linked to externally present stimuli or tasks. The fact that the human default system is involved in such a variety of mental operations as autobiographical memory, envisioning the future, theory of mind, or moral decision making, among many others (for a good review, see Buckner et al., 2008), suggests that this system can eventually apply to circumstances that can be visualized or externally performed. If we apply the same reasoning as we did above for the semantic system, the parallelisms between both systems are more apparent, as situations supported by the human default system should also involve the occasional recruitment of more primary or secondary perceptual or motor cortical areas in order to imagine specific perceptions and actions. This is a very plausible scenario (see, e.g., Kosslyn & Thompson, 2003 for fMRI evidence of primary visual areas activated in visual imagery).

The main purpose of language comprehension is nevertheless not the understanding of single words within a given utterance, but rather the specific relationships between those words. Helping to determine these relationships is the main role of syntax, which in turn contributes to elucidate the semantic structure of the sentence. The latter is a semantic frame representing the actual relationships between the different entities (objects, persons, places, and so on) mentioned in a sentence. Brain activations related to these combinatorial or propositional semantic processes are normally obtained in experiments in which grammatically correct but semantically incongruent sentences are compared with semantically congruent or plausible sentences. As an example, compare "*She spreads the warm bread with shoes*" and the same sentence ending with "*butter*" instead. In other occasions, the activations produced by normal sentences have been compared with the activations produced by sentences composed of pseudowords, or "jabberwocky" sentences, in which a syntactic structure can still be determined but -given that pseudowords have no semantic content as they are not real words-, no semantic structure can theoretically be extracted. As an example, here is a portion of the poem by Lewis Carroll that gave birth to the name of this type of paradigm: "*Twas brillig, and the slithy toves / Did gyre and gimble in the wabe; / All mimsy were the borogoves, /And the mome raths outgrabe*". Overall, the activations observed with these experimental paradigms tap on several places within the "more general" or heteromodal semantic system for words commented so far. Two of these places locate within the parieto-temporal junction and the temporal pole (Mashal et al., 2009; Obleser & Kotz, 2010; Pallier et al., 2011), that is, two portions within the posterior heteromodal association areas of the system used for words. Another portion of the semantic brain system for words that seems also importantly involved in the combination of semantic information is the posterior cingulate/precuneus (Mashal et al., 2009; Whitney et al., 2009). Finally, an area within the IFG belonging to the frontal heteromodal association areas of the semantic system -BA 47, eventually spreading to BA 45-, has also been seen implied in combinatorial semantic operations (reviewed in Hagoort, 2007). As can be seen, most of these loci have been implied in the processing of the semantic content of words; a few of them (BA 45, posterior cingulate/precuneus) have been occasionally observed in syntactic operations as well (particularly BA 45; see above). Interestingly, several of these regions also play a relevant role in discourse processing, as we will see in the next section.

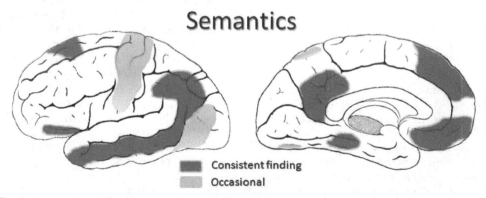

Semantics

Consistent finding
Occasional

Fig. 3. Approximate locations of the semantic system

6. The meaning of language (II)

Human language normally extends beyond sentences, most often consisting of longer messages usually known as discourses, narratives, stories, or –simply- texts. The global or unitary comprehension of a group of sentences would involve even more associative areas than simpler levels, namely because additional processes, known to demand higher levels of association, play a relevant role in discourse comprehension. Among these additional processes, the most outstanding appear to be the achievement of *inferences* and *pragmatic interpretations*, obtained by using world-knowledge and discourse context constantly in interaction. Finally, according to the so-called "situational models" (Zwaan, 2004), it is also assumed that reading or hearing long linguistic messages or discourses conveys, when feasible, the recreation of the situation depicted in the text, normally by simulating or recreating the events described in the story. Results from the fMRI studies reported so far in this topic seem to support this overall depiction.

Experiments studying text comprehension have been very varied in their designs and procedures. In principle, whenever we have two or more sentences, the same processes presumably involved in text comprehension should be already in play, as linking two sentences would be sufficient to activate inferential and interpretive processes. Accordingly, if two sentences, as "*The telephone was ringing*" and "*My brother wanted to tell me the news*", are uttered consecutively, one understands that the second is an idea related to the first sentence; in this case, that it is my brother who was calling, and that the reason for his call was that my brother wanted to tell me something of interest. Without these inferences, performed easily and automatically and based on our world-knowledge, the two sentences would be just two senseless isolated emissions. A good example of the study of the coherence we normally achieve during text comprehension is extracted from Ferstl and von Cramon (2001), where coherence was compared with cohesion, that is, the linkage of two sentences by means of a cohesive element as "*therefore*" in the following pair of sentences: "*Mary's exam was about to start. Therefore, her palms were sweaty*". These two sentences are cohesive, due to the presence of a linking element, as well as coherent, since our world-knowledge tells us that sweaty palms are a possible consequence of being nervous, the latter being a normal consequence of an examination situation. In fact, both sentences are coherent even without the cohesive element. Now read the following pair of sentences: "*Mary's exam was about to start. Therefore, the pizza arrived*". Even with the cohesive element, these two sentences are not coherent; our knowledge of the world cannot help us to infer a possible logical link between these two utterances.

In other occasions, discourse processing has been studied using loosely structured passages rendered coherent only by providing a title or an illustration. As a good example, consider a portion of a classical ambiguous paragraph from Bransford and Johnson (1972): "*A newspaper is better than a magazine. The seashore is a better place than the street. At first it is better to run than to walk but walking is fine after a while. You may have to try several times, it takes skill but it's easy to learn. Even young children can enjoy it. Once successful there are very few complications. Birds seldom get too close. [...]*". This paragraph is noticeably better understood - and remembered- when preceded by the title: "*Making and flying a kite*". Comparing the processing of this type of paragraphs preceded by the title and the same paragraphs without the title would yield, for the former, the activation of brain areas supplying global coherence and, for the latter, the attempts to attain it (Martín-Loeches et al., 2008).

Two recent reviews by Evelyn C. Ferstl and colleagues (Ferstl, 2010; Ferstl et al., 2008) -the first one using similar statistical methods as in Binder et al. (2009) for the semantic system-provide an unbeatable account of the topic. Overall, and interestingly, the main results suggest that most of the areas supporting discourse comprehension overlap with the semantic system activated by words (see above), also comprising regions used as well for other more basic linguistic processes. There also exist brain regions specific for discourse processing, a remarkable finding that will be discussed later in detail.

The reviews by Ferstl et al. (2008) and Ferstl (2010) outline a number of results that could –in our view- be grouped into four principal regions. One of the most consistent findings appears to involve the anterior temporal lobes, bilaterally, particularly the temporal poles. As mentioned, this is part of the semantic system for words proposed by Binder et al., (2009), and we have seen it is also involved when sentences have to be interpreted semantically. Nonetheless, a remarkable particularity is that in discourse processing both anterior temporal poles, bilaterally, are involved whereas semantics for words was rather left-lateralized. Another distinctiveness is that the area of the anterior temporal poles involved in discourse processing is larger than the portion used for words, the former spreading ventrally and dorsally covering the whole temporal poles. Accordingly, the anterior temporal lobes, and especially the temporal poles, seem crucial for understanding the meaning of words, sentences, and paragraphs, seemingly constituting a main hub of the semantic system used in language processing. Fertl et al. (2008) propose that a main role for this area in *propositionalization*, the process required for combining words into semantically based content units. Together with the temporal poles, discourses seem also to consistently activate other region that is also crucial for word and sentence semantics: the parieto-temporal junction. This is yet a portion of the posterior heteromodal association cortex already clustered with the temporal poles when we reviewed sentence semantics.

A second group of results would comprise the left IFG and STS/STG, spreading to part of the MTG. Ferstl et al. (2008) suggest that at least part of this "fronto-temporal network", substantiate language perception, integration, and interpretation. On the other hand, these activations are not present in a number of studies, being therefore less consistent than other areas contributing to discourse processing. As we have seen earlier, the left IFG seems to exhibit a functional gradient in language processing where syntax appears to be central but phonological and semantic processes are also importantly present; additionally, the role of the STG in syntax analysis is also a consistent finding, but again phonological processes are also observed in this region. Accordingly, even if activated during discourse processing, the role of these perisylvian areas might be not so specific of longer texts. However, this issue may still need further clarification. Recent studies of very slow brain blood flow fluctuations (around 0.1 Hz) have shown that regions in the posterior part of the left superior temporal sulcus/gyrus are consistently correlated at these frequencies with left IFG, particularly within BA 44 or the *pars opercularis* (Lohman et al., 2010). This type of fluctuations might thus reflect processes clearly beyond sentences, in the range of discourse or very large language emissions. The role of these very slow fluctuations for overall language comprehension is still unknown, but the fact that this fronto-temporal network participates, to a larger or a lesser degree, in apparently all the language processes studied so far (even if mainly in phonological and syntactic) emerges as a revealing cue to better understand human language and its possible evolutionary origins.

A third group of findings outlined in Ferstl et al. (2008) and Ferstl (2010) reviews relates to mid-parietal areas, namely the posterior cingulate/precuneus. Acccordingly, apart from participating in syntactic analysis (though very occasionally) and semantics of words and sentences, this region appears of relevance for discourse processing. Indeed, this is a very consistent finding.

The fourth and last region involved in discourse processing comprises the fronto-medial prefrontal cortex (dorso-medial and ventromedial prefrontal cortex), including large portions of the medial side of BAs 8, 9, 10, and 11. To some degree, all of these areas have been mentioned before as mainly implied in the semantic analysis of words. Even though, this grouping here is somewhat different. The main divergence is that the system comprising these areas for discourse processing complements with substantial additions of neural tissue. One addition is the involvement of the entire BA 10, including not only the medial parts, but also the lateral parts -even spreading to BA 46-, which was not the case in word semantics. The other addition conveys the whole anterior cingulate gyrus (in semantics for words, only a very small ventral anterior portion of this gyrus appeared involved). The involvement of these additional portions in discourse processing may convey important consequences. First, BA 10 is the largest cytoarchitectonic area in the human brain, having increased its size substantially during human evolution, as is the case for its connections (Semendeferi et al., 2001). Second, most of these connections seem to affect the anterior cingulate particularly (Allman et al., 2002), which is another milestone in human brain evolution. In fact, the anterior cingulate is so peculiar in the human brain that it is the main structure containing a special type of neurons, the spindle or Von Economo cells. Only the great apes within the primate order posses this type of neurons presumably related with complex social behaviour, humans exhibiting a disproportionate larger number of them (Allman et al., 2011). Third, BA 10 has recently revealed as the single region showing a significant effect unique to *g*, the psychometric construct of *general intelligence* (Gläscher et al., 2010). Consequently, although this is a group of areas directly involved in language processing, its language-specificity does not appear evident.

The same appears to be the case of the posterior cingulate/precuneus region, the third group of findings involved in discourse processing. The concrete role of the posterior cingulate/precuneus has yet to be elucidated. This region participates in many linguistic processes, but also in a number of other non-linguistic operations. As mentioned earlier, it appears a certainly polyvalent region, involved in emotion, memory, and imagery; it also belongs to the human default system, and it is one of the very few regions connected reciprocally with most other cortical regions. Indeed, this part of the brain is one of the main hubs of the "human core system", the anatomical counterpart of the human default system (Chudek et al., 2008). On the other hand, the anterior medial regions also involved in discourse processing are again largely overlapping with corresponding portions of the human default system. This outstanding overlap between brain systems for word semantics and, particularly, discourse processing and the human default system has been already raised by Binder et al. (2009) and Speer et al. (2009). Ferstl et al. (2008) and Ferstl (2010) focused on the similarities of the discourse-processing system and the system supporting theory of mind. However, considering that the circuits for theory of mind and the human default system have been seen to be largely equivalent (e.g. Buckner et al., 2008), Ferstl and colleagues' suggestion could surely be reworded to imply the default system. Overall, the human default system appears to be such a general and abstract-coded system that it can apply to a considerable number of situations and circunstances, including word semantics and discourse processing in language. Eventually, the recruitment of more primary and secondary perceptual or motor areas would also be necessary in order to visualize or imagine specific perceptions, actions, or any type of situations outlined in a text.

Discourse

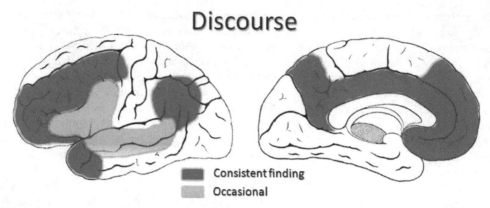

■ Consistent finding
■ Occasional

Fig. 4. Approximate locations of the system to process discourse

7. All together

Recent developments in brain imaging techniques include brain *tractography* with MRI, which has been promptly used to study human language. Brain tactography can be achieved through *diffusion tensor* and *diffusion spectrum* techniques. The main difference between the two of them depends on the deterministic vs. probabilistic approaches used to analyze the movement of water molecules within the main tracts substantiating cortico-cortical connections (de Schotten et al., 2011). It must be noted here, however, that the novelty and the relative scarcity of studies approaching language with this technique may explain certain inconsistencies between studies (for an extensive review, see Friederici, 2009).

Although it is well known after Karl Wernicke, the relevance for human language of the *arquate fasciculus* (AF) connecting Broca's and Wernicke's areas appears largely strengthened by tractographic techniques. The data also stress the relevance for language processing of other fascicles connecting anterior and posterior brain areas. A detailed description of all these connections is also emerging.

One of the first studies applying tractography to approach language was developed by Catani et al. (2005). These authors reported a direct strong connection between Broca's and Wernicke's areas through the FA, but given the fact that the areas actually connected covered a wider territory than the classical Broca's and Wernicke's areas (though, as shown earlier, the precise limits for these two areas may vary depending on the author), Catani and colleagues suggested to call them Broca's and Wernicke's *territories*, respectively. Their results also revealed the existence of two additional but indirect pathways connecting Broca's and Wernicke's territories. One would run laterally, consisting of an anterior segment connecting Broca's territory and the inferior parietal cortex. The other would be a posterior segment connecting the inferior parietal cortex with Wernicke's territory. Given the apparent relevance of these two indirect segments, and the fact that the inferior parietal cortex appears the main meeting point for these indirect connections, Catani et al. (2005) suggested to call this region the *Geschwind's territory*, in the memory of Norman Geschwind, who already proposed a relevant role of the inferior parietal cortex in language. This region largely overlaps with semantic areas involved in word and discourse processing, as we have seen.

The AF seems to have evolved substantially in the human brain from tiny tracts connecting the IFG with the posterior part of BA 22 and the inferior parietal regions, already present in the macaque brain. These connections appear more robust and abundant in the chimpanzee, thereafter reaching the plainest robustness of the human brain (Rilling et al., 2008). Actually, one of the main differences between the human and the chimpanzee brains in this regard is the notable expansion of the posterior ramifications of the AF, which spread not only to involve Wernicke's area and surrounding parietal regions, but also posterior portions of the MTG. The development of these connections, occurring particularly and noticeably within the left hemisphere, seem to have played a critical role in the evolution of human language.

Interestingly, two other tracts connecting anterior and posterior regions seem relevant in language processing. One is the superior longitudinal fasciculus (SLF), connecting Broca's area (particularly, BA 44) with the posterior temporal lobe, namely in the STG and the MTG and also involving portions of BA 40. As this tract runs parallel to the AF, several authors (e.g., Rilling et al., 2008) consider both as representing together a functional unit called the *dorsal stream*. The other connection is more primitive; part of it is actually the most developed fronto-temporal connection in the macaque brain and conveys the ventral portion of the extreme capsule and the uncinate fasciculus. Through these connections, the IFG is connected with the anterior and posterior STG (Frey et al., 2008; Rilling et al., 2008), and it is indeed possible that at least part of this *ventral stream* is preferentially used in simpler grammar such as finite-state, relatively accessible to other non-human primates (Friederici et al., 2006).

Finally, there are evidences for an additional number of connections importantly involved in language, most of them located locally within the IFG and the STG (Friederici, 2009).

8. Conclusions

The moment arrives to summarize and interpret the major milestones that could be elucidated from the preceding exposition. In the following, we will also express a number of reflections on human language using brain function as a main perspective.

A first and relatively robust conclusion that can be extracted so far is that the human brain contains at least two major "centers of gravity", or main hubs in the networks devoted to language processing. These foci are, on the one hand, the left inferior frontal gyrus (IFG) and, on the other, the left superior temporal gyrus (STG), the latter probably spreading to the superior temporal sulcus (STS) and posterior portions of the middle temporal gyrus (MTG) as well as to some parts of the inferior parietal cortex. Both foci are highly and densely interconnected by means of several tracts, the most outstanding one being the arquate fasciculus (AF). Most of the primary functions and processes involving these foci are seemingly phonological/articulatory and syntactic in nature. These two main hubs are located in perisylvian areas and appear critical for human language. Actually, the main loci of the cerebral lesions yielding core symptoms highly specific of language are the perisylvian areas; the most conspicuous aphasias are usually the consequence of lesions affecting either these regions or the AF (e.g., LaPointe, 2011).

If the depiction in the preceding paragraph can be taken as relatively robust, the same is not the case when we attempt to subdivide each hub (IFG and STG). An approximate depiction seems that as we move from more posterior/dorsal regions to more anterior/ventral in the left IFG, a gradient of activations can be found to be specifically involved (in this order) in phonology/articulation, syntax, and semantics. A similar gradient could be found in the STG when moving from the primary auditory association areas in or around Hesch's gyrus, spreading widely to both anterior and posterior regions in the STG, probably covering also parts of the inferior parietal cortex. In the latter case, the gradient seems to cover, following this order, phonology/articulation and syntax. If we want to expand these functions to semantic processes, then STS and at least several portions of the MTG should be included.

From there, the system spreads to notably many other brain regions, comprising, posteriorly, large portions of the whole temporal lobes, including the temporal poles and part of the basal regions, as well as significant portions of the parietal cortex. Frontally, the system spreads to more anterior regions, including large extensions of the prefrontal cortex; among them, an area showing the most substantial increase in size in humans when compared to other primates and importantly involved in general intelligence. Significant medial regions, both in the prefrontal cortex and in the parietal cortex, are also included in this system. This *extended language network* (using an expression coined by Ferstl et al., 2008) largely overlaps with the *human default system*, a bilateral network in the human brain active when we are involved in "internal" mental tasks. If the linguistic message implies the visualization or representation of a given situation, then the corresponding primary or secondary areas of the neocortex can be activated, either motor or perceptual.

The system can therefore be viewed as a continuous flux of information spreading from perisylvian areas toward multiple, distant areas. In turn, it also seems that the limits between linguistic and non-linguistic processes within this system appear blurred. An overall rule seems to be that the closer we move toward the sylvian fissure, the more specifically linguistic the process is. But even in this case (as we have seen), these regions are not exclusively linguistic.

Finally, that the flux of information spreads from perisylvian areas toward extensive regions of the cerebral cortex (actually, nearly all portions of the cortex appear susceptible of being involved) does not necessarily mean that this spreading strictly follows a temporal (sequential) order. Actually, brain networks continuously fire at different frequencies (e.g., Buzsáki, 2006), and it is plausible that information fluxes continuously in a reciprocal way and almost simultaneously between perysilvian and more distant areas. This would be a possible underlying mechanism explaining the large number of mutual influences from one structural layer of language (phonology, syntax, and semantics) to each other, as reported in the literature (e.g., Pulvermüller et al., 2009b). Indeed, considering that there are about 10.000 connections per neuron in the cerebral cortex, firing up to 1.000 times per second and therefore performing a comparable number of calculations (Previc, 2009), a parallel or at least cascade mode of operation of the whole (extended) language network emerges as a very plausible picture. On the other hand, the centrality of auditory/verbal (i.e., phonological/articulatory) information in human language would be consistent with the position of the two main hubs involved in language processing and the direction of the information flux spreading from them as primary receptors of language information to widespread areas, even if the overall processes largely unfold in parallel.

9. Acknowledgements

The authors are funded by grant PSI2010-19619 from Ministerio de Ciencia e Innovacion, Spain (MICINN).

10. References

Allman, J., Hakeem, A. & Watson, K., (2002). Two Phylogenetic Specializations in the Human Brain. *Neuroscientist*, Vol. 8, No. 4, (August 2002), pp. 335-346, ISSN 1073-8584.

Allman, J.M.; Tetreault, N.A.; Hakeem, A.Y. & Park, S. (2011). The Von Economo Neurons in Apes and hHumans. *American Journal of Human Biology*, Vol. 23, No. 1, (January 2011), pp. 5-21, ISSN 1520-6300.

Bahlmann,J.; Schubotz,R.I.; Mueller,J.L.; Koester,D. & Friederici,A.D. (2009). Neural Circuits of Hierarchical Visuo-Spatial Sequence Processing. *Brain Research*, Vol. 1298, (November 200), pp. 161-170, ISSN 1872-6240.

Binder,J.R.; Desai,R.H.; Graves,W.W. & Conant,L.L. (2009). Where is the Semantic System? A Critical Review and Meta-Analysis of 120 Functional Neuroimaging Studies. *Cerebral Cortex*, Vol., 19, No. 12, (December 2009), pp. 2767-2796, ISSN 1460-2199.

Binkofski, F.; Buccino, G.; Stephan, K.M.; Rizzolatti, G.; Seitz, R.J. & Freund, H.J. (1999). A Parieto-Premotor Network for Object Manipulation: Evidence from Neuroimaging. *Experimental Brain Research*, Vol. 128, No. 1-2, (September 1999), pp. 210-213, ISSN 0014-4819.

Bookheimer, S., Zeffiro, T., Blaxton, T., Gaillard, W. & Theodore, W. (1995). Regional Cerebral Blood Flow Changes During Object Naming and Word Reading. *Human Brain Mapping*, Vol. 3, No. 2, (April 1995), pp. 93-106, ISSN 1097-0193.

Bornkessel-Schlesewsky, I.; Schlesewsky, M. & von Cramon, D. Yves (2009). Word order and Broca's region: Evidence for a Supra-Syntactic Perspective. *Brain and Language*, Vol. 11, No. 3, (December 2009), pp. 1255-139, ISSN 1090-2155.

Boulenger, V.; Hauk, O. & Pulvermüller, F. (2009). Grasping Ideas with the Motor System: Semantic Somatotopy in Idiom Comprehension. *Cerebral Cortex*, Vol. 19, No. 8, (August 2009), pp. 1905-1914, ISSN 1047-3211.

Bozic,M.; Tyler,L.K.; Ives,D.T.; Randall,B. & Marslen-Wilson,W.D. (2010). Bihemispheric Foundations for Human Speech Comprehension. *Proceedings of the National Academy of Sciences USA*, Vol. 107, No. 40, (November 2010), pp. 2458-2473, ISSN 17439-17444.

Bransford, J.D. & Johnson, M.K. (1972). Contextual Prerequisites for Understanding: Some Investigations on Comprehension and Recall. *Journal of Verbal Learning and Verbal Behavior*, Vol. 11, No. 6, (December 1972), pp. 717-726, ISSN 0749-596X.

Brodmann, K. (1909/1994) *Localisation in the Cerebral Cortex*, Smith-Gordon, ISBN 1-85463-028-8, London, UK.

Buckner, R.L., Andrews-Hanna, J.R., & Schacter, D.L. (2008). The Brain's Default Network: Anatomy, Function, and Relevance to Disease. *Annals of the New York Academy of Sciences*, Vol. 1124, (March 2008), pp. 1-38, ISSN 0077-8923.

Burgess, N. (2008). Spatial Cognition and the Brain. *Annals of the New York Academy of Sciences*, Vol. 1124, (March 2008), pp. 77-97, ISSN 0077-8923.

Buzsáki, G. (2006). *Rhythms of the Brain*. Oxford University Press, ISBN: 978-0-19-530106-9, New York, USA.

Catani,M.; Jones,D.K. & ffytche,D.H. (2005). Perisylvian Language Networks of the Human Brain. *Annals of Neurology*, Vol. 57, No. 1, (January 2005), pp. 8-16, ISSN 0364-5134.

Christensen, K.R (2010). Syntactic Reconstruction and Reanalysis, Semantic Dead Ends, and Prefrontal Cortex. *Brain and Cognition*, Vol. 73, No., 1, (June 2010), pp. 41-50, ISSN 1090-2147.

Ciumas, C.; Lindström, P.; Aoun, B.; Savic, I. (2008) Imaging of Odor Perception Delineates Functional Disintegration of the Limbic Circuits in Mesial Temporal Lobe Epilepsy. *Neuroimage*, Vol. 39, No. 2, (January 2008), pp. 578-592, ISSN 10538119.

Cohen, L.; Jobert, A.; Le Bihan, D. & Dehaene, S. (2004) Distinct Unimodal and Crossmodal Regions for Word Processing in the Left Temporal Cortex. *NeuroImage*, Vol. 23, No. 4, (December 2004), pp. 1256-1270, ISSN 1053-8119.

Davis, M.H.; Coleman, M.R.; Absalom, A.R.; Rodd, J.M.; Johnsrude, I.S.; Matta, B.F.; Owen, A.M. & Menon, D.K. (2007). Dissociating Speech Perception and Comprehension at Reduced Levels of Awareness. *Proceedings of the National Academie of Science USA*, Vol. 104, No. 41, (October 2007), pp. 16032-16037, ISSN 0077-8923.

de Schotten, M.T.; ffytche, D.H.; Bizzi, A.; Dell'Acqua, F.; Allin, M.; Walshe, M.; Murray, R.; Williams, S.C.; Murphy, D.G.M. & Catani, M. (2011) Atlasing Location, Asymmetry and Inter-Subject Variability of White Matter Tracts in the Human Brain with MR Diffusion Tractography. *NeuroImage*, Vol. 54, No. 1, (January 2011), pp 49-59, ISSN 1053-8119.

de Vega, M.; Glenberg, A.M.; Graesser, A.C. (2008) *Symbols and Embodiment. Debates on Meaning and Cognition*. Oxford University Press, ISBN 978-0-19-921727-4, Oxford, UK.

de Waele, C.; Baudonnière, P.M.; Lepecq, J.C.; Tran Ba Huy, P. & Vidal, P.P. (2001). Vestibular Projections in the Human Cortex. *Experimental Brain Research*, Vol. 141, No. 4, (December 2001), pp. 541-551, ISSN 0014-4819.

Dehaene, S. (2009). *Reading in the Brain*. Penguin Viking, ISBN 978-0-670-02110-9, New York, USA.

Dehaene, S., Le Clec'H, G., Poline, J.B., Le Bihan, D. & Cohen, L. (2002). The Visual Word Form Area: A Prelexical Representation of Visual Words in the Fusiform Gyrus. *NeuroReport*, Vol. 13, No. 3, (March 2002), 321–325, ISSN 0959-4965.

Démonet, J.F.; Chollet, F.; Ramsay, S., Cardebat, D.; Nespoulous, J.L.; Wise, R.; Rascol, A. & Frackowiak, R. (1992). The Anatomy of Phonological and Semantic Processing in Normal Subjects. *Brain*, Vol. 115, No. 6, (December 1992), pp. 1753–1768, ISSN 0006-8950.

Epstein, R.A.; Parker, W.E. & Feiler, A.M. (2007). Where Am I Now? Distinct Roles for Parahippocampal and Retrosplenial Cortices in Place Recognition. *Journal of Neuroscience*, Vol. 27, No. 23, (June 2007), pp. 6141-61149, ISSN 1529-2401.

Ernst, M., Nelson, E.E.; McClure, E.B.; Monk, C.S.; Munson, S.; Eshel, N.; Zarahn, E.; Leibenluft, E.; Zametkin, A.; Towbin, K.; Blair, J.; Charney, D. & Pine, D.S. (2004). Choice Selection and Reward Anticipation: An fMRI Study. *Neuropsychologia*, Vol. 42, No. 12, (December 2004), pp. 1585-1597, ISSN 0028-3932.

Ferstl, E.C. (2010). Neuroimaging of Text Comprehension: Where are We Now? *Italian Journal of Linguistics*, Vol. 22, Vol. 1, pp. 61-88, ISSN N/A.

Ferstl,E.C. & von Cramon,D.Y. (2001). The Role of Coherence and Cohesion in Text Comprehension: An Event-Related fMRI Study. *Cognitive Brain Research*, Vol. 11, No. 3, (June 2001), pp. 325-340, ISSN 0926-6410.

Ferstl,E.C.; Neumann,J.; Bogler,C. & von Cramon,D.Y. (2008). The Extended Language Network: A Meta-Analysis of Neuroimaging Studies on Text Comprehension. *Human Brain Mapping*, Vol. 29, No. 5, (May 2008), pp. 581-593, ISSN 1097-0193.

Frey,S.; Campbell,J.S.; Pike,G.B. & Petrides,M. (2008). Dissociating the Human Language Pathways with High Angular Resolution Diffusion Fiber Tractography. *Journal of Neuroscience*, Vol. 28, No. 45, (November 2008), pp. 11435-11444, ISSN 1529-2401.

Friederici, A.D.; Kotz, S.A.; Scott, S.K. & Obleser, J. (2009). Disentangling Syntax and Intelligibility in Auditory Language Comprehension. *Human Brain Mapping*, Vol. 31, No. 3, (March 2009), pp. 448-457, ISSN 1097-0193.

Friederici,A.D. (2002). Towards a Neural Basis of Auditory Sentence Processing. *Trends in Cognitive Sciences*, Vol. 6, No. 2, (February 2002), pp. 78-84, ISSN 1879-307X.

Friederici,A.D. (2009). Pathways to language: fiber tracts in the human brain. *Trends in Cognitive Sciences*, Vol. 13, No. 4, (April 2009), pp. 175-181, ISSN 1879-307X.

Friederici,A.D.; Bahlmann,J.; Heim,S.; Schubotz,R.I. & Anwander,A. (2006). The Brain Differentiates Human and Non-Human Grammars: Functional Localization and Structural Connectivity. *Proceedings of the National Academy of Sciences USA*, Vol. 103, No. 7, (February 2006), pp. 2458-2473, ISSN 1091-6490.

Fuster, J.M. (1999). *Memory in the Cerebral Cortex: An Empirical Approach to Neural Networks in the Human and Nonhuman Primate*. The MIT Press, ISBN: 978-0262561242, Cambridge, MA, USA.

Gläscher, J.; Rudrau, D.; Colom, R.; Paula, L. K.; Tranel, D.; Damasio, H. & Adolphs, R. (2010) Distributed Neural System for General Intelligence Revealed by Lesion Mapping. *Proceedings of the National Academie of Science USA*, Vol. 107, No. 10, (February 2010), pp. 4705–4709, ISSN 0077-8923.

Gray, H. (1918/2000) *Anatomy of the Human Body*. Lea & Febiger, Philadelphia, USA, Available from http.//www.bartleby.com.

Hagmann, P.; Cammoun, L.; Gigandet, X.; Meuli, R.; Honey, C.J.; Wedeen. V.J. & Sporns, O. (2008). Mapping the Structural Core of Human Cerebral Cortex. *PLoS Biology*, Vol. 6, No. 7, (July 2008), doi:10.1371/journal.pbio.0060159, ISSN-1544-9173.

Hagoort, P. (2007). The Memory, Unification, and Control (MUC) Model of Language. In: *Automaticity and control in language processing*, A. S. Meyer, L. Wheeldon & A. Krott (Eds.), pp. 243-270, Psychology Press, 0-203-96851-4, Hove, UK.

Hauser,M.D.; Chomsky,N.; Fitch,W.T. (2002) The Faculty of Language: What Is It, Who Has It, and How Did It Evolve? *Science*, Vol., 298, No. 5598, (November 2002), pp. 1569-1579, ISSN 0036-8075.

Heim, S.; van Ermingen, M.; Huber, W. & Amunts, K. (2010). Left Cytoarchitectonic BA 44 Processes Syntactic Gender Violations in Determiner Phrases. *Human Brain Mapping*, Vol. 31, No. 10, (October 2010), pp. 1532–1541, ISSN: 1097-0193.

Heine, B. & Kuteva, T. (2007) *The Genesis of Grammar. A Reconstruction*. Oxford University Press, ISBN 978-0-19-922777-8, Oxford, UK.

Jackendoff, R. (2002). *Foundations of Language: Brain, Meaning, Grammar, Evolution*. Oxford University Press, ISBN 978-0198270126, New York, USA.

Koelsch, S.; Schulze, K.; Sammler, D.; Fritz, T.; Muller, K. & Gruber, O. (2009). Functional Architecture of Verbal and Tonal Working Memory: An fMRI Study. *Human Brain Mapping*, Vol. 30, No. 3, (March 2009), pp. 859-873, ISSN 1097-0193.

Koelsch, S; Fritz, T.; Von Cramon, D.Y.; Müller, K. & Friederici, A.D. (2006) Investigating Emotion with Music: An fMRI Study. *Human Brain Mapping*, Vol. 27, No. 3, (March 2006), pp. 239-250, ISSN: 1097-0193.

Kosslym, S.M. & Thompson, W.L. (2003). When Is Early Visual Cortex Activated During Visual Mental Imagery? *Psychological Bulletin*, Vol. 129, No. 5, (September 2003), pp. 723–746, ISSN 0033-2909.

Kotz,S.A.; Schwartze,M. (2010). Cortical Speech Processing Unplugged: a Timely Subcortico-Cortical Framework. *Trends in Cognitive Sciences*, Vol. 14, No. 9, (September 2010), pp. 392-399, ISSN 1879-307X.

Kübler, A.; Dixon, V. & Garavan, H. (2006). Automaticity and Reestablishment of Executive Control - An fMRI Study. *Journal Cognitive Neuroscience*, Vol. 18, No. 8, (August 2006), pp. 1331-1342, ISSN 0898-929X.

Kuperberg, G.R.; Sitnikova, T.; Lakshmanan, B.M. (2008). Neuroanatomical Distinctions within the Semantic System During Sentence Comprehension: Evidence from Functional Magnetic Resonance Imaging. *Neuroimage*, Vol. 40, No. 1, (March 2008), pp. 367-388, ISSN 10538119.

LaPointe, L. (2011). *Aphasia and Related Neurogenic Language Disorders, 4th edition*, Thieme, ISBN 978-1604062618, Stuttgart, Germany.

Leff,A.P.; Iverson,P.; Schofield,T.M.; Kilner,J.M.; Crinion,J.T.; Friston,K.J. & Price,C.J. (2009). Vowel-Specific Mismatch Responses in the Anterior Superior Temporal Gyrus: An fMRI Study. *Cortex*, Vol., 45, No. 4, (April 2009), pp 517-526, ISSN 0010-9452.

Leube, D.T.; Erb, M.; Grodd, W.; Bartels, M.; Kircher, T.T. (2001). Differential Activation in Parahippocampal and Prefrontal Cortex During Word and Face Encoding Tasks. *Neuroreport*, Vol. 12, No. 12, (August 2001), pp. 2773-7, ISSN 1460-9568.

Lieberman, P. (2000). *Human Language and Our Reptilian Brain*. Harvard University Press, ISBN 0674002265, Cambridge, MA, USA.

Lohmann, G.; Hoehl, S.; Brauer, J.; Danielmeier, C.; Bornkessel-Schlesewsky, I.; Bahlmann, J.; Turner, R. & Friederici, A. (2010) Setting the Frame: The Human Brain Activates a Basic Low-Frequency Network for Language Processing. *Cerebral Cortex*, Vol. 20, No. 6, (September 2010), pp. 1286-1292, ISSN 1047-3211.

MacDonald, M.C. & Christiansen, M.H. (2002). Reassessing Working Memory: Comment on Just and Carpenter (1992) and Waters and Caplan (1996). *Psychological Review*, 109, Vol. 1, (January 2002), pp. 35-54, ISSN 0033295X.

Maddock, R.J. (1999) The Retrosplenial Cortex and Emotion: New Insights from Functional Neuroimaging of the Human Brain. *Trends in Neurosciences*, Vol. 22, No. 7, (July 1999), pp. 310-316, ISSN 0166-2236.

Makuuchi, M.; Bahlmann, A.; Anwander, A. & Friederici, A.D. (2009). Segregating the Core Computational Faculty of Human Language from Working Memory. *Proceedings of the National Academy of Sciences USA*, Vol. 106, No. 20, (May 2009), pp. 8362-8367, ISSN 1091-6490.

Malouin, F.; Richards, C.L.; Jackson, P.L.; Dumas, F. & Doyon, J. (2003). Brain Activations During Motor Imagery of Locomotor-Related Tasks: A PET Study. *Human Brain Mapping*, Vol. 19, No. 1, (May 2003), pp. 47-62, ISSN 1097-0193.

Martin,A. & Chao,L.L. (2001). Semantic Memory and the Brain: Structure and Processes. *Current Opinion in Neurobiology*, Vol. 11, No. 2, (April 2001), pp. 194-201, ISSN 0959-4388.

Martin-Loeches,M.; Casado,P.; Hernandez-Tamames,J.A. & Alvarez-Linera,J. (2008). Brain Activation in Discourse Comprehension: A 3t fMRI Study. *NuroImage*, Vol. 41, No. 2, (June 2008), pp. 614-622, ISSN 1095-9572.

Mashal,N.; Faust,M.; Hendler,T. & Jung-Beeman,M. (2009). An fMRI Study of Processing Novel Metaphoric Sentences. *Laterality*, Vol. 14, No. 1, (January 2009), pp. 30–54, ISSN 1464-0678.

Matsumura, M.; Sadato, N.; Kochiyama, T.; Nakamura, S.; Naito, E.; Matsunami, K; Kawashima, R.; Fukuda, H. & Yonekura, Y. (2004). Role of the Cerebellum in Implicit Motor Skill Learning: A PET Study. *Brain Research Bulletin*, Vol. 63, No. 6, (July 2004), pp. 471-83, ISSN 0361-9230.

Meltzer,J.A.; McArdle,J.J.; Schafer,R.J. & Braun,A.R. (2010). Neural Aspects of Sentence Comprehension: Syntactic Complexity, Reversibility, and Reanalysis. *Cerebral Cortex*, Vol. 20, No. 8, (August 2010), pp. 1853-1864.

Mesulam, M.M. (1998). From Sensation to Cognition. *Brain*, Vol. 121, No. 6, (June 1998), pp. 1013–1052, ISSN 0006-8950.

Meyer,M.; Steinhauer,K.; Alter,K.; Friederici,A.D. & von Cramon,D.Y. (2004). Brain Activity Varies with Modulation of Dynamic Pitch Variance in Sentence Melody. *Brain and Language*, Vol. 89, No. 2, (May 2004), pp. 277-289, ISSN 0093-934X.

Newman, S.D.; Lee, D. & Ratliff, K.L. (2009). Off-Line Sentence Processing: What Is Involved in Answering a Comprehension Probe? *Human Brain Mapping*, Vol. 30, No. 8, (August 2009), pp. 2499-2511, ISSN 1097-0193.

Obleser, J. & Kotz, S.A. (2010). Expectancy Constraints in Degraded Speech Modulate the Language Comprehension Network. *Cerebral Cortex*, Vol. 20, No. 3, (March 2010), pp. 633-640, ISSN 1047-3211.

Pallier,C.; Devauchelle,A.D.; Dehaene,S. (2011). Cortical Representation of the Constituent Structure of Sentences. *Proceedings of the National Academy of Sciences USA*, Vol. 108, No. 6, (February 2011), pp. 2522-2527, ISSN 17439-17444.

Pinker, S. (2007). *The Stuff of Thought*, Penguin, ISBN 978-0-670-06327-7, New York, USA.

Previc, F.H. (2009) *The dopaminergic mind in human evolution and history*, Cambridge University Press, ISBN 978-0-521-51699-0, Cambridge, UK.

Price, C.J. (2000). The Anatomy of Language: Contributions from Functional Neuroimaging. *Journal of Anatomy*, Vol. 197, No. 3, (October 2000), pp. 335-359, ISSN 1469-7580.

Price, C.J. (2010). The Anatomy of Language: A Review of 100 fMRI Studies Published in 2009. *Annals of the New York Academy of Sciences*, Vol. 1191, (December 2010), pp. 62-88, ISSN 0077-8923.

Price, C.J.; Winterburn, D.; Giraud, A. L.; Moore, C. J. & Noppeney, U. (2003). Cortical Localisation of the Visual and Auditory Word Form Areas: A Reconsideration of The Evidence. *Brain and Language*, Vol. 86, No. 2, (August 2003), Pages 272-286, ISSN 0093-934X.

Pulvermüller, F. & Fadiga, L. (2010). Active Perception: Sensorimotor Circuits as a Cortical Basis for Language. *Nature Reviews Neuroscience*, Vol. 11, No. 5, (May 2010), pp. 351-360, ISSN 1471-0048.

Pulvermüller, F. (2010). Brain Embodiment of Syntax and Grammar: Discrete Combinatorial Mechanisms Spelt Out in Neuronal Circuits. *Brain and Language,* Vol. 112, No. 3, (March 2010), pp. 167-179, ISSN 0093-934X.

Pulvermüller, F.; Kherif, F.; Hauk, O.; Mohr, B. & Nimmo-Smith, I. (2009a). Distributed Cell Assemblies for General Lexical and Category-Specific Semantic Processing as Revealed by fMRI Cluster Analysis. *Human Brain Mapping*, Vol. 30, No. 12, (December 2009), pp. 3837–3850, ISSN 1097-0193.

Pulvermuller, F.; Shtyrov, Y. & Hauk, O. (2009b) Understanding in an Instant: Neurophysiological Evidence for Mechanistic Language Circuits in the Brain. *Brain and Language*, Vol. 110, No. 2, (August 2009), pp. 81-94 ISSN 0093-934X.

Raettig, T.; Frisch, S.; Friederici, A.D. & Kotz, S.A. (2010). Neural Correlates of Morphosyntactic and Verb-Argument Structure Processing: An EfMRI Study. *Cortex*, Vol., 46, No.5, (May 2010), pp 613-620, ISSN 0010-9452.

Rilling,J.K.; Glasser,M.F.; Preuss,T.M.; Ma,X.; Zhao,T.; Hu,X.& Behrens,T.E. (2008). The Evolution of the Arcuate Fasciculus Revealed with Comparative DTI. *Nature Neuroscience*, Vol. 11, No. 4, (April 2008), pp. 426-428, ISBN 1097-6256.

Rizzolatti, G. & Craighero, L. (2004). The Mirror-Neuron System. *Annual Review of Neuroscience*, Vol. 27, (July 2004), pp. 169–192, ISSN 0147-006X.

Rodd, J.M.; Longe, O.A.; Randall, B.; Tyler, L.K. (2010). The Functional Organisation of the Fronto-Temporal Language System: Evidence from Syntactic and Semantic Ambiguity. *Neuropsychologia*, Vol. 48, No. 5, (April 2010), pp. 1324-1335, ISSN 1873-3514.

Rogalsky, C.; Matchin W.; Hickok, G. (2008). Broca's Area, Sentence Comprehension, and Working Memory: An fMRI Study. *Frontiers in Human Neuroscience*, Vol. 2, Art. 14, (October 2008), doi: 10.3389/neuro.09.014.2008, ISSN 1662-5161.

Royet, J.P.; Koenig, O.; Gregoire, M.C.; Cinotti, L.; Lavenne, F.; Le Bars, D.; Costes, N.; Vigouroux, M.; Farget, V.; Sicard, G.; Holley, A.; Mauguière, F.; Comar, D. & Froment, J.C. (1999). Functional Anatomy of Perceptual and Semantic Processing for Odors. *Journal Cognitive Neuroscience*, Vol. 11, No. 1, (January 1999), pp. 94-109, ISSN 0898-929X.

Schon,D.; Gordon,R.; Campagne,A.; Magne,C.; Astesano,C.; Anton,J.L. & Besson,M. (2010). Similar Cerebral Networks in Language, Music and Song Perception. *NuroImage*, Vol. 51, No. 1, (May 2010), pp. 450-461, ISSN 1095-9572.

Semendeferi, K.; Armstrong, E.; Schleicher, A.; Zilles, K.; Van Hoesen, G.W. (2001). Prefrontal Cortex in Humans and Apes: A Comparative Study of Area 10. *American Journal of Physical Anthropology*, Vol. 114, No. 3, (March 2001), pp. 224-41, ISSN 1096-8644.

Shetreet,E.; Friedmann,N. & Hadar,U. (2009). An fMRI study of syntactic layers: sentential and lexical aspects of embedding. *NuroImage*, Vol. 48, No. 4, (December 2009), pp. 707-716, ISSN 1095-9572.

Snedeker, J. (2008). Effects of Prosodic and Lexical Constraints on Parsing in Young Children (and Adults). *Journal of Memory and Language*, Vol. 58, No. 2, (February 2008), pp. 574-608, ISSN 1096-0821.

Specht,K.; Osnes,B.; Hugdahl,K. (2009). Detection of Differential Speech-Specific Processes in the Temporal Lobe Using fMRI and a Dynamic "Sound Morphing" Technique. *Human Brain Mapping*, Vol. 30, No. 10, (October 2009), pp. 3436–3444, ISSN: 1097-0193.

Speer, N.S.; Reynolds, J.R.; Swallow, K.M. & Zacks, J.M. (2009). Reading Stories Activates Neural Representations of Visual and Motor Experiences. *Psychological Science*, Vol. 20, No. 8, (August 2009), pp 989-999, ISSN 0956-7976.

Tettamenti, M.; Rotondi, I. & Perani, D. (2009) Syntax Without Language: Neurobiological Evidence for Cross-Domain Syntactic Computations. *Cortex*, Vol. 45, No. 7, (July 2009), pp. 825-838, ISSN 0010-9452.

Tomasino, B.; Werner, C.J.; Weiss, P.H. & Fink, G.R. (2007). Stimulus Properties Matter More than Perspective: An fMRI Study of Mental Imagery and Silent Reading of Action Phrases. *Neuroimage*, Vol. 36, Suppl. 2, (May 2007), pp. T128– 141, ISSN 10538119.

Uylings, H.B.M.; Malofeeva, L.I.; Bogolepova. I.N.; Amunts, K. & Zilles, K. (1999). Broca's Language Area From a Neuroanatomical and Developmental Perspective. In: *The Neurocognition of Language*. C A.T. Brown & P. Hagoort (Eds.), 319-336, Oxford, ISBN 9780198507932, Oxford University Press.

Whitney,C.; Huber,W.; Klann,J.; Weis,S.; Krach,S. & Kircher,T. (2009). Neural Correlates of Narrative Shifts During Auditory Story Comprehension. *NeuroImage*, Vol. 47, No. 1, (August 2009), pp. 360–366, ISSN 1095-9572.

Wise, R.J.S.; Scott, S.K.; Blank, C.; Mummery, C.J.; Murphy, K.; Warburton, E.A. (2001). Separate Neural Subsystems Within `Wernicke's Area'. *Brain*, Vol. 124, No. 1, (January 2001), pp. 83-95, ISSN 0006-8950.

Yoo, S.S.; Freeman, D.K.; McCarthy, J.J. 3rd; Jolesz, F.A. (2003). Neural Substrates of Tactile
       Imagery: A Functional MRI Study. *Neuroreport*, Vol. 14, No. 4, (March 2003), pp.
       581-585, ISSN 0959-4965.
Zwaan, R.A. (2004). The Immersed Experiencer: Toward an Embodied Theory of Language
       Comprehension. In: *The Psychology of Learning and Motivation, Vol. 44*, B.H. Ross
       (Ed.), 35-62, Academic Press, ISBN 0-12-543344-1, San Diego, USA.

Neuronal Networks Observed with Resting State Functional Magnetic Resonance Imaging in Clinical Populations

Gioacchino Tedeschi[1,2] and Fabrizio Esposito[2,3,4]
[1]*Department of Neurological Sciences, Second University of Naples,*
[2]*Neurological Institute for Diagnosis and Care "Hermitage Capodimonte",*
[3]*Department of Neuroscience, University of Naples "Federico II",*
[4]*Department of Cognitive Neuroscience, Maastricht University*
[1,2,3]*Italy*
[4]*The Netherlands*

1. Introduction

Functional Magnetic resonance imaging (fMRI, (Ogawa et al., 1990)) in the absence of experimental tasks and behavioral responses, performed with the patient in a relaxed "resting" state (rs-fMRI), takes advantage of the neural origin of spontaneous blood-oxygen-level-dependent (BOLD) signal fluctuations (Biswal et al., 1995) to represent the rate and timing of activity synchronization across the entire brain (Damoiseaux et al., 2006; Mantini et al., 2007; van de Ven et al., 2004).

Independent component analysis (ICA) (Hyvarinen et al., 2001), when applied to whole-brain rs-fMRI, allows extracting from each individual patient data set a series of activation images describing the BOLD signal temporal correlations within and between functionally connected brain regions, forming highly reproducible neural networks called resting state networks (RSN) (Damoiseaux et al., 2006; Mantini et al., 2007). Particularly, ICA transforms individual patient rs-fMRI data sets into series of RSN maps, allowing for a voxel-based population analysis of whole-brain functional connectivity without the need to specify "a priori" the regions of interest constituting the layout of the neural network (McKeown et al., 1998; van de Ven et al., 2004).

In normal volunteers there are at least six RSNs consistently found whose neurological significance has been established according to the functional specialization and anatomical connectivity of the constituent regions (Greicius et al., 2009; van den Heuvel et al., 2009) as well as to the possible association with neuro-electrical rhythms (Mantini et al., 2007). Altogether the functional connectivity of these RSNs represents a basic physiological condition of the human resting brain (Gusnard & Raichle, 2001).

While the number, role, meaning and potential of RSNs in representing and interpreting the functional architecture of the human brain is still debated and sometimes controversial (Morcom & Fletcher, 2007), a number of voxel-based population rs-fMRI studies have uncovered significant differences between normal and clinical populations in various neurological disorders, and a particular attention has been given to cognitive decline as a primary or secondary aspect of neurodegeneration (Bonavita et al., 2011; Cherkassky et al., 2006; Greicius et al., 2007; Greicius et al., 2004; Mohammadi et al., 2009; Nakamura et al., 2009; Rocca et al., 2010; Rombouts et al., 2005; Roosendaal et al., 2010; Sorg et al., 2007; Sorg et al., 2009; Tedeschi et al., 2010).

In this chapter we will review the physiological and technical background of resting state neural networks and the ICA methodology currently used for observing and analyzing RSNs in normal and clinical populations. The main physiological RSNs will be illustrated and discussed with special emphasis to those exhibiting functional abnormalities in neurological disorders. In addition, two clinical applications will be presented, where this methodology showed pathological changes in amyotrophic lateral sclerosis (ALS) and multiple sclerosis (MS) patients in comparison to normal subjects.

2. Physiology and anatomy of the resting-state networks

In a functional connectivity study, the active human brain is conveniently represented in terms of independent functional networks of mutually interacting regions (Friston et al., 1996). Anatomically, these regions can be either distant from each other or result from a fine segregation of bigger into smaller neuronal assemblies. Functionally, two imaging voxels or regions exhibiting neural signals highly correlated in time (synchronized) are conceptually part of the same network.

When measuring the brain with fMRI over prolonged intervals of time (e. g. from two to ten minutes), it is possible to detect throughout the brain characteristic spontaneous fluctuations in the BOLD signal which occur at relatively low frequencies (<0.1 Hz) and are not of technical (artifactual) origin (Biswal et al., 1995; Damoiseaux et al., 2006; Mantini et al., 2007; Smith et al., 1999; van de Ven et al., 2004). When assessing the functional connectivity of these fluctuations across regions, a series of networks can be built, that clearly resemble the same functional networks activated during the performance of active tasks, even if the participant is not performing any specific task and is simply instructed to remain still, with eyes closed and without thinking to anything specific. In other words, under simple resting conditions, the brain is engaged in spontaneous activity which is not attributable to specific inputs or to the generation of specific output, but is intrinsically originated.

A possible link between functional connectivity and spontaneous synchrony of brain signals was already proposed in early electroencephalography (EEG) studies (French & Beaumont, 1984), suggesting that long-range EEG coherencies across cortical regions and between hemispheres could be originated from a relatively small number of interacting regions and processes (see, also, e.g., (Koenig et al., 2005; Locatelli et al., 1998)). Even if EEG and fMRI signals have very different spatial and temporal scales, it has been later demonstrated that a tight correspondence exists between the spatial distribution of low-frequency BOLD signal fluctuations and the main EEG rhythms, for at least six reproducible RSNs (Mantini et al., 2007), in line with the idea that the two modalities share a common neurophysiological origin, represented by the local field potential (LFP) (Logothetis & Pfeuffer, 2004). More specifically, it has been hypothesized that the low-frequency BOLD signal fluctuations are themselves due to low-frequency LFPs or to low frequency modulations of high-frequency LFPs (Raichle, 2010).

The most frequently and consistently reported RSNs, which are also correlated with EEG rhythms, include the default-mode network (DMN), functionally connecting the posterior and anterior cingulate cortex (PCC and ACC) and, bilaterally, the inferior parietal lobules

(Greicius et al., 2003; Raichle et al., 2001); the visual network (VIS) involving bilaterally the retinotopic occipital cortex up to the temporal-occipital junctions and middle temporal gyri (Lowe et al., 1998; Wang et al., 2008); the fronto-parietal network (FPN) including, bilaterally, the intra-parietal cortex and the superior-lateral frontal cortex (Corbetta & Shulman, 2002); the sensori-motor network (SMN) involving, bilaterally, the pre- and post-central gyri, the medial frontal gyrus, the primary and supplementary motor and the primary and secondary sensory areas (Biswal et al., 1995); the auditory network (AUD), involving, bilaterally, the superior and middle temporal cortex (Seifritz et al., 2002) and the self-referential network (SRN) involving the ventro-medial prefrontal cortex and the perigenual anterior cingulate cortex (D'Argembeau et al., 2007). The brain maps of these six typical RSNs in a normal population are exemplarily shown in figure 1 using different colors for the different networks.

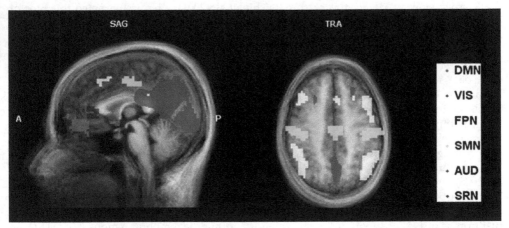

Fig. 1. Typical RSN maps. Visual network (VIS), default-mode network (DMN), fronto-parietal network (FPN), sensori-motor network (SMN), auditory network (AUD) self-referential (SRN) network.

As anticipated (and exemplified in figure 1), all the RSNs consist of anatomically separated, but functionally connected regions, sharing and supporting the same sensitive, motor or cognitive functions (Cordes et al., 2000). The RSNs reported in the normative literature have generally resulted to be quite consistent across studies, despite some differences in data acquisition and analysis techniques that partially account for the variability observed in the number and lay out of the networks. For instance, the DMN has been sometimes distinguished into two separate subnetworks, the anterior and posterior DMN (see, e. g., (Damoiseaux et al., 2008)), and the FPN as two lateralized networks (right and left FPNs, RFPN and LFPN) (see, e. g., (Damoiseaux et al., 2006; Tedeschi et al., 2010)). The auditory and visual networks have been presented in terms of a one single network (see, e. g., (Mantini et al., 2007)), two (see, e. g., (Damoiseaux et al., 2006)) or even three (see, e. g., (Rocca et al., 2011)) subnetworks.

Understanding the functional correlate of a given RSN under normal physiological conditions is crucial to correctly address any possible link between altered rs-fMRI patterns and behavioral and clinical variables. However, it should also be recognized that cytoarchitectonically distinct brain regions are kept functionally connected by white matter connections that directly (monosynaptically) or indirectly (multisynaptically) make the ongoing communication physically possible (Greicius et al., 2009; van den Heuvel et al., 2009). Thereby, it is equally important to clarify whether the observed RSN functional connectivity is mediated by direct or indirect structural connections, e. g. by combining rs-fMRI with diffusion tensor imaging (DTI), an MRI technique that allows the study of white matter fiber bundles.

By far, the most studied RSN in the clinical and research neuroimaging community is the DMN (Greicius et al., 2003; Raichle et al., 2001). This network has attracted considerable interest in the neuroscience community for its possible role as the baseline cognitive state of a subject and its link to memory and executive functions in normal and pathological conditions. In fact, the DMN normally includes the ACC and PCC regions, known to be involved in attention-related processes (Badgaiyan & Posner, 1998) and often detectable as transiently or consistently deactivated during many different types of cognitive tasks (McKiernan et al., 2003). For this reason, Raichle et al. (2001), who first targeted this type of brain activity with positron emission tomography (PET) imaging, have introduced the concept of "default-mode" activity and attempted to differentiate a "cognitive" baseline state from a "general" resting state in human brain. Thereafter (Greicius et al., 2003) the DMN has been often conceptualized as a "stand-alone" function or system to be analyzed with data models specifically oriented to functional connectivity (Bullmore et al., 1996). Within the DMN, the PCC node, one of the most intensively interconnected regions in the whole brain (Cavanna & Trimble, 2006; Hagmann et al., 2008), seems to mediate all the intrinsic functional connectivity of the brain (Fransson & Marrelec, 2008). Indeed, the PCC plays an essential role in all types of introspective mental activity, ranging from immediate suppressing of distracting thoughts to avoid mistakes (Li et al., 2007; Weissman et al., 2006) up to modulating rethinking about the past to imagine the future and awareness (Buckner et al., 2008).

The VIS network involves regions in the striate, peri-striate and extra-striate visual cortex, which are normally activated by a visual task. This network extends from the lingual and fusiform gyri (i. e. V1 to V4) up to the occipito- and middle temporal regions (i. e. MT/V5), even if, in some reports, regions belonging to the primary and secondary visual system are shown to belong to separate visual RSNs (see, e. g., (Rocca et al., 2011)).

The fronto-parietal (or "executive-attention") network (FPN), sometimes found to be lateralized (i.e., right and left FPN), is also relevant for cognition. Particularly, the FPNs seem to be central for cognitive processing as they involve regions such as the dorsal frontal and parietal cortices potentially overlapping with the dorsal attention network which is known to mediate executive control processing (Corbetta & Shulman, 2002).

The SMN includes regions in the precentral and postcentral gyrus and in the supplementary motor area, all regions that both anatomically and functionally correspond well to motor and sensory areas, e. g. activated during a finger tapping task (Biswal et al., 1995).

The AUD network involves regions in the auditory cortex, which are normally activated by an auditory task. This network extends from the Heschl's gyrus to the superior temporal gyrus and the insula and has been also reported as one or two RSNs (see, e. g., (Damoiseaux et al., 2006)).

3. Methodology for the analysis of the resting-state networks

RSN can be observed using several functional connectivity analysis tools. A straightforward approach entails extracting the extracting the time-course of the BOLD signal from a predefined region-of-interest (ROI) and subsequently searching all regions whose time-course significantly correlates with the ROI time-course. This method produces RSN maps that are extremely simple to interpret (Fox & Raichle, 2007; Greicius et al., 2003), but has the important drawback that the resulting functional connectivity maps will depend on the location, extension and order of the "seed" regions chosen, and on how these are defined in advance of the analysis. By contrast, "component-based" statistical techniques (Andersen et al., 1999; Friston et al., 1993), that do not require a-priori assumptions on the regions involved, enable the observation of multiple neural networks from whole-brain resting state data sets, thereby avoiding the possibility of bias.

ICA (Hyvarinen et al., 2001) has been successfully applied to neuroimaging data of diverse imaging modalities for generating convenient representations of activated brain networks in single subjects and groups. Particularly, in fMRI, ICA is commonly applied in its spatial variant (Calhoun et al., 2001b; McKeown et al., 1998) where each statistically independent component process corresponds to a spatial map distributed over all voxels of the imaging slab. Besides separating many types of structured dynamic artefacts from fMRI time series (see, e. g., (De Martino et al., 2007)), spatial ICA can provide a meaningful representation of function-related BOLD signals and unravel the whole-brain distributed functional connectivity under different experimental and clinical conditions. Particularly, spatial ICA is commonly applied in rs-fMRI to model the spontaneous low-frequency BOLD signals in terms of whole-brain distributed maps (Mantini et al., 2007).

When exploring fMRI data with spatial ICA, it is always necessary to decide how many ICA components to extract and, among these, select those components that can be consistently and reliably associated with functional connectivity networks of interest for a given application. The number of components is basically a "free choice" parameter (Calhoun et al., 2009), typically ranging between 20 and 60, even if potential changes in the layout of certain ICA generated RSN maps, such as splitting of a network into multiple networks, may result from the extraction of substantially more components than the minimum needed for a stable decomposition (Abou-Elseoud et al., 2010; Kiviniemi et al., 2009).

After fMRI data preparation and preprocessing, a group statistical analysis is typically required to summarize RSN functional connectivity in one or more populations of interest and to search for possible regional differences between populations within selected RSNs.

In many cases, population-level studies based on ICA use a two-level approach, first running single-subject ICA and then combining the components into a second-level group (random effects) analysis; in order to match components between subjects clustering and spatial correlation techniques are used (Esposito et al., 2005; Schopf et al., 2011; Wang & Peterson, 2008). This strategy provides maximal power to model subject-level structured noise (Cole et al., 2010) and has the important advantage of capturing unique spatial and temporal features of the subjects' data set even if the signal to noise ratio (SNR) is substantially lower in some subjects compared to other subjects. The disadvantage of this approach is that the components that are matched across subjects are not necessarily extracted in the same way for each subject of a group (Erhardt et al., 2010).

As an alternative to clustering, temporal (Calhoun et al., 2001a; Varoquaux et al., 2010) and spatial (Svensen et al., 2002) concatenation as well as "tensorial" (Beckmann & Smith, 2005; Guo & Pagnoni, 2008) data aggregation schemes have been previously examined to perform only one ICA decomposition, thereby circumventing the problem of a "first-level" component matching. The most used aggregate group ICA approaches (Calhoun et al.,

2001a; Zuo et al., 2010) are based on temporal concatenation and assume "common" ICA maps for all subjects in the first level analysis. A population analysis is then performed retrospectively determining the individual ICA components from the group ICA components. Thereby, all these methods implicitly assume that a given component is really present with exactly the same layout in all the subjects.

4. Resting state networks in clinical populations

The observational study of RSN functional connectivity in normal and clinical populations allows generating a comprehensive picture of brain functions and dysfunctions by the sole analysis of resting state fMRI activity, i. e. without relying on an active performance or engagement of the patient. This aspect is particularly attractive when studying uncooperative populations, but is generally suited to all cases where behaviors and performances are pathologically impaired. For this reason many research groups have studied RSN functional connectivity in different neurological and psychiatry disorders, detected differences between patients and controls and correlated these measures to clinical variables.

The largest numbers of studies and the most consistent results have been obtained for disorders like Alzheimer disease (AD) (Greicius et al., 2004; Petrella et al., 2011; Rombouts et al., 2005; Sorg et al., 2007; Supekar et al., 2008; Wang et al., 2007; Wang et al., 2006; Zhang et al., 2010; Zhang et al., 2009) and schizophrenia (Bates et al., 2009; Bluhm et al., 2007; Foucher et al., 2005; Greicius, 2008; Hoptman et al., 2010; Jang et al., 2011; Lagioia et al., 2010; Lynall et al., 2010; Mannell et al., ; Ongur et al., 2010; Repovs et al., 2011; Rotarska-Jagiela et al., 2010; Shen et al., ; Skudlarski et al., ; van den Heuvel & Hulshoff Pol, ; Woodward et al., 2011; Zhou et al., 2008). In this chapter, we present two examples of clinical RSN study, applied to ALS and MS.

4.1 Resting state networks in Amyotrophic Lateral Sclerosis

ALS is a chronic progressive disease that predominantly affects the motor system (Turner et al., 2009b), but neurodegeneration may also extend beyond motor areas (Geser et al., 2008; Geser et al., 2009; Murphy et al., 2007; Turner et al., 2009a). In fact, ALS patients often exhibit variable degrees of cognitive impairment with rather typical involvement of frontal executive functions (Grossman et al., 2008; Murphy et al., 2007). Thereby, studying the SMN, but also the DMN and the FPN, is crucially important to elucidate both motor and extra-motor involvement in ALS, to examine the possible interaction between physiologically sensitive and disease modified rs-fMRI parameters and to compare these functional measures with the clinical and MRI structural aspects of the neurodegenerative process.

The fact that rs-fMRI allows exploring whole-brain functional connectivity in all these RSNs with minimal bias towards a specific motor or cognitive function is particularly attractive for studying ALS patients, whose degree of cooperation normally introduces substantial variability in their performances.

The rs-FMRI fluctuations within the SMN network are reduced or even suppressed in ALS patients compared to age- and sex-matched normal controls (Mohammadi et al., 2009; Tedeschi et al., 2010). For instance, comparing the SMN maps on a voxel by voxel basis has shown statistically significant group differences bilaterally in the primary motor cortex (PMC) (figure 2).

ALS has long been characterized as a neurodegenerative disorder affecting the motor system, therefore, the observation that the coherent RS-fMRI fluctuations within the SMN are strongly reduced can be easily linked to most existing animal models of ALS explaining motor neuron degeneration both at the cellular and molecular levels (Dal Canto et al., 1995; Wong et al., 1995; Wils et al., 2010).

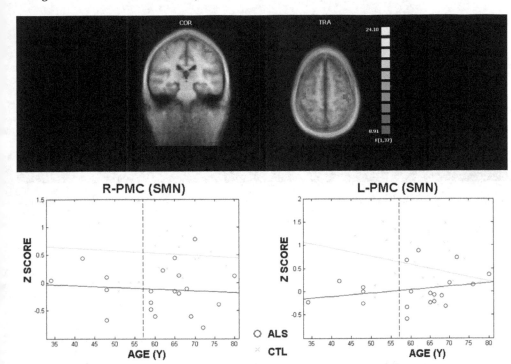

Fig. 2. ALS disease effects in the SMN. Upper panel: F-map of statistically significant disease effects within the SMN network (P=0.05, cluster-level corrected) overlaid on the average Talairach-transformed T1 image (coronal and axial cuts). Lower panel: Scatter plots of the regional ICA z-scores vs age in the R-PMC (left) and in the L-PMC (right). PMC = primary motor cortex. ALS = amyotrophic lateral sclerosis patients. CTL = control subjects.

The RFPN network is also partially suppressed in ALS patients. Figure 3 shows the localization of two regions within this network, in the superior frontal gyrus (SFG) and in the supra-marginal gyrus (SMG), where the network-specific RS-fMRI fluctuations resulted suppressed in ALS compared to controls. These effects in a cognitive executive network like the RFPN likely reflect a rather typical frontal cortex dysfunction observed in ALS patients (Abrahams et al., 1996; Hatazawa et al., 1988; Rule et al., 2010; Vercelletto et al., 1999).

Observing RSNs in ALS patients over an extended range of age has highlighted the possible interaction between aging and neurodegeneration (Tedeschi et al., 2010). Previous work has reported a significant effect of aging on DMN regions in the normal population (Esposito et al., 2008; Grady et al., 2006; Greicius et al., 2004; Koch et al., 2009; Persson et al., 2007). In ALS patients, the DMN network has shown an age-by-disease interaction effect in the PCC (figure 4), with the strength of the RS-fMRI fluctuations relatively increased rather than reduced with increasing age (and disease duration). In addition, there was also a group-by-age interaction effect in RFPN, and more precisely the middle frontal gyrus (MFG) (figure

4), further reflecting a possible attempt of the ALS brain to compensate the motor neuron degeneration by reorganizing the functional connectivity in cognitive networks within unaffected (or less affected) domains.

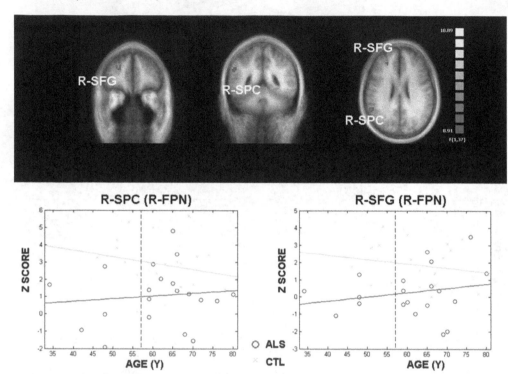

Fig. 3. ALS disease effects in the RFPN network. Upper panel: F-map of statistically significant disease effects within the R-FPN network (P=0.05, cluster-level corrected) overlaid on the average Talairach-transformed T1 image (two right sagittal cuts and one axial cut). Lower panel: Scatter plot of the regional ICA z-scores vs age in the SMG (left) and in the SFG (right). SMG = supramarginal gyrus. SFG = superior frontal gyrus. ALS = amyotrophic lateral sclerosis patients. CTL = control subjects.

This age compensatory effect on the functional connectivity can also be linked to biological processes of neuronal aging and degeneration. In fact, a few studies based on animal and cellular models of ALS pathophysiology (see, e. g., (Madeo et al., 2009)) have linked neurodegeneration and aging to specific strategies of neuroprotection by which the cell damage is contrasted with adaptive mechanisms against the physiological stress implied by aging. Thereby, these interaction patterns might represent the functional expression of the interaction between a widespread brain neurodegeneration and a physiological mechanism activated by aging. Particularly, the observed positive correlation between aging and spontaneous functional connectivity might be the result of a specific change in the default system to counteract the physiologically driven decline with age, given that ALS patients continuously alert the default system for performing any task potentially requested and made possible by the residual motor capabilities.

4.2 Default-mode network dysfunction in Multiple Sclerosis

Cognitive impairment is frequently observed in MS pathology (Benedict et al., 2006; Rao et al., 1991) and fMRI activation studies in MS patients with cognitive impairment have suggested that cerebral reorganisation (Filippi & Rocca, 2004; Mainero et al., 2004) and recruitment of non impaired cortical regions may occur as a compensatory mechanism to limit the cognitive consequences of tissue damage (Filippi & Rocca, 2004; Wishart et al., 2004).

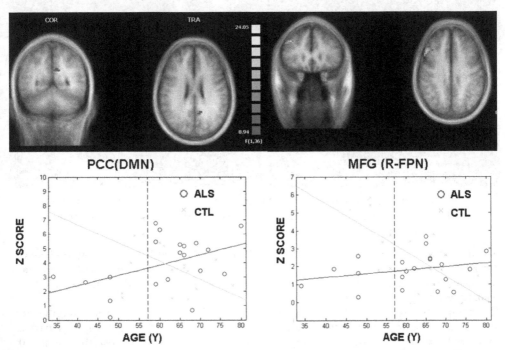

Fig. 4. ALS disease-by-age interaction in the DMN (left panel) and RFPN (right panel). Upper panels: F-map of disease by age interaction effects (P=0.05, cluster-level corrected) overlaid on the average Talairach-transformed T1 image (coronal and axial cuts). Lower panels: Regional ICA z-scores vs age in the PCC (left) and in the MFG (right).

Thereby, rs-fMRI is an attractive way to explore the spatio-temporal distribution of the spontaneous coherent fluctuations of BOLD signals within and between different regions throughout the entire human brain in different functional domains.

RS-FMRI studies have reported DMN alterations in both relapsing-remitting (RR) and progressive MS patients, when comparing MS patient groups with age and sex-matched healthy controls (Bonavita et al., 2011; Rocca et al., 2010).

The DMN connectivity distribution in RR MS patients may deviate from the control group both in the anterior node (in the ACC), that is substantially suppressed in the RR MS patient groups, and in the posterior nodes (in the PCC and, bilaterally, in the IPC), where a more distributed spatial re-organization seems to occur. Figure 5 shows a DMN comparisons map between a group of RR MS patients and a control group which clearly indicates that rs-fMRI coherent fluctuations within the DMN are reduced in RR MS patients close to the midline, both in the ACC and in the PCC, but also that, RR MS patients exhibit spots of more coherent fluctuations far from the midline, at the periphery of the PCC and toward the parieto-occipital regions of the DMN.

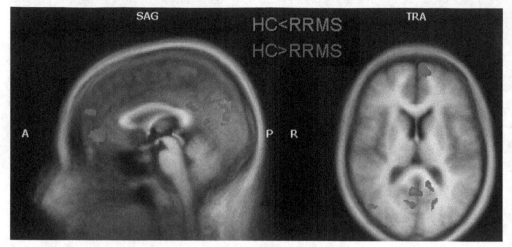

Fig. 5. Comparison between a group of RR MS patients and healthy controls (HCs). The clusters of significant differential activity are overlaid on two orthogonal slices of the averaged normalized anatomy.

A better display of the differences in the DMN functional connectivity distribution between the RR-MS and control groups is visible in figure 6, where all clusters with statistically significant differential effects are reconstructed as 3D volumes with separate colours in relation to the sign of the differences.

The comparison between RR-MS patients and normal controls becomes certainly more interesting if cognitive impaired (CI) and cognitive preserved (CP) subgroups are separately compared. Figure 7 shows this comparison and the 3D maps suggest that, while the suppression of the ACC node is a common aspect to both CI and CP RR MS patients, the re-organization of the functional connectivity in the posterior DMN can be different depending on the cognitive impairment of RR MS patients.

In summary, RR MS patients, regardless of their cognitive status exhibit a weaker DMN connectivity at the level of the ACC and the central/midline region of the PCC, together with an expanded connectivity at the level of the peripheral portions of the PCC and bilateral IPC. However, distribution changes in the posterior DMN appear with different lay outs in CI and CP patients and may thus be associated with the cognitive status of RRMS patients.

As for the other MS forms, progressive MS patients also exhibit reduced DMN connectivity, but mainly in the anterior part of the DMN (Rocca et al., 2011), where as clinically isolated syndrome (CIS) suggestive of MS seem to have increased DMN connectivity in the PCC node when compared to RR MS patients (Roosendaal et al., 2010), thus suggesting that the possible compensatory mechanism observed in the posterior DMN might be visible quite early in the disease course.

With respect to the selective involvement of the ACC in MS, one should consider that the ACC has extensive associative connections with other areas (Paus, 2001). Thereby, if cortico-cortical functional connectivity reduction is the result of axonal transection by white matter lesions, then highly connected (and distant) regions like ACC should be more vulnerable than regions with relatively fewer connections. Actually, there is evidence from histopathological studies that the cingulate gyrus shows a higher prevalence of cortical demyelinated lesions than other areas (Bo et al., 2003; Kutzelnigg & Lassmann, 2006) and therefore it is likely that these regions are intrinsically more vulnerable and more directly involved by the disease.

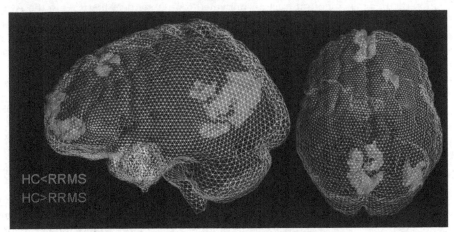

Fig. 6. Comparison between a group of RR MS patients and healthy controls (HCs). The clusters of significant differential activity are displayed as reconstructed as 3D volumes.

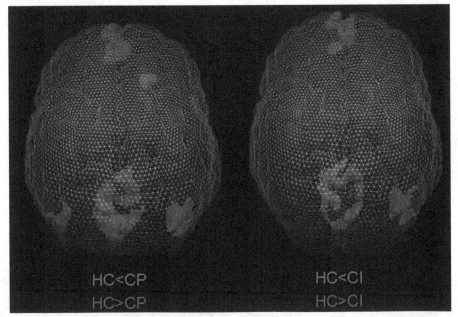

Fig. 7. Comparison between the separate groups of cognitive preserved (CP) (left) and cognitive impaired (CI) (right) RR MS patients and healthy controls (HC). The clusters of significant activity are displayed reconstructed as 3D volumes.

Van den Heuvel et al. (van den Heuvel et al., 2008) have investigated the structural connection of the DMN by combining diffusion tensor imaging and rs-fMRI data and found that the microstructural organization of the interconnecting cingulum tract, as measured by fractional anisotropy, is directly associated with the level of functional connectivity of the DMN, in particular the cingulum tract is confirmed to interconnect the PCC to the ACC of the DMN. This direct anatomical connection reflects a vast number of axonal connections between the posterior node/PCC and anterior node/ACC, responsible for the facilitation of neuronal communication between these regions. The cingulum tract is a thin white matter association bundle that is located just above and all along the corpus callosum, therefore it is expected to be frequently involved by WM lesions of MS. Thereby, if white matter MS plaques significantly contribute in determining the disconnection phenomena observed between the PCC and the ACC with the net functional loss of the ACC in the DMN of RRMS subjects, it is likely that DMN distribution changes in the posterior node represent a compensatory mechanism to sustain cognitive performances.

5. Conclusion

The present chapter has highlighted the importance of observing RSN in clinical populations in relation to both physiological and pathological factors and the potential impact of rs-fMRI as a non-invasive technique to explore whole-brain functional connectivity in neurological diseases for which the biological mechanisms are not completely understood. Particularly, since rs-fMRI does not require patient interaction, it will be possible to apply the present functional neuroimaging methodology to patients at highly advanced stages of the disease and eventually allow for longitudinal investigations.

Besides potentially shedding light on the pathological mechanisms occurring in certain neurological disorders, the clinical applications may also favor a better understanding of RSN functional connectivity in the context of brain neurophysiology, especially when the rs-fMRI patterns are carefully examined in relation to physiological and anatomical factors and to the possible interaction between these and the temporal course of a disease.

6. References

Abou-Elseoud, A., Starck, T., Remes, J., Nikkinen, J., Tervonen, O. & Kiviniemi, V. (2010): The effect of model order selection in group PICA. *Hum Brain Mapp*, Vol.31, No.8, pp. 1207-16.

Abrahams, S., Goldstein, L. H., Kew, J. J., Brooks, D. J., Lloyd, C. M., Frith, C. D. & Leigh, P. N. (1996): Frontal lobe dysfunction in amyotrophic lateral sclerosis. A PET study. *Brain*, Vol.119 (Pt 6), pp. 2105-20.

Andersen, A. H., Gash, D. M. & Avison, M. J. (1999): Principal component analysis of the dynamic response measured by fMRI: a generalized linear systems framework. *Magn Reson Imaging*, Vol.17, No.6, pp. 795-815.

Badgaiyan, R. D. & Posner, M. I. (1998): Mapping the cingulate cortex in response selection and monitoring. *Neuroimage*, Vol.7, No.3, pp. 255-60.

Bates, A. T., Kiehl, K. A., Laurens, K. R. & Liddle, P. F. (2009): Low-frequency EEG oscillations associated with information processing in schizophrenia. *Schizophr Res*, Vol.115, No.2-3, pp. 222-30.

Beckmann, C. F. & Smith, S. M. (2005): Tensorial extensions of independent component analysis for multisubject FMRI analysis. *Neuroimage*, Vol.25, No.1, pp. 294-311.

Benedict, R. H., Cookfair, D., Gavett, R., Gunther, M., Munschauer, F., Garg, N. & Weinstock-Guttman, B. (2006): Validity of the minimal assessment of cognitive function in multiple sclerosis (MACFIMS). *J Int Neuropsychol Soc*, Vol.12, No.4, pp. 549-58.

Biswal, B., Yetkin, F. Z., Haughton, V. M. & Hyde, J. S. (1995): Functional connectivity in the motor cortex of resting human brain using echo-planar MRI. *Magn Reson Med*, Vol.34, No.4, pp. 537-41.

Bluhm, R. L., Miller, J., Lanius, R. A., Osuch, E. A., Boksman, K., Neufeld, R. W., Theberge, J., Schaefer, B. & Williamson, P. (2007): Spontaneous low-frequency fluctuations in the BOLD signal in schizophrenic patients: anomalies in the default network. *Schizophr Bull*, Vol.33, No.4, pp. 1004-12.

Bo, L., Vedeler, C. A., Nyland, H. I., Trapp, B. D. & Mork, S. J. (2003): Subpial demyelination in the cerebral cortex of multiple sclerosis patients. *J Neuropathol Exp Neurol*, Vol.62, No.7, pp. 723-32.

Bonavita, S., Gallo, A., Sacco, R., Della Corte, M., Bisecco, A., Docimo, R., Lavorgna, L., Corbo, D., Di Costanzo, A., Tortora, F., Cirillo, M., Esposito, F. & Tedeschi, G. (2011): Distributed changes in default-mode resting-state connectivity in multiple sclerosis. *Mult Scler*, Vol.17, No.4, pp. 411-422.

Buckner, R. L., Andrews-Hanna, J. R. & Schacter, D. L. (2008): The brain's default network: anatomy, function, and relevance to disease. *Ann N Y Acad Sci*, Vol.1124, pp. 1-38.

Bullmore, E. T., Rabe-Hesketh, S., Morris, R. G., Williams, S. C., Gregory, L., Gray, J. A. & Brammer, M. J. (1996): Functional magnetic resonance image analysis of a large-scale neurocognitive network. *Neuroimage*, Vol.4, No.1, pp. 16-33.

Calhoun, V. D., Adali, T., Pearlson, G. D. & Pekar, J. J. (2001a): A method for making group inferences from functional MRI data using independent component analysis. *Hum Brain Mapp*, Vol.14, No.3, pp. 140-51.

Calhoun, V. D., Adali, T., Pearlson, G. D. & Pekar, J. J. (2001b): Spatial and temporal independent component analysis of functional MRI data containing a pair of task-related waveforms. *Hum Brain Mapp*, Vol.13, No.1, pp. 43-53.

Calhoun, V. D., Liu, J. & Adali, T. (2009): A review of group ICA for fMRI data and ICA for joint inference of imaging, genetic, and ERP data. *Neuroimage*, Vol.45, No.1 Suppl, pp. S163-72.

Cavanna, A. E. & Trimble, M. R. (2006): The precuneus: a review of its functional anatomy and behavioural correlates. *Brain*, Vol.129, No.Pt 3, pp. 564-83.

Cherkassky, V. L., Kana, R. K., Keller, T. A. & Just, M. A. (2006): Functional connectivity in a baseline resting-state network in autism. *Neuroreport*, Vol.17, No.16, pp. 1687-90.

Cole, D. M., Smith, S. M. & Beckmann, C. F. (2010): Advances and pitfalls in the analysis and interpretation of resting-state FMRI data. *Front Syst Neurosci*, Vol.4, pp. 8.

Corbetta, M. & Shulman, G. L. (2002): Control of goal-directed and stimulus-driven attention in the brain. *Nat Rev Neurosci*, Vol.3, No.3, pp. 201-15.

Cordes, D., Haughton, V. M., Arfanakis, K., Wendt, G. J., Turski, P. A., Moritz, C. H., Quigley, M. A. & Meyerand, M. E. (2000): Mapping functionally related regions of brain with functional connectivity MR imaging. *AJNR Am J Neuroradiol*, Vol.21, No.9, pp. 1636-44.

D'Argembeau, A., Ruby, P., Collette, F., Degueldre, C., Balteau, E., Luxen, A., Maquet, P. & Salmon, E. (2007): Distinct regions of the medial prefrontal cortex are associated with self-referential processing and perspective taking. *J Cogn Neurosci*, Vol.19, No.6, pp. 935-44.

Damoiseaux, J. S., Beckmann, C. F., Arigita, E. J., Barkhof, F., Scheltens, P., Stam, C. J., Smith, S. M. & Rombouts, S. A. (2008): Reduced resting-state brain activity in the "default network" in normal aging. *Cereb Cortex*, Vol.18, No.8, pp. 1856-64.

Damoiseaux, J. S., Rombouts, S. A., Barkhof, F., Scheltens, P., Stam, C. J., Smith, S. M. & Beckmann, C. F. (2006): Consistent resting-state networks across healthy subjects. *Proc Natl Acad Sci U S A*, Vol.103, No.37, pp. 13848-53.

De Martino, F., Gentile, F., Esposito, F., Balsi, M., Di Salle, F., Goebel, R. & Formisano, E. (2007): Classification of fMRI independent components using IC-fingerprints and support vector machine classifiers. *Neuroimage*, Vol.34, No.1, pp. 177-94.

Erhardt, E. B., Rachakonda, S., Bedrick, E. J., Allen, E. A., Adali, T. & Calhoun, V. D. (2010): Comparison of multi-subject ICA methods for analysis of fMRI data. *Hum Brain Mapp*, Vol.pp.

Esposito, F., Aragri, A., Pesaresi, I., Cirillo, S., Tedeschi, G., Marciano, E., Goebel, R. & Di Salle, F. (2008): Independent component model of the default-mode brain function: combining individual-level and population-level analyses in resting-state fMRI. *Magn Reson Imaging*, Vol.26, No.7, pp. 905-13.

Esposito, F., Scarabino, T., Hyvarinen, A., Himberg, J., Formisano, E., Comani, S., Tedeschi, G., Goebel, R., Seifritz, E. & Di Salle, F. (2005): Independent component analysis of fMRI group studies by self-organizing clustering. *Neuroimage*, Vol.25, No.1, pp. 193-205.

Filippi, M. & Rocca, M. A. (2004): Cortical reorganisation in patients with MS. *J Neurol Neurosurg Psychiatry*, Vol.75, No.8, pp. 1087-9.

Foucher, J. R., Vidailhet, P., Chanraud, S., Gounot, D., Grucker, D., Pins, D., Damsa, C. & Danion, J. M. (2005): Functional integration in schizophrenia: too little or too much? Preliminary results on fMRI data. *Neuroimage*, Vol.26, No.2, pp. 374-88.

Fox, M. D. & Raichle, M. E. (2007): Spontaneous fluctuations in brain activity observed with functional magnetic resonance imaging. *Nat Rev Neurosci*, Vol.8, No.9, pp. 700-11.

Fransson, P. & Marrelec, G. (2008): The precuneus/posterior cingulate cortex plays a pivotal role in the default mode network: Evidence from a partial correlation network analysis. *Neuroimage*, Vol.42, No.3, pp. 1178-84.

French, C. C. & Beaumont, J. G. (1984): A critical review of EEG coherence studies of hemisphere function. *Int J Psychophysiol*, Vol.1, No.3, pp. 241-54.

Friston, K. J., Frith, C. D., Fletcher, P., Liddle, P. F. & Frackowiak, R. S. (1996): Functional topography: multidimensional scaling and functional connectivity in the brain. *Cereb Cortex*, Vol.6, No.2, pp. 156-64.

Friston, K. J., Frith, C. D. & Frackowiak, R. S. (1993): Principal component analysis learning algorithms: a neurobiological analysis. *Proc Biol Sci*, Vol.254, No.1339, pp. 47-54.

Geser, F., Brandmeir, N. J., Kwong, L. K., Martinez-Lage, M., Elman, L., McCluskey, L., Xie, S. X., Lee, V. M. & Trojanowski, J. Q. (2008): Evidence of multisystem disorder in whole-brain map of pathological TDP-43 in amyotrophic lateral sclerosis. *Arch Neurol*, Vol.65, No.5, pp. 636-41.

Geser, F., Martinez-Lage, M., Kwong, L. K., Lee, V. M. & Trojanowski, J. Q. (2009): Amyotrophic lateral sclerosis, frontotemporal dementia and beyond: the TDP-43 diseases. *J Neurol*, Vol.256, No.8, pp. 1205-14.

Grady, C. L., Springer, M. V., Hongwanishkul, D., McIntosh, A. R. & Winocur, G. (2006): Age-related changes in brain activity across the adult lifespan. *J Cogn Neurosci*, Vol.18, No.2, pp. 227-41.

Greicius, M. (2008): Resting-state functional connectivity in neuropsychiatric disorders. *Curr Opin Neurol*, Vol.21, No.4, pp. 424-30.

Greicius, M. D., Flores, B. H., Menon, V., Glover, G. H., Solvason, H. B., Kenna, H., Reiss, A. L. & Schatzberg, A. F. (2007): Resting-state functional connectivity in major depression: abnormally increased contributions from subgenual cingulate cortex and thalamus. *Biol Psychiatry*, Vol.62, No.5, pp. 429-37.

Greicius, M. D., Krasnow, B., Reiss, A. L. & Menon, V. (2003): Functional connectivity in the resting brain: a network analysis of the default mode hypothesis. *Proc Natl Acad Sci U S A*, Vol.100, No.1, pp. 253-8.

Greicius, M. D., Srivastava, G., Reiss, A. L. & Menon, V. (2004): Default-mode network activity distinguishes Alzheimer's disease from healthy aging: evidence from functional MRI. *Proc Natl Acad Sci U S A*, Vol.101, No.13, pp. 4637-42.

Greicius, M. D., Supekar, K., Menon, V. & Dougherty, R. F. (2009): Resting-state functional connectivity reflects structural connectivity in the default mode network. *Cereb Cortex*, Vol.19, No.1, pp. 72-8.

Grossman, M., Anderson, C., Khan, A., Avants, B., Elman, L. & McCluskey, L. (2008): Impaired action knowledge in amyotrophic lateral sclerosis. *Neurology*, Vol.71, No.18, pp. 1396-401.

Guo, Y. & Pagnoni, G. (2008): A unified framework for group independent component analysis for multi-subject fMRI data. *Neuroimage*, Vol.42, No.3, pp. 1078-93.

Gusnard, D. A. & Raichle, M. E. (2001): Searching for a baseline: functional imaging and the resting human brain. *Nat Rev Neurosci*, Vol.2, No.10, pp. 685-94.

Hagmann, P., Cammoun, L., Gigandet, X., Meuli, R., Honey, C. J., Wedeen, V. J. & Sporns, O. (2008): Mapping the structural core of human cerebral cortex. *PLoS Biol*, Vol.6, No.7, pp. e159.

Hatazawa, J., Brooks, R. A., Dalakas, M. C., Mansi, L. & Di Chiro, G. (1988): Cortical motor-sensory hypometabolism in amyotrophic lateral sclerosis: a PET study. *J Comput Assist Tomogr*, Vol.12, No.4, pp. 630-6.

Hoptman, M. J., Zuo, X. N., Butler, P. D., Javitt, D. C., D'Angelo, D., Mauro, C. J. & Milham, M. P. (2010): Amplitude of low-frequency oscillations in schizophrenia: a resting state fMRI study. *Schizophr Res*, Vol.117, No.1, pp. 13-20.

Hyvarinen, A., Karhunen, J. & Oja, E. 2001. Independent Component Analysis. New York: John Wiley & Sons, Inc.

Jang, J. H., Jung, W. H., Choi, J. S., Choi, C. H., Kang, D. H., Shin, N. Y., Hong, K. S. & Kwon, J. S. (2011): Reduced prefrontal functional connectivity in the default mode network is related to greater psychopathology in subjects with high genetic loading for schizophrenia. *Schizophr Res*, Vol.127, No.1-3, pp. 58-65.

Kiviniemi, V., Starck, T., Remes, J., Long, X., Nikkinen, J., Haapea, M., Veijola, J., Moilanen, I., Isohanni, M., Zang, Y. F. & Tervonen, O. (2009): Functional segmentation of the brain cortex using high model order group PICA. *Hum Brain Mapp*, Vol.30, No.12, pp. 3865-86.

Koch, W., Teipel, S., Mueller, S., Buerger, K., Bokde, A. L., Hampel, H., Coates, U., Reiser, M. & Meindl, T. (2009): Effects of aging on default mode network activity in resting state fMRI: Does the method of analysis matter? *Neuroimage*, Vol.pp.

Koenig, T., Studer, D., Hubl, D., Melie, L. & Strik, W. K. (2005): Brain connectivity at different time-scales measured with EEG. *Philos Trans R Soc Lond B Biol Sci*, Vol.360, No.1457, pp. 1015-23.

Kutzelnigg, A. & Lassmann, H. (2006): Cortical demyelination in multiple sclerosis: a substrate for cognitive deficits? *J Neurol Sci*, Vol.245, No.1-2, pp. 123-6.

Lagioia, A., Van De Ville, D., Debbane, M., Lazeyras, F. & Eliez, S. (2010): Adolescent resting state networks and their associations with schizotypal trait expression. *Front Syst Neurosci*, Vol.4, pp.

Li, C. S., Yan, P., Bergquist, K. L. & Sinha, R. (2007): Greater activation of the "default" brain regions predicts stop signal errors. *Neuroimage*, Vol.38, No.3, pp. 640-8.

Locatelli, T., Cursi, M., Liberati, D., Franceschi, M. & Comi, G. (1998): EEG coherence in Alzheimer's disease. *Electroencephalogr Clin Neurophysiol*, Vol.106, No.3, pp. 229-37.

Logothetis, N. K. & Pfeuffer, J. (2004): On the nature of the BOLD fMRI contrast mechanism. *Magn Reson Imaging*, Vol.22, No.10, pp. 1517-31.

Lowe, M. J., Mock, B. J. & Sorenson, J. A. (1998): Functional connectivity in single and multislice echoplanar imaging using resting-state fluctuations. *Neuroimage*, Vol.7, No.2, pp. 119-32.

Lynall, M. E., Bassett, D. S., Kerwin, R., McKenna, P. J., Kitzbichler, M., Muller, U. & Bullmore, E. (2010): Functional connectivity and brain networks in schizophrenia. *J Neurosci*, Vol.30, No.28, pp. 9477-87.

Madeo, F., Eisenberg, T. & Kroemer, G. (2009): Autophagy for the avoidance of neurodegeneration. *Genes Dev*, Vol.23, No.19, pp. 2253-9.

Mainero, C., Caramia, F., Pozzilli, C., Pisani, A., Pestalozza, I., Borriello, G., Bozzao, L. & Pantano, P. (2004): fMRI evidence of brain reorganization during attention and memory tasks in multiple sclerosis. *Neuroimage*, Vol.21, No.3, pp. 858-67.

Mannell, M. V., Franco, A. R., Calhoun, V. D., Canive, J. M., Thoma, R. J. & Mayer, A. R. Resting state and task-induced deactivation: A methodological comparison in patients with schizophrenia and healthy controls. *Hum Brain Mapp*, Vol.31, No.3, pp. 424-37.

Mantini, D., Perrucci, M. G., Del Gratta, C., Romani, G. L. & Corbetta, M. (2007): Electrophysiological signatures of resting state networks in the human brain. *Proc Natl Acad Sci U S A*, Vol.104, No.32, pp. 13170-5.

McKeown, M. J., Makeig, S., Brown, G. G., Jung, T. P., Kindermann, S. S., Bell, A. J. & Sejnowski, T. J. (1998): Analysis of fMRI data by blind separation into independent spatial components. *Hum Brain Mapp*, Vol.6, No.3, pp. 160-88.

McKiernan, K. A., Kaufman, J. N., Kucera-Thompson, J. & Binder, J. R. (2003): A parametric manipulation of factors affecting task-induced deactivation in functional neuroimaging. *J Cogn Neurosci*, Vol.15, No.3, pp. 394-408.

Mohammadi, B., Kollewe, K., Samii, A., Krampfl, K., Dengler, R. & Munte, T. F. (2009): Changes of resting state brain networks in amyotrophic lateral sclerosis. *Exp Neurol*, Vol.217, No.1, pp. 147-53.

Morcom, A. M. & Fletcher, P. C. (2007): Does the brain have a baseline? Why we should be resisting a rest. *Neuroimage*, Vol.37, No.4, pp. 1073-82.

Murphy, J. M., Henry, R. G., Langmore, S., Kramer, J. H., Miller, B. L. & Lomen-Hoerth, C. (2007): Continuum of frontal lobe impairment in amyotrophic lateral sclerosis. *Arch Neurol*, Vol.64, No.4, pp. 530-4.

Nakamura, T., Hillary, F. G. & Biswal, B. B. (2009): Resting network plasticity following brain injury. *PLoS One*, Vol.4, No.12, pp. e8220.

Ogawa, S., Lee, T. M., Kay, A. R. & Tank, D. W. (1990): Brain magnetic resonance imaging with contrast dependent on blood oxygenation. *Proc Natl Acad Sci U S A*, Vol.87, No.24, pp. 9868-72.

Ongur, D., Lundy, M., Greenhouse, I., Shinn, A. K., Menon, V., Cohen, B. M. & Renshaw, P. F. (2010): Default mode network abnormalities in bipolar disorder and schizophrenia. *Psychiatry Res*, Vol.183, No.1, pp. 59-68.

Paus, T. (2001): Primate anterior cingulate cortex: where motor control, drive and cognition interface. *Nat Rev Neurosci*, Vol.2, No.6, pp. 417-24.

Persson, J., Lustig, C., Nelson, J. K. & Reuter-Lorenz, P. A. (2007): Age differences in deactivation: a link to cognitive control? *J Cogn Neurosci*, Vol.19, No.6, pp. 1021-32.

Petrella, J. R., Sheldon, F. C., Prince, S. E., Calhoun, V. D. & Doraiswamy, P. M. (2011): Default mode network connectivity in stable vs progressive mild cognitive impairment. *Neurology*, Vol.76, No.6, pp. 511-7.

Raichle, M. E. (2010): Two views of brain function. *Trends Cogn Sci*, Vol.14, No.4, pp. 180-90.

Raichle, M. E., MacLeod, A. M., Snyder, A. Z., Powers, W. J., Gusnard, D. A. & Shulman, G. L. (2001): A default mode of brain function. *Proc Natl Acad Sci U S A*, Vol.98, No.2, pp. 676-82.

Rao, S. M., Leo, G. J., Bernardin, L. & Unverzagt, F. (1991): Cognitive dysfunction in multiple sclerosis. I. Frequency, patterns, and prediction. *Neurology*, Vol.41, No.5, pp. 685-91.

Repovs, G., Csernansky, J. G. & Barch, D. M. (2011): Brain Network Connectivity in Individuals with Schizophrenia and Their Siblings. *Biol Psychiatry*, Vol.69, No.10, pp. 967-973.

Rocca, M. A., Valsasina, P., Absinta, M., Riccitelli, G., Rodegher, M. E., Misci, P., Rossi, P., Falini, A., Comi, G. & Filippi, M. (2010): Default-mode network dysfunction and cognitive impairment in progressive MS. *Neurology*, Vol.74, No.16, pp. 1252-9.

Rocca, M. A., Valsasina, P., Pagani, E., Bianchi-Marzoli, S., Milesi, J., Falini, A., Comi, G. & Filippi, M. (2011): Extra-visual functional and structural connection abnormalities in Leber's hereditary optic neuropathy. *PLoS One*, Vol.6, No.2, pp. e17081.

Rombouts, S. A., Barkhof, F., Goekoop, R., Stam, C. J. & Scheltens, P. (2005): Altered resting state networks in mild cognitive impairment and mild Alzheimer's disease: an fMRI study. *Hum Brain Mapp*, Vol.26, No.4, pp. 231-9.

Roosendaal, S. D., Schoonheim, M. M., Hulst, H. E., Sanz-Arigita, E. J., Smith, S. M., Geurts, J. J. & Barkhof, F. (2010): Resting state networks change in clinically isolated syndrome. *Brain*, Vol.133, No.Pt 6, pp. 1612-21.

Rotarska-Jagiela, A., van de Ven, V., Oertel-Knochel, V., Uhlhaas, P. J., Vogeley, K. & Linden, D. E. (2010): Resting-state functional network correlates of psychotic symptoms in schizophrenia. *Schizophr Res*, Vol.117, No.1, pp. 21-30.

Rule, R. R., Schuff, N., Miller, R. G. & Weiner, M. W. (2010): Gray matter perfusion correlates with disease severity in ALS. *Neurology*, Vol.74, No.10, pp. 821-7.

Schopf, V., Windischberger, C., Robinson, S., Kasess, C. H., Fischmeister, F. P., Lanzenberger, R., Albrecht, J., Kleemann, A. M., Kopietz, R., Wiesmann, M. & Moser, E. (2011): Model-free fMRI group analysis using FENICA. *Neuroimage*, Vol.55, No.1, pp. 185-93.

Seifritz, E., Esposito, F., Hennel, F., Mustovic, H., Neuhoff, J. G., Bilecen, D., Tedeschi, G., Scheffler, K. & Di Salle, F. (2002): Spatiotemporal pattern of neural processing in the human auditory cortex. *Science*, Vol.297, No.5587, pp. 1706-8.

Shen, H., Wang, L., Liu, Y. & Hu, D. Discriminative analysis of resting-state functional connectivity patterns of schizophrenia using low dimensional embedding of fMRI. *Neuroimage*, Vol.49, No.4, pp. 3110-21.

Skudlarski, P., Jagannathan, K., Anderson, K., Stevens, M. C., Calhoun, V. D., Skudlarska, B. A. & Pearlson, G. Brain connectivity is not only lower but different in schizophrenia: a combined anatomical and functional approach. *Biol Psychiatry*, Vol.68, No.1, pp. 61-9.

Smith, A. M., Lewis, B. K., Ruttimann, U. E., Ye, F. Q., Sinnwell, T. M., Yang, Y., Duyn, J. H. & Frank, J. A. (1999): Investigation of low frequency drift in fMRI signal. *Neuroimage*, Vol.9, No.5, pp. 526-33.

Sorg, C., Riedl, V., Muhlau, M., Calhoun, V. D., Eichele, T., Laer, L., Drzezga, A., Forstl, H., Kurz, A., Zimmer, C. & Wohlschlager, A. M. (2007): Selective changes of resting-state networks in individuals at risk for Alzheimer's disease. *Proc Natl Acad Sci U S A*, Vol.104, No.47, pp. 18760-5.

Sorg, C., Riedl, V., Perneczky, R., Kurz, A. & Wohlschlager, A. M. (2009): Impact of Alzheimer's disease on the functional connectivity of spontaneous brain activity. *Curr Alzheimer Res*, Vol.6, No.6, pp. 541-53.

Supekar, K., Menon, V., Rubin, D., Musen, M. & Greicius, M. D. (2008): Network analysis of intrinsic functional brain connectivity in Alzheimer's disease. *PLoS Comput Biol*, Vol.4, No.6, pp. e1000100.

Svensen, M., Kruggel, F. & Benali, H. (2002): ICA of fMRI group study data. *Neuroimage*, Vol.16, No.3 Pt 1, pp. 551-63.

Tedeschi, G., Trojsi, F., Tessitore, A., Corbo, D., Sagnelli, A., Paccone, A., D'Ambrosio, A., Piccirillo, G., Cirillo, M., Cirillo, S., Monsurro, M. R. & Esposito, F. (2010): Interaction between aging and neurodegeneration in amyotrophic lateral sclerosis. *Neurobiol Aging*, Vol.pp.

Turner, B. J., Parkinson, N. J., Davies, K. E. & Talbot, K. (2009a): Survival motor neuron deficiency enhances progression in an amyotrophic lateral sclerosis mouse model. *Neurobiol Dis*, Vol.34, No.3, pp. 511-7.

Turner, M. R., Kiernan, M. C., Leigh, P. N. & Talbot, K. (2009b): Biomarkers in amyotrophic lateral sclerosis. *Lancet Neurol*, Vol.8, No.1, pp. 94-109.

van de Ven, V. G., Formisano, E., Prvulovic, D., Roeder, C. H. & Linden, D. E. (2004): Functional connectivity as revealed by spatial independent component analysis of fMRI measurements during rest. *Hum Brain Mapp*, Vol.22, No.3, pp. 165-78.

van den Heuvel, M., Mandl, R., Luigjes, J. & Hulshoff Pol, H. (2008): Microstructural organization of the cingulum tract and the level of default mode functional connectivity. *J Neurosci*, Vol.28, No.43, pp. 10844-51.

van den Heuvel, M. P. & Hulshoff Pol, H. E. Exploring the brain network: a review on resting-state fMRI functional connectivity. *Eur Neuropsychopharmacol*, Vol.20, No.8, pp. 519-34.

van den Heuvel, M. P., Mandl, R. C., Kahn, R. S. & Hulshoff Pol, H. E. (2009): Functionally linked resting-state networks reflect the underlying structural connectivity architecture of the human brain. *Hum Brain Mapp*, Vol.30, No.10, pp. 3127-41.

Varoquaux, G., Sadaghiani, S., Pinel, P., Kleinschmidt, A., Poline, J. B. & Thirion, B. (2010): A group model for stable multi-subject ICA on fMRI datasets. *Neuroimage*, Vol.51, No.1, pp. 288-99.

Vercelletto, M., Ronin, M., Huvet, M., Magne, C. & Feve, J. R. (1999): Frontal type dementia preceding amyotrophic lateral sclerosis: a neuropsychological and SPECT study of five clinical cases. *Eur J Neurol*, Vol.6, No.3, pp. 295-9.

Wang, K., Jiang, T., Yu, C., Tian, L., Li, J., Liu, Y., Zhou, Y., Xu, L., Song, M. & Li, K. (2008): Spontaneous activity associated with primary visual cortex: a resting-state FMRI study. *Cereb Cortex*, Vol.18, No.3, pp. 697-704.

Wang, K., Liang, M., Wang, L., Tian, L., Zhang, X., Li, K. & Jiang, T. (2007): Altered functional connectivity in early Alzheimer's disease: a resting-state fMRI study. *Hum Brain Mapp*, Vol.28, No.10, pp. 967-78.

Wang, L., Zang, Y., He, Y., Liang, M., Zhang, X., Tian, L., Wu, T., Jiang, T. & Li, K. (2006): Changes in hippocampal connectivity in the early stages of Alzheimer's disease: evidence from resting state fMRI. *Neuroimage*, Vol.31, No.2, pp. 496-504.

Wang, Z. & Peterson, B. S. (2008): Partner-matching for the automated identification of reproducible ICA components from fMRI datasets: algorithm and validation. *Hum Brain Mapp*, Vol.29, No.8, pp. 875-93.

Weissman, D. H., Roberts, K. C., Visscher, K. M. & Woldorff, M. G. (2006): The neural bases of momentary lapses in attention. *Nat Neurosci*, Vol.9, No.7, pp. 971-8.

Wishart, H. A., Saykin, A. J., McDonald, B. C., Mamourian, A. C., Flashman, L. A., Schuschu, K. R., Ryan, K. A., Fadul, C. E. & Kasper, L. H. (2004): Brain activation patterns associated with working memory in relapsing-remitting MS. *Neurology*, Vol.62, No.2, pp. 234-8.

Woodward, N. D., Rogers, B. & Heckers, S. (2011): Functional resting-state networks are differentially affected in schizophrenia. *Schizophr Res*, Vol.pp.

Zhang, H. Y., Wang, S. J., Liu, B., Ma, Z. L., Yang, M., Zhang, Z. J. & Teng, G. J. (2010): Resting brain connectivity: changes during the progress of Alzheimer disease. *Radiology*, Vol.256, No.2, pp. 598-606.

Zhang, H. Y., Wang, S. J., Xing, J., Liu, B., Ma, Z. L., Yang, M., Zhang, Z. J. & Teng, G. J. (2009): Detection of PCC functional connectivity characteristics in resting-state fMRI in mild Alzheimer's disease. *Behav Brain Res*, Vol.197, No.1, pp. 103-8.

Zhou, Y., Shu, N., Liu, Y., Song, M., Hao, Y., Liu, H., Yu, C., Liu, Z. & Jiang, T. (2008): Altered resting-state functional connectivity and anatomical connectivity of hippocampus in schizophrenia. *Schizophr Res*, Vol.100, No.1-3, pp. 120-32.

Zuo, X. N., Kelly, C., Adelstein, J. S., Klein, D. F., Castellanos, F. X. & Milham, M. P. (2010): Reliable intrinsic connectivity networks: test-retest evaluation using ICA and dual regression approach. *Neuroimage*, Vol.49, No.3, pp. 2163-77.

5

Neuro-Anatomical Overlap Between Language and Memory Functions in the Human Brain

Satoru Yokoyama
Tohoku University
Japan

1. Introduction

In the nineteenth century, two studies in aphasiology comprise a turning point for research of brain-language relationships: Broca, 1861 and Wernicke, 1874. Based on these two studies, it was claimed that Broca's area (i.e., the pars triangularis and pars opercularis of the left inferior frontal gyrus) and Wernicke's area (i.e., the posterior part of the left superior/middle temporal gyrus, but in some situations including a part of the inferior parietal lobule) were involved in language production and comprehension, respectively (Geschwind, 1970). Recently, due to the development of functional brain imaging techniques (e.g., PET and fMRI), normal brains have been measured to examine the neuro-cognitive architecture of language processing. In particular, both Broca's and Wernicke's areas have been shown to be responsible for several language functions, such as single word processing and sentence processing (Fig. 1).

However, these two important regions are also activated for working memory-related processes, at least, including executive functions and short term memory processes of linguistic information, and the processes of storage and access to long term memory of linguistic information. This memory system could be assumed essential for language comprehension. For example, in order to comprehend a word, we have to first identify a series of sounds or letters as a certain word and to access its semantic information from long term memory. For sentence comprehension, we have to tentatively memorize several words comprising the sentence to compute the syntactic and semantic structure of the sentence. For example, it is clear that if we do not tentatively memorize words comprising the sentence, we cannot comprehend the sentence, since we have to compute the syntactic/semantic information of the sentence by using these words. Hence, in order to understand a language expression, we need the involvement of both the short and long term memory systems. In previous studies, there were essentially two types of standpoints regarding the involvement of the memory system in language comprehension. The first is that of the „specialist", who assumes that the syntactic processing system of the language processing system exists in our brain and is independent from other congnitive functions. The second is that of the „generalist", who assumes that the syntactic processing system has neural substrates in common with other cognitive functions, mainly the working memory system.

In this chapter, recent neuroimaging studies of the neuro-cognitive architecture of single word and sentence processing will be briefly reviewed and the relationships between language and memory in the human brain will be discussed in the context of functional neuroimaging evidence.

Broca's area   Wernicke's area

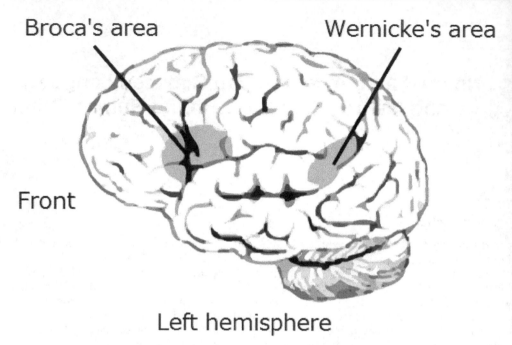

Front

Left hemisphere

Fig. 1. Broca's area and Wernicke's area.

2. Neural basis of language comprehension

2.1 Neural basis of single word processing

There is a wealth of evidence that auditory and visual word processing have at least partly independent neural bases, particularly in the early stages of stimulus processing. While these two processes have been reported to utilize different brain regions in the early stages of processing (i.e., modality-related processes and the processing of non-linguistic to linguistic information translation), a common word recognition system exists in the late stages of processing (i.e., phonological processing and semantic processing) (e.g., Chee et al., 1999; Booth et al., 2003). Chee et al. study used semantic concreteness judgment task, non-semantic syllable counting control task for auditory stimuli, and case size judgement control task for visual stimuli, while Booth et al. study used semantic relation judgment task and rhyming control task. Both studies reported that the left inferior frontal and middle temporal gyri were commonly activated for both auditory and visual word processing. In contrast, while visual word processing activated visual-related areas including the occipital lobe, the ventral part of inferior temporal gyrus, and the fusiform gyrus, auditory word processing activated auditory-related areas including the superior temporal gyri.

2.2 Phonological working memory involvement in single-word processing

It is known that phonological working memory is essential for processing words. It is assumed that the anterior part of the left inferior frontal gyrus (i.e., the pars triangularis of the inferior frontal gyrus/Brodomann area 45) and the left inferior parietal region (i.e., the supramarginal gyrus) comprise the verbal working memory circuit (for a recent meta-analysis see Vigneau et al., 2006). The former area is thought to be involved in articulatory rehearsal and the latter in phonological storage (e.g., Poldrack et al., 1999; Warburton et al., 1996; McGuire et al., 1996; Paulesu et al., 2000; Jessen et al., 1999; Zattore et al., 1996; Price et al., 1996). These two areas have often been reported to be active during single word processing (e.g., Hautzel et al., 2002; Jonides et al., 1998; Rypma et al., 1999; Cohen et al., 1997). The neuroimaging results are compatible with the working memory theory proposed by Baddeley, since the correlation between the sub-functions and locations of the involved brain regions reported in these neuroimaging studies is in line with the assumption of this model (e.g., Baddeley, 2003).

2.3 Lexico-semantic processing
The left inferior frontal region, the left lateral and ventral middle/inferior temporal regions, and the left inferior parietal region are activated during semantic processing tasks. It is still unclear whether the left inferior frontal region is actived by single word semantic processing per se. Demb et al. (1995) have reported that brain activity in this region is greater for more difficult semantic processing tasks than for corresponding less difficult semantic processing tasks. Similarly, the left inferior frontal region was modulated by the frequency of words (Fiebach et al., 2002). It is common knowledge that low frequency words are more difficult to process than high frequency ones. Hence, in single word semantic processing, there exists the possibility that modulation of the left inferior frontal region by word frequency is explained by access to lexico-semantic information stored in long term memory. In contrast, it has been claimed that only the orbital part of the left inferior frontal gyrus is associated with the processing of semantic information retrieval. Several meta-analysis results in particular have supported this claim (Fiez, 1997; Bookheimer, 2002; Binder et al., 2009). A meta-analysis (Vigneau et al., 2006) has also supported the report that the left parietal lobe contributes to semantic processing regardless of the difference between pictures and words (Vandenberghe et al., 1996).

While the temporal lobe plays a role in storing long term memory, the role of the left posterior part of superior/middle temporal gyri is still unclear. As evidence, most neuroimaging studies using comparisons between real word and pseudoword comprehension have reported that this region is more active for real word comprehension than for pseudoword comprehension (e.g., Pugh et al., 1996; Price et al., 1997; Friederici et al., 2000; Booth et al., 2002; Fiebach et al., 2002; Perani et al., 1999; Yokoyama et al., 2006b, and others). In contrast, Fiebach et al. (2002) showed that the left inferior frontal region is modulated by word frequency while the left posterior part of the middle temporal gyrus is not. Hence, at least the role of the left posterior part of the middle (and/or superior) temporal gyrus differs from that of the left inferior frontal region in lexico-semantic processing.

It has been made clear that the left inferior temporal region contributes to semantic processing. The inferior temporal region is commonly known to be involved in the storage or the long term memory of word information. Lesion studies have reported that damage to the temporal lobe cause category-related deficits (Kapur et al., 1994; Gitelman et al., 2001; Lambon Ralph et al., 2007; Noppeney et al., 2007; Warrington, 1975; Hodges et al., 1992, 1995; Mummery et al., 2000). Patients with anterior temporal damage show more difficulty processing the concept of living things than that of artifacts, while patients with posterior temporal and parietal damage show the opposite pattern (Warrington & Shallice, 1984; Warrington & McCarthy, 1987; Forde & Humphreys, 1999; Gainotti, 2000; Lambon Ralph et al., 2007; Warrington & McCarthy, 1987, 1994; Hillis & Caramazza, 1991). Functional brain imaging studies have replicated such results from lesion studies (Cappa et al., 1998; Moore & Price, 1999; Perani et al., 1999; Grossman et al., 2002; Kable et al., 2002; Tyler et al., 2003; Davis et al., 2004; Kable et al., 2005).

2.4 The role of sensorimotor areas on language comprehension

It has recently been reported that sensorimotor areas are active during language comprehension. Even in language or picture comprehension without sensorimotor input, sensorimotor areas are active (Pulvermuller, 1999; Malach et al., 2002; Gainotti, 2004; Kable et al., 2002; Grossmann et al., 2002; Hauk et al., 2004; Pulvermuller et al., 2005; Tettamanti et al., 2005; Kemmerer et al., 2008; Desai et al., 2009; Hwang et al., 2009). Hauk et al. (2004) reported that the silent reading of action words related to face, arm, and leg movements activates the motor areas related to the movement of the tongue, fingers, and feet. Such sensorimotor activation has also been found during sentence listening stimuli describing hand movements and visual events (Desai et al., 2010). According to sensorimotor theories, sensorimotor areas play a role in category-related long term memory through the encoding process of sensorimotor experiences (e.g., Martin, 2007). Hence, it has been assumed that concepts are wholly or partially organized by sensorimotor experience (Barsalou et al., 2003; Gallese & Lakoff, 2005; Pulvermmuller, 1999).

2.5 Grammatical category

Regarding grammatical category, the neural dissociation between nouns and verbs in the brain has been investigated by neuroimaging techniques. However, there exists some discrepancy at this time. In lesion studies, it has been reported that nouns and verbs are distinctly processed in the human brain (e.g., Bates et al., 1991; Miceli et al., 1988; Shapiro & Caramazza, 2003). In contrast, in neuroimaging studies, while several studies reported that different brain activations exist between noun and verb processing (Perani et al., 1999; Tyler et al., 2004; Yokoyama et al., 2006b), others find no difference between them (Tyler et al., 2001; Li et al., 2004). Based on the reported findings, several possibilities are proposed at this time. One possibility is that a cross-linguistic difference influences such discrepancy as the reported neuroimaging studies used different languages as stimuli (Yokoyama et al., 2006b). Still, despite the discrepancy among languages, the reported brain activations were located in the left inferior frontal gyrus and posterior superior/middle temporal gyrus. Hence, at least the word information related to grammatical category information, such as nouns and verbs, and is consistent with the hypothesis that long term memory of word information is stored in the temporal lobe.

2.6 Morphological processing of words

Regarding the morphological processing of words, one plausible hypothesis exists, namely that of „rule and memory" (Pinker, 1999; Ullman, 2001; 2004). However, actual neuroimaging results have not completely support this hypothesis. In this hypothesis, while rule-based morphological processing of words (e.g., "-ed" past tense form) would be processed as a procedural memory circuit in the left inferior frontal region and basal ganglia, words with irregular morphological changes would be stored in an independent form in the temporal lobe (Ullman, 2001; 2004). Since rule-based computation is reflected by task difficulty or task performance, this hypothesis is consistent with the above results in neuroimaging studies reporting that the left inferior frontal gyrus is related to task performance or working memory load. Also, since the temporal lobe plays a role in the storage of word information, this hypothesis is fully in line with the results of neuroimaging studies on the long term memory of semantic information, as described in section 2.3.

Additionally, Yokoyama et al. (2006b) showed partially supportive evidence that the left inferior frontal gyrus (and also the left premotor area) are active during the morphological processing of verbs. Yokoyama et al. (2009a) further showed that the developmental change of brain activity in L2 verb acquisition is observed, not in the temporal region which would be related to semantic memory, but in the inferior frontal gyrus which would be related to procedural memory. These results are in line with the above hypothesis. Also, fMRI results reported in Beretta et al. (2003) support the rule and memory hypothesis but show no clear dissociation in the brain activation between rule processing and memory processing of words. Hence, while supportive evidence at this time has been reported in several previous neuroimaging studies, it remains unclear whether the rule and computation hypothesis is correct or not.

2.7 Neural basis of sentence processing

One of the main issues regarding sentence processing in cognitive neuroscience is whether lexico-semantic and syntactic processing are dissociable or not in the human brain (e.g., Firederici et al., 2003). In particular, it is controversial what role Broca's area and the inferior frontal gyrus play in sentence processing. Some researchers have reported that the neural basis for the syntactic computation system overlaps that of workload related to working memory (e.g., Just et al., 1996), workload related to task performance (Love et al., 2006), the phonological working memory system (Rogalsky et al., 2009), the cognitive control system for resolving competition etc. (January et al., 2008; Yokoyama et al., 2009b), or other interpretation (e.g., Bornkessel et al., 2005). These overlapped brain regions basically include the left inferior frontal gyrus (Broca's area) and the posterior part of the left superior/middle temporal gyrus (Wernicke's area). The pars opercularis (Brodomann area 44) and pars triangularis (Brodomann area 45) of the inferior frontal gyrus, which are corresponding to Broca's area (Fig. 2), were commonly activated for lexico-semantic and syntactic processing in the most recent meta-analysis study (Vigneau et al., 2006).

In contrast, other studies have reported that the neural basis for syntactic processing of sentence comprehension is independent from other cognitive systems. Yet to claim such dissociation, we have to pay careful attention to other confounding factors and interpretations. For example, since the left dorsal prefrontal cortex, or middle frontal gyrus, was active for sentence comprehension independent of phonological short term memory load, this region is specific to sentence comprehension (Hashimoto & Sakai, 2002). However in Baddeley's working memory theory, the working memory system has a modality-free executive processing system and modality-dependent short term memory systems. To claim that the observed brain activation is independent from the working memory system, it is necessary to compare brain activities, not only between sentence comprehension and short term memory process, but also between sentence comprehension and the executive process. Indeed, in neuroimaging studies of executive process, the left dorsal prefrontal cortex was active (e.g., Eldreth et al., 2007). This region was close to the brain region observed in

Hashimoto and Sakai (2002). Contrastively, the left posterior part of the temporal region was specifically active for sentence reading independent of phonological short term memory (Cutting et al., 2006). However, it is unfortunate that only the sentence comprehension condition included verbs in this study and the phonological short term memory condition did not. The comprehension of verbs has been reported to activate the left posterior superior/middle temporal gyrus (Perani et al., 1999; Yokoyama et al., 2006b). Therefore, the comprehension of verbs would cause brain activation in the left posterior temporal region in the sentence comprehension condition in Cutting et al. (2006). Makuuchi et al. (2009) has reported that the pars opercularis of the inferior frontal gyrus is specifically active for syntactic computation regardless of syntactic difficulty. This study did not directly consider the executive process in working memory, similar to Hashimoto and Sakai (2002). Hence future studies are necessary to at least consider each aspect of the working memory system in order to propose that the neural substrate for sentence comprehension or its syntactic computation is independent from other cognitive processes, including the working memory system.

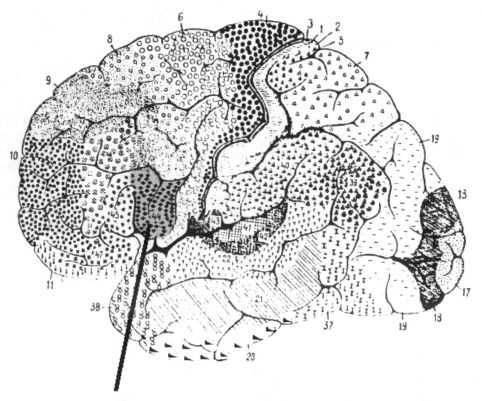

The pars opercularis of the inferior frontal gyrus

= Brodmann area 44

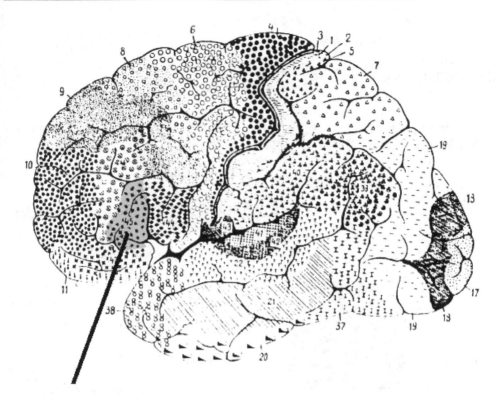

The pars triangularis of the inferior frontal gyrus

= Brodmann area 45

Fig. 2. The pars opercularis (Brodomann area 44) and pars triangularis (Brodmann area 45) of the inferior frontal gyrus.

Furthermore, in such previous neuroimaging studies, experimental stimuli using sentences with highly complex syntactic structures tended to be used to manipulate working memory load in the experimental design. In our daily lives we would not often use such complex sentences with long embedded clauses or relative clauses. Since such complex sentences are thought to be incomprehensible without intentional monitoring, additional intentional cognitive control or monitoring processes would affect brain activation compared to cases using simple sentences. It is necessary to test whether a hypothesis built using such complex sentences can be applicable to cases using simplex sentences or not.

3. Regional overlap between language comprehension and memory system

According to the above review, most sub-processes for language comprehension can be observed in the frontal, temporal, and parietal lobes (Fig. 3).

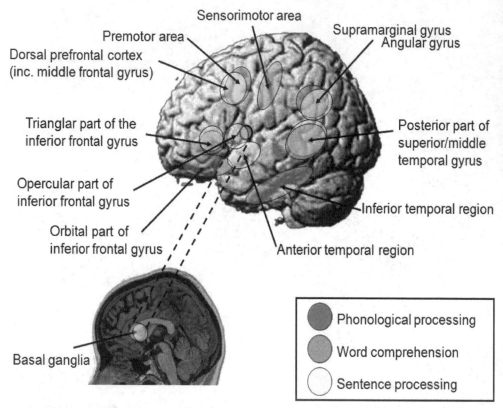

Fig. 3. Brain mapping of language function.

While different processing systems are utilized in the early stages of the language process (i.e., modality-related processes (i.e., visual and auditory input) and the processing of non-linguistic to linguistic information translation), a common word recognition system exists in the late stages of the process (i.e., phonological processing, semantic processing, and sentence processing). Findings suggest that the inferior frontal and inferior parietal regions are associated with working memory load and/or phonological processing to perform experimental tasks for single word processing. The left inferior frontal region is malso suggested to be associated with intended acts, planning, and/or cognitive control to resolve competition, which have common processes with other cognitive functions (Owen et al., 2005; January et al., 2008; Yokoyama et al., 2009b). Thought to be involved in the semantic processing of words are the orbito-frontal and parietal "retrieval" system, and the temporal "storage" system (i.e., long term memory). Also, sensorimotor areas have been shown to be activated during word and sentence comprehension tasks. Their activation may be due to sensorimotor experiences which induce the storage of long term memories in the sensorimotor areas. While sentence comprehension activates the left inferior frontal and dorsal prefrontal cortex, these activations are thought to be based on phonological working memory and executive functions. Taken together, language comprehension would be supported by the neural substrates of the working memory and

long term memory systems, as well as other cognitive function systems (e.g., intended act, planning, and cognitive control).
While the above mentioned results reported in previous studies at least indicate that a common neural substrate supports language comprehension and memory-related processes which are functionally similar, observation of the overlapped activation between other cognitive processes might not necessarily indicate a functional overlapping of these processes. Even if both language comprehension and memory processes utilize the same brain region, the roles of the brain region are thought to be different between them. Hence, the simple subtraction analysis used in previous neuroimaging studies may not be enough to resolve this issue and functional and/or effective connectivity analysis methods might be useful or necessary in future studies. Such methods would be able to test whether a commonly activated area is connected with different regions between different conditions. If this is the case, it would mean that both language comprehension and other cognitive processes utilize common neural substrates, though the roles of the commonly activated brain regions would be different between them.

4. Conclusion

Through a review of the literature we find that, since the neural basis of language comprehension overlaps that of other cognitive systems, mainly the memory system regionwise, most previous neuroimaging studies support the „generalist" view. However, it is to be noted that the overlaps of the neural substrate may not indicate a functional overlap since there exists a possibility that, while a brain region is commonly activated for both processes, the brain region plays different roles between them. In future studies, to clarify which brain region or cognitive process is common for language comprehension and other cognitive systems, and which is different between them, it will be necessary to develop a new experimental paradigm and also a new data analysis method, such as the functional/effective connectivity and multi-voxel pattern analysis. These methods should then be applied to language comprehension studies. Additionally, it will be necessary to consider the relationship between language and memory functions in language acquisition (i.e., Yokoyama et al., 2006a; 2009a), since, at this time, findings in neuroimaging studies regarding this issue are very few. Examination of whether or not and how semantic memory is related to the acquisition of lexico-semantic information, as well as whether or not and how procedural memory is responsible for proficienct gramatical processes such as morphological processing and sentence structure computation, might also be necessary.

5. References

Baddeley, A.D. (2003). Working memory: Looking back and looking forward. *Nature Reviews: Neuroscience*, Vol. 4, pp.829-839

Barsalou L.W.; Kyle Simmons W.; Barbey A.K. & Wilson C.D. (2003). Grounding conceptual knowledge in modality-specific systems. *Trends in Cognitive Sciences*, Vol. 7 No. 2, pp. 84-91.

Bates, E.; Chen, S.; Tzeng, O.; Li, P.& Opie, M. (1991). The noun–verb problem in Chinese aphasia. *Brain and Language*, Vol. 41, pp.203-233.

Beretta, A.; Campbell, C.; Carr, T.H.; Huang, J.; Schmitt, LM.; Christianson, K. & Cao, Y. (2003). An ER-fMRI investigation of morphological inflection in German reveals that the brain makes a distinction between regular and irregular forms. *Brain and Language*, pp.8567–8592.

Binder, J.R.; Desai, R.H.; Graves, W.W. & Conant, LL. (2009). Where is the semantic system? A critical review and meta-analysis of 120 functional neuroimaging studies. *Cerebral cortex*, Vol. 19, pp.2767-2796.

Bookheimer, S. (2002). Functional MRI of language: New approaches to understanding the cortical organization of semantic processing. *Annual Review of Neuroscience*, Vol. 25, pp. 151-188.

Bornkessel, I.; Zysset, S.; Friederici, A.D.; von Cramon, D.Y. & Schlesewsky, M. (2005). Who did what to whom? The neural basis of argument hierarchies during language comprehension. *Neuroimage*, Vol. 26, pp. 221-233.

Broca, P. (1861). Remarques sur le siége de la faculté du langage articulé, suivies d'une observation d'aphémie (perte de la parole), *Bulletin de la Société Anatomique de Paris*. Vol. 6, pp. 330–357.

Cappa, S.F.; Perani, D.; Schnur, T.; Tettamanti, M. & Fazio F. (1998). The effects of semantic category and knowledge type on lexical-semantic access: a PET study. *Neuroimage*. Vol. 8, No.4: pp.350-359.

Chee, M.W.; Caplan, D.; Soon,C.S.; Sriram, N.; Tan, E.W.; Thiel, T. & Weekes B. (1999). P rocessing of visually presented sentences in Mandarin and English studied with fMRI. *Neuron*, Vol. 23 No.1: pp.127-37.

Cohen, LG.; Celnik, P.; Pascual-Leone, A.; Corwell, B.; Falz, L.; Dambrosia, J.; Honda, M.; Sadato, N.; Gerloff, C.; Catala MD. & Hallett M. (1997). Functional relevance of cross-modal plasticity in blind humans. *Nature*, Vol. 389, pp.180-183.

Cutting, LE.; Clements, AM.; Courtney, S.; Rimrodt, SL.; Schafer, JG.; Bisesi, J.; Pekar, JJ. & Pugh, KR. (2006). Differential components of sentence comprehension: Beyond single word reading and memory, *NeuroImage*, Vol. 29, pp.429-438.

Davis, M.H.; Meunier, F. & Marslen–Wilson, W.D. (2004). Neural responses to morphological, syntactic, and semantic properties of single words: An fMRI study. *Brain and Language*, Vol. 89, pp.439–449.

Demb, J.B.; Desmond, J.E.; Wagner, A.D.; Vaidya, C.J.; Glover, G.H. & Gabrieli, J.D.E. (1995). Semantic encoding and retrieval in the left inferior prefrontal cortex: a functional MRI study of task difficulty and process specificity. *Journal of Neuroscience*, Vol. 15, pp.5870- 5878.

Desai, R.H.; Binder, J.R.; Conant L.L. & Seidenberg M.S. (2010). Activation of sensory-motor areas in sentence comprehension. *Cerebral Cortex*. Vol. 20, pp.468-78.

Eldreth, DA.; Patterson, MD.; Porcelli, AJ.; Biswal, BB.; Rebbechi, D. & Rypma, B.(2006) Evidence for multiple manipulation processes in prefrontal cortex. *Brain Res*. Vol. 1123, No.1, pp.145-56.

Fiebach, C.J.; Friederici, A.D.; Müller, K.von. & Cramon, D.Y. (2002). fMRI evidence for dual routes to the mental lexicon in visual word recognition. *Journal of Cognitive Neuroscience*, Vol. 14, pp.11-23.

Fiez, JA. (1997). Phonology, semantics, and the role of the left inferior prefrontal cortex. *Human Brain Mapping*, Vol. 5, pp.79-83.

Forde, E.; M. E. & Humphreys, G. W. (1999).Category-specific recognition impairments: A review of important case studies and influential theories. *Aphasiology*, Vol. 13, pp.169–193.

Friederici, A. D.; Opitz, B. & von Cramon, D. Y. (2000). Segregating semantic and syntactic aspects of processing in the human brain: An fMRI investigation of different word types. *Cerebral Cortex*, Vol. 10, pp.698–705.

Friederici, A.D.; Ruschemeyer, S.A.; Hahne, A. & Fiebach, C.J. (2003). The role of the left inferior frontal and superior temporal cortex in sentence comprehension: localizing syntactic and semantic processing. *Cerebral Cortex*, Vol. 13, pp. 170–177.

Gainotti G. (2000).What the locus of brain lesion tells us about the nature of the cognitive defect underlying category-specific disorders: a review. *Cortex*, Vol. 36 No.4, pp.539-559.

Gainotti G.(2004).A metanalysis of impaired and spared naming for different categories of knowledge in patients with a visuo-verbal disconnection. *Neuropsychologia*, Vol. 42, No.3, pp.299-319.

Gallese, V. & Lakoff, G. (2005). The Brain's Concepts: The Role of the Sensory-Motor System in Reason and Language. *Cognitive Neuropsychology*, Vol. 22, pp.455-479.

Geschwind, N. (1970). The organization of language and the brain, *Science*, Vol. 170, No.961, pp.940–944.

Gitelman, DR.; Ashburner, J.; Friston, KJ.; Tyler, LK. & Price, CJ.(2001) Voxel-based morphometry of herpes simplex encephalitis. *Neuroimage*, Vol. 13, No.4, pp.623- 631.

Grossman, M.; Smith, E.E.; Koenig, P.; Glosser, G.; De Vita, C. & Moore, P. (2002). The neural basis for categorization in semantic memory. *Neuroimage*, Vol. 17, pp.1549-1561.

Hashimoto, R. & Sakai, K.L. (2002) Specialization in the left prefrontal cortex for sentence comprehension, *Neuron*, Vol. 35, pp.589-597.

Hauk, O.; Johnsrude, I. & Pulvermüller, F. (2004). Somatotopic representation of action words in human motor and premotor cortex. *Neuron*, Vol. 41, pp.301-307.

Hautzel, H.; Mottaghy, FM.; Schmidt, D.; Zemb, M.; Shah, NJ.; Muller-Gartner, HW. & Krause BJ. (2002). Topographic segregation and convergence of verbal, object, shape and spatial working memory in humans. *Neuroscience Letters*, Vol. 323, pp.156-160.

Hillis, A.E. & Caramazza, A. (1991). Category-specific naming and comprehension impairment: a double dissociation. *Brain*, Vol. 14, No.5, pp.2081-94.

Hodges, J.R.; Patterson, K.; Oxbury, S. & Funnell, E. (1992). Semantic dementia. Progressive fluent aphasia with temporal lobe atrophy. *Brain*, Vol. 115, No. 6, pp.1783-806.

Hodges, J.R.; Graham, N. & Patterson K. (1995). Charting the progression in semantic dementia: implications for the organisation of semantic memory. *Memory*. - Vol. 3, No. 34, pp.463-95.

Hwang, K.; Palmer, ED.; Basho, S.; Zadra, JR. & Müller, RA. (2009). Category-specific activations during word generation reflect experiential sensorimotor modalities. *Neuroimage*, Vol. 48, No. 4, pp.717-725.

January, D.; Trueswell. JC. & Thompson-Schill, SL. (2009). Co-localization of stroop and syntactic ambiguity resolution in Broca's area: implications for the neural basis of sentence processing. *Journal of Cognitive Neuroscience*, Vol. 21, pp.2434-2444.

Jessen, F.; Erb, M.; Klose, U.; Lotz, M.; Grodd, W. & Heun, R. (1999). Activation of human language processing brain regions after the presentation of random letter strings demonstrated with eventrelated functional magnetic resonance imaging. *Neuroscience Letters*, Vol. 270, pp.13-16.

Jonides, J.; Smith, EE.; Marshuetz, C.; Koeppe, RA. & Reuter-Lorenz, PA.; (1998). Inhibition in verbal working memory revealed by brain activation. *Proceedings of the National Academy of Science of the United States of America*, Vol. 95, pp. 8410- 8413.

Just, M.A.; Carpenter, P.A.; Keller, T.A.; Eddy, W.F. & Thulborn, K.R. (1996). Brain activation modulated by sentence comprehension. *Science*, Vol. 274, pp.114-116.

Kable, JW.; Lease-Spellmeyer, J. & Chatterjee, A. (2002). Neural substrates for action event knowledge. *Journal of Cognitive Neuroscience*, Vol. 14, pp. 795-805.

Kable, JW.; Kan, IP.; Wilson, A.; Thompson-Schill, SL. & Chatterjee, A.(2005). Conceptual representations of action in the lateral temporal cortex. *J Cogn Neurosci.* Vol. 17, No. 12, pp.1855-1870.

Kapur, S.; Rose, R.; Liddle, PF.; Zipursky, RB.; Brown, GM.; Stuss, D.; Houle, S. & Tulving E. (1994) The role of the left prefrontal cortex in verbal processing: semantic processing or willed action? *Neuroreport*, Vol. 5, No. 16, pp.2193-2196.

Kemmerer, D.; Gonzalez-Castillo, J.; Talavage, T.; Patterson, S. & Wiley, C. (2008) Neuroanatomical distribution of five semantic components of verbs: Evidence from fMRI. *Brain and Language*, Vol. 107, pp.16-43.

Lambon Ralph, M.A.; Lowe, C. & Rogers, T.T. (2007) Neural basis of category-specific semantic deficits for living things: evidence from semantic dementia, *HSVE and a neural Brain*, Vol. 130, No. 4, pp.1127-1137.

Li, P.; Jin, Z. & Tan, LH. (2004). Neural representations of nouns and verbs in Chinese: an fMRI study. *NeuroImage*, Vol. 21, pp.1533-1541.

Love, T.; Haist, F.; Nicol. J. & Swinney, D. (2006). A functional neuroimaging investigation of the roles of structural complexity and task-demand during auditory sentence processing. *Cortex*, Vol. 42, pp.577-590

Makuuchi, M.; Bahlmann, J.; Anwander, A. & Friederici, AD. (2009). Segregating the core computational faculty of human language from working memory. *PNAS*, Vol. 106, pp.8362-8367.

Malach, R.; Levy, I. & Hasson, U. (2002). The topography of high-order human object areas. *Trends in Cognitive Science*, Vol. 6, pp.176-184.

Martin, R.C. (2007). Semantic short-term memory, language processing, and inhibition. In A. S. Meyer, L. R. Wheeldon, and A. Knott (Eds.), *Automaticity and control in language processing*, pp.161-191, Psychology Press.

McGuire, P.K.; Silbersweig, DA.; Murray, RM.; David, AS.; Frackowiak, RSJ. & Frith, CD. (1996). Functional anatomy of inner speech and auditory verbal imagery. *Psychological Medicine*, Vol. 26, pp.29-38.

Miceli, G., Silveri, C., Nocentini, U., & Caramazza, A., (1988). Patterns of dissociation in c omprehension and production of nouns and verbs. *Aphasiology*, Vol. 2, pp.351-358.

Moore, CJ. & Price, CJ. (1999). Three distinct ventral occipitotemporal regions for reading and object naming. *Neuroimage*, Vol. 10, No. 2, pp.181-92.

Moore, CJ. & Price, Cj. 1999). A functional neuroimaging study of the variables that generate category-specific object processing differences. *Brain*, Vol. 122, No. 5, pp.943-62.

Mummery, C.J.; Patterson, K.; Price, C.J.; Ashburner, J.; Frackowiak, R.S. & Hodges, J.R. (2000) A voxel-based morphometry study of semantic dementia: relationship between temporal lobe atrophy and semantic memory. *Ann Neurol*, Vol. 47, No. 1, pp.36-45.

Noppeney, U.; Patterson, K.; Tyler, L.K.; Moss, H.; Stamatakis, E.A.; Bright, P.; Mummery, C. & Price, C.J. (2007). Temporal lobe lesions and semantic impairment: a comparison of herpes simplex virus encephalitis and semantic dementia. *Brain*, Vol. 130, No, 4 pp.138-47.

Owen, A.M.; McMillan, K.M.: Laird, A.R. & Bullmore, E. (2005). N-back working memory paradigm: a meta-analysis of normative functional neuroimaging studies. *Hum. Brain Mapp*, Vol. 25, pp.46– 59.

Paulesu, E.; McCrory, E.; Fazio, F.; Menoncello, L.; Brunswick, N.; Cappa, S.F.; Cotelli, M.; Cossu, G.; Corte, F.; Lorusso, M.; Pesenti, S.; Gallagher, A.; Perani, D.; Price, C.J.; Frith. & Frith, CD. (2000). A cultural effect on brain function. *Nature Neuroscience*, Vol. 3, pp.91-96.

Perani, D.; Cappa, SF.; Schnur, T.; Tettamanti, M.; Collina, S.; Rosa, M.M. & Fazio, F. (1999). The neural correlates of verb and noun processing: a PET study. *Brain*, Vol. 122, pp.2337- 2344.

Perani, D.; Schnur, T.; Tettamanti, M.; Gorno-Tempini, M.; Cappa, S. & Fazio, F. (1999). Word and picture matching: a PET study of semantic category effects. *Neuropsychologia*, Vol. 37, No. 3, pp.293-306.

Pinker, S. (1999). Words and Rules. *Basic Books.*

Poldrack, RA.; Wagner, AD.; Prull, MW.; Desmond, JE.; Glover, GH. & Gabrieli, JD. (1999). Functional specialization for semantic and phonological processing in the left inferior prefrontal cortex. *Neuroimage*, Vol. 10, pp.15-35.

Price, C.J.; Wise, R.J. & Frackowiak, R.S. (1996). Demonstrating the implicit processing of visually presented words and pseudowords. *Cerebral Cortex*, Vol. 6, pp.62-70.

Price, C. J.; Moore, C. J.; Humphreys, G. W. & Wise, R. J. S. (1997). Segregating semantic from phonological processes during reading. *Journal of Cognitive Neuroscience*, Vol. 9, pp.727–733.

Pugh, K. R.; Shaywitz, B. A.; Shaywitz, S. E.; Constable, R. T.; Skudlarski, P.; Fulbright, R. K.; Bronen, R. A.; Shankweiler, D. P.; Katz, L.; Fletcher, J. M. & Gore, J. C. (1996). Cerebral organization of component processes in reading. *Brain*, Vol. 119, pp.1221– 1238.

Pulvermüller, F. (1999) Words in the brain's language.Behav *Brain Sci*, Vol. 22, No. 2, pp.253-79.

Pulvermüller, F.; Hauk, O.; Nikulin, VV. & Ilmoniemi, RJ. (2005). Functional links between motor and language systems. *European Journal of Neuroscience*, Vol. 21, pp.793-797.

Rogalsky, C. & Hickok, G. (2009). Selective attention to semantic and syntactic features modulates sentence processing networks in anterior temporal cortex. *Cerebral Cortex*, Vol. 19, No. 4, pp.786-796.

Rypma, B.; Prabhakaran, V.; Desmond, J.E.; Glover, G.H. & Gabrieli, J.D. (1999). Load-dependent roles of frontal brain regions in the maintenance of working memory. *NeuroImage*, Vol. 9, pp.216-226.

Shapiro, K. & Caramazza, A.,(2003). Grammatical processing of nouns and verbs in the left frontal cortex. *Neuropsychologia*, Vol. 41, pp.1189-1198.

Tettamanti, M.; Moro, A.; Messa, C.; Moresco, R.M.; Rizzo, G.; Carpinelli, A.; Matarrese, M.; Fazio, F. & Perani, D. (2005). Basal ganglia and language: phonology modulates dopaminergic release. *NeuroReport*, Vol. 16, pp.397-401.

Tyler, L.K.; Russell, R.; Fadili, J. & Moss, HE. (2001). The neural representation of nouns and verbs: PET studies. *Brain*, Vol. 124, pp.1619-1634.

Tyler, L.K.; Bright, P.; Fletcher, P. & Stamatakis, E.A. (2004). Neural processing of nouns and verbs: the role of inflectional morphology. *Neuropsychologia,* Vol. 42, pp.512-523.

Tyler, L.K.; Stamatakis, E.A.; Dick, E.; Bright, P.; Fletcher, P. & Moss, H. (2003). Objects and their actions : evidence for a neurally distributed semantic system. *Neuroimage,* Vol. 18, No. 2, pp.542-57.

Ullman, MT. (2001). The declarative/procedural model of lexicon and grammar. *Journal of Psycholinguistic Research,* Vol. 30, pp.37-69.

Ullman, MT. (2004). Contributions of memory circuits to language: the declarative/procedural model. *Cognition,* Vol. 92, pp.231-70.

Vandenberghe, R.; Price, CJ.; Wise, R.; Josephs, O. & Frackowiak, RS. (1996). Functional anatomy of a common semantic system for words and pictures. *Nature,* Vol. 383, pp. 254-256.

Vigneau, M.; Beaucousin, V.; Herve, PY.; Duffau, H.; Crivello, F.; Houde, O.; Mazoyer, B. & - TzourioMazoyer, N. (2006). Meta-analyzing left hemisphere language areas: phonology, semantics, and sentence processing. *Neuroimage,* Vol. 30, pp.1414-1432.

Warburton, EA.; Wise, RJS.; Price, CJ.; Weiller, C.; Hadar, U.; Ramsay, S. & Frackowiak, RSJ. (1996). Noun and verb retrieval by normal subjects. Studies with PET. *Brain,* Vol. 119, pp.159-179.

Warrington, E.K. & McCarthy, R.A. (1987). Categories of knowledge. Further fractionations and an attempted integration. *Brain,* Vol. 110, No. 5, pp.1273-96.

Warrington, E.K. (1984) Shallice T. Category specific semantic impairments. *Brain,* Vol. 107 No. 3, pp.829-54.

Warrington, E.K. (1975). The selective impairment of semantic memory. *Q J Exp Psychol,* Vol. 27, No. 4, pp.635-57.

Warrington, E.K. & McCarthy, R.A.(1987). Categories of knowledge. Further fractionations and an attempted integration. *Brain,* Vol. 110, No. 5, pp.1273-1296.

Warrington, E.K. & McCarthy, R.A. (1994). Multiple meaning systems in the brain: a case for visual semantics. *Neuropsychologia,* Vol. 32, No. 12, pp.1465-1473.

Wernicke, C. (1874). Der aphasische Symptomencomplex, *Cohn & Weigert, Breslau.*

Yokoyama, S.; Miyamoto, T.; Riera, J.; Kim, J.; Akitsuki, Y.; Iwata, K.; Yoshimoto, K.; Horie, K.; Sato, S. & Kawashima, R. (2006a). Cortical mechanisms involved in the processing of verbs: An fMRI study. *Journal of Cognitive Neuroscience,* Vol. 18, No. 8, pp. 1304-1313.

Yokoyama, S.; Okamoto, H.; Miyamoto, T.; Yoshimoto, K.; Kim, J.; Iwata, K.; Jeong, H.; Uchida, S.; Ikuta, N.; Sassa, Y.; Nakamura, W.; Horie, K.; Sato, S. & Kawashima R. (2006b). Cortical activation in the processing of passive sentences in L1 and L2: An fMRI study. *Neuroimage,* Vol 30, pp. 570-579.

Yokoyama, S.; Miyamoto, T.; Kim, J.; Uchida, S.; Yoshimoto, K. & Kawashima, R. (2009a). Learning effect of L2 words in non-fluent second language learners: an fMRI study. *Second Languages: Teaching, Learning and Assessment.* pp.147-156.

Yokoyama, S.; Yoshimoto, K.; Miyamoto, T. & Kawashima, R. (2009b). Neuro-physiological evidence of linguistic empathy processing in the human brain: a functional magnetic resonance imaging study. *Journal of Neurolinguistics,* Vol. 22, pp. 605-615.

Zatorre, R.J.; Halpern, A.R.; Perry, D.W.; Meyer, E. & Evans, E.C. (1996). Hearing in the mind's ear: A PET investigation of musical imagery and perception. *Journal of Cognitive Neuroscience,* Vol. 8, pp.29-46.

6

Images of the Cognitive Brain Across Age and Culture

Joshua Goh[1] and Chih-Mao Huang[2]
[1]National Institute on Aging, Baltimore, MD
[2]University of Illinois, Urbana-Champaign, IL
USA

1. Introduction

While structural and functional characteristics of the brain are largely similar across individuals, there is also evidence that much neural heterogeneity, both structural and functional, is present between different groups of people. For example, some individuals have greater regional brain volumes and thicknesses than others, and neural activity in response to the same stimuli varies across different individuals as well. Moreover, neural structure and function are temporally dynamic, showing changes across the human lifespan. Understanding how such neural heterogeneity arises between different individuals over the human lifespan is important for uncovering factors that influence developmental trajectories from adulthood to advanced age. In this article, we consider two general sources that contribute to neural heterogeneity over the adult lifespan – age-related biological changes and culture-related differences in external experience.

Over the human lifespan, biological processes related to brain structural integrity and neurobiological function change from adulthood to advanced aging (Goh, 2011; Goh & Park, 2009a; Park & Goh, 2009; Park & Reuter-Lorenz, 2009). In brief, aging has been associated with shrinkage of gray matter volume and thickness, reductions in white matter integrity, reductions in neurogenesis, and dysregulation of neuromodulatory mechanisms such as neurotransmitter action and synaptic communication. These age-related neurobiological changes have been associated with age-related changes in cognitive processing that is generally characterized by lower performance in tests of cognitive flexibility, fidelity, and speed in older adults compared to younger adults. Functionally, aging is associated with a decrease in the selectivity of brain responses to different types of stimuli as well as an increase in engagement of frontal regions. Importantly, it has been suggested that because age-related neurobiological changes tend to level off individual differences, neural differences between older adult individuals may be reduced compared to younger adult individuals (Baltes & Lindenberger, 1997; Park & Gutchess, 2002; Park et al., 1999; Park et al., 2004; Park & Gutchess, 2006). Thus, along with lower cognitive behavioral performance, aging may also be associated with greater, albeit compromised, similarity in brain structure and function across individuals.

Over the lifespan as well, individuals undergo different life experiences such as culturally different social and cognitive environments that emphasize dissociable ways of processing information (Nisbett, 2003; Nisbett & Masuda, 2003; Nisbett et al., 2001). For example,

Western culture has been associated with an emphasis on independence and individualism as important societal values. In addition, studies have shown that these values may bias Westerners towards a more analytic cognitive processing style, reflected as greater attention to objects and the features associated with an object. In contrast, East Asian culture tends to emphasize societal interdependence and collectivism, which are reflected in a bias towards a more holistic style of cognitive processing, involving greater attention to contextual relationships between different objects. Importantly, neuroimaging studies have shown that there are neural differences between Western and East Asian samples that are associated with these culture-related differences in individualistic-collectivistic values and analytic-holistic cognitive processing biases, respectively (Goh & Park, 2009b; Han & Northoff, 2008; Park & Huang, 2010). These neuroimaging findings suggest that culture-related differences in external experience may result in dissociable neural structural and functional development over the lifespan.

A key question that arises when considering the influences of age and culture on the brain is how they interact with each other over the human lifespan (Park & Gutchess, 2002; Park et al., 1999; Park & Gutchess, 2006). Three possible cases arise with respect to this interaction between age and culture. First, culture-related neural differences across individuals may accentuate with increasing age. With increasing age, and assuming that individuals remain in the same cultural environment, individuals gain greater experience in their cultural environment. Such prolonged cultural exposure may result in more engrained psychological biases and also increasingly divergent expression of neural structural and functional development between different cultural groups. Second, culture-related neural differences, once attained, may remain at the same level throughout the lifespan. This case may arise because external cultural factors reach an asymptotic level of influence on neurocognitive processing, such that further experience does not increase the biases. This cap on the influence of external experience may be necessary to maintain a homeostatic level of neural processing important for adaptive function in the environment. For example, it would be detrimental for Westerners to become so completely attentive to objects and lose all attention to contextual information (and vice versa for East Asians) the more experience they accrue in their analytic processing style. In addition, the maintenance of cultural neural differences over the lifespan may also arise because neurobiological effects of age in reducing individual neural differences dampen the diverging effects of cultural experiences. Third, culture-related neural differences may be reduced with increasing age. It is possible that age-related neurobiological changes impact all individuals to such a degree that differences in brain structure and function across older individuals is diminished relative to younger adults. Overall, these first two cases of age by culture interactions (or lack thereof) suggest that the neurobiological effects of age do not completely diminish individual differences in brain structure and function that arise from external experience, at least those associated with cultural influences. In contrast, the third case of an attenuation of culture-related neural differences with aging would suggest that the neurobiological effects of age exert a stronger influence on brain structure and function than external experiences related to culture.

To characterize how age and culture influence brain structure and function, this article reviews recent neuroimaging studies from both these fields, and considers the evidence for the above three cases of interaction between age and culture. In the following section, we provide an overview of neuroimaging findings pertaining to cognitive aging. We show that, due to changes in neurobiological structure and function, aging is generally associated with a reduction in the distinctiveness of neurocognitive representations as well as increases in the neural effort involved in cognitive processing perhaps to compensate for the age-related declines. Next, we provide an overview of findings pertaining to cultural differences in cognition. We cover the evidence for cultural differences in behavior and functional brain responses related to perceptual processing and attention that are consistent with an analytic-holistic dichotomy in processing styles between Westerners and East Asians. We then consider some findings in children and older adults that relate to the development of cultural biases over the lifespan. These studies are few, but they provide an initial platform for understanding how neurobiological changes with aging and culture-related external experiences interact in the brain. Finally, we evaluate some important methodological issues that limit the extent to which current data can be interpreted and applied to other samples.

Overall, the findings reviewed below will show that culture-related behavioral and neural differences are quite evident and seem to be present from a very young age during childhood. Moreover, these culture-related neural differences appear to be present even in older adulthood. Thus, the evidence suggests that aging does not disproportionately diminish the influence of experience on neural processing in the brain, at least for those sensitive to culture-related experiences.

2. Age-related functional imaging findings

There is a wealth of literature that documents age-related changes in fundamental cognitive processes across the lifespan (Park et al., 2002). The speed at which information is processed (Salthouse, 1996), the capacity of working memory (Park et al., 1996; Park et al., 2002), the ability to selectively attend to relevant information (Hasher & Zacks, 1988), and the efficiency of sentence processing (Wlotko et al., 2010) - all of these behavioral measurements of cognitive functions show age-related declines in many older adults (Figure 1). At the same time, studies have shown age-related reductions in gray matter regional brain volumes and thickness (Fjell et al., 2009; Raz et al., 2005; Raz & Rodrigue, 2006; Salat et al.,

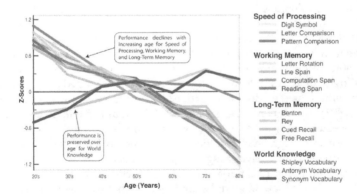

Fig. 1. Age-related cognitive changes in fluid and crystallized abilities in normal aging. Cross-sectional aging data show gradual age-related declines on the cognitive mechanisms of speed processing, working memory and long-term memory, beginning in young adulthood. But verbal-crystallized knowledge is protected from age differences. Copyright © 2002 by the American Psychological Association. Adapted with permission from Park et al. (2002). Models of visuospatial and verbal memory across the adult life span. *Psychology and Aging*, 17(2), 299-320.

2004), reductions in white matter integrity (Davis et al., 2009; Head et al., 2004; Kennedy & Raz, 2009a, 2009b), slower rates of neurogenesis and proliferation of new neuron (Kempermann & Gage, 1999; Kempermann et al., 2002; Kempermann et al., 1998), and dysregulation of neurotransmitter and synaptic action (Burke & Barnes, 2006; Burke & Barnes, 2010; Kaasinen et al., 2000; Li & Sikström, 2002), that may be underlying bases for cognitive declines observed in older adults (Goh, 2011; Goh & Park, 2009a; Greenwood, 2007; Park & Goh, 2009; Park & Reuter-Lorenz, 2009;   Reuter-Lorenz & Park, 2010). However, despite such universal age-related declines in neurobiology and cognition, cognitive aging studies using functional magnetic resonance imaging (fMRI) and positron emission tomography (PET) have revealed a more mixed picture. These studies, which we now review, show that the functional brain ages in a dynamic way, declining in some respects but maintaining the ability to engage adaptive neural functions even in advanced age (Dennis & Cabeza, 2008; Park & Reuter-Lorenz, 2009).

2.1 Reduced distinctiveness of cognitive representations
Studies have shown that young adults have a high degree of functional specialization in the ventral visual cortex for different categories of visual stimuli (for review, see Grill-Spector & Malach, 2004; Grill-Spector et al., 2008; Spiridon & Kanwisher, 2002). Briefly, the ventral visual cortex is a broad region encompassing the infero-medio-temporal and occipital regions that are specialized for processing the identity of objects—the "what" pathway (Mishkin et al., 1983), with many structures within this region characterized by a high specificity of neural responses. These functionally distinct subregions that respond selectively to categories of visual input include (1) the "fusiform face area (FFA)" within the fusiform gyrus that is specialized to process faces but not other categories of stimuli (Kanwisher et al., 1997), (2) the "parahippocampal place area (PPA)" in the parahippocampal gyrus that is specialized to selectively respond to outdoor scenes, places, and houses (Epstein & Kanwisher, 1998), (3) the lateral occipital complex (LOC) that is specialized to recognize objects (Grill-Spector et al., 1998; Malach et al., 1995), and (4) the left visual word form area (VWFA) located in the fusiform gyrus that is specialized for letters and words (Polk et al., 2002). Note that these visual categories elicit responses across a network of ventral visual regions (Haxby et al., 2001; Haxby et al., 2000), but these specialized regions respond most preferentially to these respective categories.
It has been shown that, relative to young adults, there is a reduced distinctiveness of cognitive representations (i.e., dedifferentiation) in perceptual function with age. Baltes & Lindenberger (1997) and Lindenberger & Baltes (1994) examined a large lifespan sample and reported that measures of visual and auditory perception explained most of the age-related variance on measures of high-level cognition such as memory and reasoning. This suggests that whereas younger adults have a high degree of specificity across different cognitive domains, a dedifferentiation of different cognitive functions occurs with age. In addition, some studies have shown that older adults are less able than younger adults to behaviorally distinguish between stimuli that are close in perceptual resemblance (Bartlett & Leslie, 1986; Betts et al., 2007; Goh et al., 2010a; Stark et al., 2010). It has been suggested that such age-related reduction in distinctiveness of cognitive representations is due to a decrease in neural specificity and a broadening of neural tuning curves such that a given region that responds selectively in young adults will respond to a wider array of inputs in older adults (Goh et al., 2010a; Leventhal et al., 2003; Park & Reuter-Lorenz, 2009; Schmolesky et al., 2000; Wang et al., 2005; Yu et al., 2006).

Indeed, Park et al. (2004) presented pictures of faces, houses, pseudowords, chairs and scrambled controls to both older and young adults and acquired functional brain data as the participants passively viewed the stimuli. The results showed markedly less neural specificity for these categories in the aging brain in the fusiform face area (FFA) and parahippocampal place area (PPA), amongst others. Whereas the FFA showed greater response to faces and less activation to other categories (i.e., places, chairs and words) in young adults, the FFA in older adults responded to faces but also with considerable activation to other categories, reflecting an age-related reduction in selective neural responses to these different visual categories. Voss et al. (2008) replicated this neural pattern of reduced selectivity of neural responses to different visual categories in older compared to younger adults, indicating the robustness of this finding across different samples of older adults.

In initial work on exploring age-related differences in functional specialization of ventral visual cortex, Goh et al. (2004) used fMRI adaptation to isolate brain regions that were involved in processing objects from those involved in processing scenes in younger adults. The fMRI adaptation paradigm allows for the evaluation of neural selectivity and specialization based on the phenomenon that neural response to repeated stimuli is typically reduced (Grill-Spector & Malach, 2001; Henson, 2003). In Goh et al., (2004), research participants passively viewed quartets of pictures that consisted of central objects embedded within background scenes (Figure 2). The objects and scenes of the picture quartets were selectively changed allowing for the identification of distinct brain regions in young adults that were clearly sensitive to object repetition only (object-processing regions in the LOC), or background scene repetition only (scene-processing regions). In subsequent studies, Goh and colleagues applied the same experiment on older adults and compared age-related differences in functional specialization of the ventral visual cortex for objects and scenes, albeit in an East Asian sample (Chee et al., 2006; Goh et al., 2007). They found a decreased specificity in older adults for object recognition within the lateral occipital cortex, suggesting that age-related reduction in distinctiveness of cognitive representation is present even in a culturally different sample of older adults.

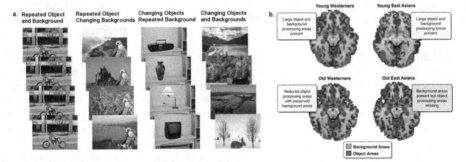

Fig. 2. Ventral visual brain regions selectively sensitive to object and background scene repetition in young and older, Westerners and East Asians, adapted from Goh et al. (2007), Age and culture modulate object processing and object-scene binding in the ventral visual area, *Cognitive, Affective & Behavioral Neuroscience*, 7(1), 44-52, copyright © 2007, with permission from Psychonomic Society Publications. a) Sample of picture quartet stimuli with selectively repeated objects and backgrounds used in that fMRI adaptation study. b) Young adults show clear object-related processing in lateral occipital regions and background-related processing in parahippocampal regions. Object processing regions are reduced in older adults with older East Asians showing disproportionately greater reduction.

Goh et al. (2010a) further demonstrated that age-related cognitive dedifferentiation is associated with reduced neural selectivity for within-category stimuli (i.e., different types of faces) as well. In this fMRI adaptation study, young and older adults were instructed to make same-different judgments to serially presented face-pairs that were Identical, Moderate (40 % difference) in similarity through morphing, or completely Different. They found that older adults showed adaptation in the fusiform face area (FFA) during the identical as well as the moderate conditions relative to the different condition (Figure 3). In contrast, young adults showed adaptation during the identical condition, but minimal adaptation to the moderate condition relative to the different condition. In addition, greater adaptation in the FFA was associated with poorer ability to discriminate faces. These findings provided clear evidence for reduced fidelity of neural representation of faces with age that was associated with poorer behavioral perceptual performance.

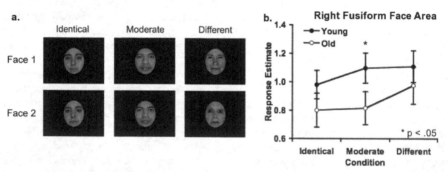

Fig. 3. Functional responses to Identical, Moderate (40% morph difference), and Different face-pairs in young and older adults, adapted from Goh et al. (2010a), Reduced neural selectivity increases fMRI adaptation with age during face discrimination, *NeuroImage*, 51(1), 336-344, copyright © 2010, with permission from Elsevier. a) Sample face-pair stimuli used in the fMRI adaptation experiment. b) Functional responses in the right fusiform face area show that younger adults treated moderately different face-pairs like they were completely different, whereas older adults treated moderately different face-pairs like they were identical.

In a different approach involving multi-voxel pattern analysis (MVPA), Carp et al. (2010) compared age differences in the distinctiveness of distributed patterns of neural activation evoked by different categories of visual images. They found that neural activation patterns within the ventral visual cortex were less distinctive among older adults, congruent with neural dedifferentiation with aging. In addition, they also showed such age-related neural dedifferentiation extend beyond the ventral visual cortex, with older adults showing decreased distinctiveness in early visual cortex, inferior parietal cortex, and prefrontal regions. Moreover, using MVPA as well, J. Park et al. (2010) investigated how well these age-related differences in neural specificity could explain individual differences in cognitive performance. They found that neural specificity significantly predicted performance on a range of fluid processing behavioral tasks (e.g., dot-comparison, digit-symbol) in older adults (~ 30% of the variance in a composite measure of fluid processing ability).

Taken together, the evidence from these different neuroimaging studies consistently demonstrate a reduced neural distinctiveness of cognitive representations with age in ventral visual cortex. Given such age-related dedifferentiation of the ventral visual cortex, which links age-related changes in behavior with brain changes, we now consider a more mixed pattern of functional responses in older adults in cognitive aging studies on the frontal regions.

2.2 Increased neural effort involved in cognitive processing

Although some studies have reported an under-recruitment of brain activity with age (e.g., Logan et al., 2002), different patterns of age-related neural over-recruitment, especially in the prefrontal cortex, have been consistently reported across several cognitive domains (Dennis & Cabeza, 2008; Grady, 2008; Park & Reuter-Lorenz, 2009; Reuter-Lorenz & Cappell, 2008). These neural patterns are such that older adults appear to (1) exhibit increased activity in similar regions engaged by young adults, (2) reveal additional activation in regions that are not activated in young adults, and (3) elicit greater bilateral activity than the more unilateral activity observed in their young counterparts (Cabeza et al., 2002; Cabeza et al., 2004; Daselaar et al., 2003; Jimura & Braver, 2010; Morcom et al., 2003) when performing equivalently or only slightly poorer relative to young adults. Prefrontal over-recruitment is so common across such a wide range of tasks that some authors have suggested that it is a general characteristic of age-related neural change (Cabeza et al., 2004; Davis et al., 2008).

A dominant observation of age-related over-recruitment is the bilateral activation of homologous prefrontal regions in older adults on tasks where their younger counterparts show unilateral activation pattern. Specifically, whereas young adults typically engage left lateralized frontal activity for tasks that involve verbal working memory, semantic processing, and recognition memory, older adults tend to show preserved left frontal activity with additional contralateral recruitment in the homologous site of the right hemisphere that is not observed in young adults (Figure 4; Cabeza et al., 1997; de Chastelaine et al., 2011; Daselaar et al., 2003; Duverne et al., 2009; Leshikar et al., 2010; Madden et al., 1999; Reuter-Lorenz et al., 2000; Schneider-Garces et al., 2010). Similarly, older adults engage both right and left prefrontal activity during tasks in which younger adults engage only right lateralized prefrontal activity, such as in tasks associated with face processing, spatial working memory, non-verbal spatial judgment, and episodic recall (Cabeza et al., 1997; Grady et al., 1995; D. Park et al., 2010; Reuter-Lorenz et al., 2000). This additional contralateral prefrontal recruitment that results in the pattern of greater bilateral activation in older adults has been described as Hemispheric Asymmetry Reduction in OLDer adults (HAROLD; Cabeza, 2002).

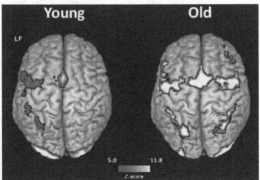

Fig. 4. Age-related over-recruitment of neural activation in verbal working memory. young adults engage unilateral frontal activity for tasks that involve verbal working memory, whereas older adults reveal preserved left frontal activity with additional contralateral recruitment in the homologous site of the right hemisphere. Adapted from Schneider-Garces et al. (2010), Span, CRUNCH, and beyond: working memory capacity and the aging brain, *Journal of Cognitive Neuroscience*, 22(4), 655-669, copyright © 2010, with permission from MIT Press.

Age-related over-recruitment of frontal regions is often interpreted as being compensatory and involved in the improvement or maintenance of performance in the face of age-related neurodegeneration (Cabeza, 2002; Davis et al., 2008; Heuninckx et al., 2008; Vallesi et al., 2011). For example, Rossi et al. (2004) reported direct evidence for the compensatory role of age-related over-recruitment in prefrontal regions by conducting a repetitive Transcranial Magnetic Stimulation (rTMS). rTMS is a technique which transiently disrupts neural function by applying repetitive magnetic stimulation to a specific area of the brain, creating a temporally artificial brain lesion. Rossi et al. (2004) showed that younger adults' memory retrieval accuracy was more affected when the rTMS was applied to the left prefrontal cortex but less affected when rTMS was applied to the right prefrontal region. In contrast, older adults' retrieval accuracy was equally affected, whether rTMS was applied to the left or right prefrontal regions, suggesting bilateral prefrontal activation has a causal link to behavioral performance in older adults. A compensatory account of age-related over-recruitment was also supported in Morcom et al. (2003) who showed that greater frontal bilaterality in older adults compared to young predicted better performance when successfully encoding subsequently remembered items.

Some studies have reported impaired behavioral performance associated with additional contralateral prefrontal recruitment, suggesting that prefrontal over-recruitment may not always be compensatory. For example, de Chastelaine et al. (2011) found that older adults' memory performance positively correlated with neural over-recruitment in the left prefrontal cortex, a region also engaged by young adults. However, the correlation was negative with respect to additional recruitment in the right prefrontal cortex of older adults, a region that was not observed in young adults, suggesting that over-recruitment in the right frontal regions in older individuals does not always contribute to memory performance (see also Duverne et al., 2009). Resolving whether age-related over-recruitment is associated with compensatory or declining function, would require studies that more effectively measure and equate differences in cognitive ability and performance across young and older adults, as well as better define what compensation means. Nevertheless, a broad number of studies are at least in agreement that there is consistent age-related over-recruitment that is generally associated with better cognitive outcomes.

In addition to being beneficial for behavioral performance, evidence also suggests that increased neural effort observed in prefrontal cortex may reflect a compensatory response to deteriorating neural systems in more posterior sites of the brain, including the medial temporal lobe (Cabeza et al., 2004; Gutchess et al., 2005; Park et al., 2003), and occipital cortex (Cabeza et al., 2004; Davis et al., 2008; Goh et al., 2010a). Park & Gutchess (2005) systematically reviewed neural activations associated with long-term memory and noted that decreased hippocampal and parahippocampal activation in medial temporal lobes are coupled with the increased frontal activation in older adults. Indeed, Gutchess et al. (2005) showed that during an incidental memory encoding task, older adults had lower activation than young adults in the left and right parahippocampus and greater activation than young adults in the middle frontal cortex. Goh et al. (2010a) also showed that increased frontal engagement was also associated lower neural selectivity in the ventral visual regions. Moreover, Cabeza et al. (2004) reported that older adults showed increased bilateral prefrontal activation and decreased occipital function compared to their young counterparts across various cognitive tasks, indicating a Posterior Anterior Shift in Aging (PASA) functional activity (Davis et al., 2008). These results suggest a neurocognitive compensatory role of prefrontal regions for age-related neural deterioration in posterior brain regions.

With this review on the pattern of age-related reductions in neural distinctiveness in cognitive representations and increases in frontal engagement, we now turn to consider the evidence for the second source of influence on brain structure and function – cultural experience.

3. Culture-related findings

In a comprehensive review of sociopolitical and historical progressions, Nisbett (2003) proposed that the value system of one's cultural environment exerts an influence on self-perceptions and even cognitive processing. That is, social and physical pressures in the cultural environment encourage certain modes of behavior and thinking and suppress others. Over time, these cultural pressures become internalized and act as a bias with which individuals process subsequent social and physical situations as well. In this article, we focus on differences between Westerners and East Asians, as there have been more studies that directly compared these two culture groups. It has been shown that whereas Western culture places more emphasis on independence and individualism, East Asian culture values interdependence and collectivism (Hofstede, 1980, 2001; Kitayama et al., 1997; Nisbett, 2003; Nisbett & Masuda, 2003; Nisbett et al., 2001; Oyserman et al., 2002; Triandis et al., 1988; Triandis, 1995). Nisbett (2003) argues that Westerners embedded in a culture of individualism tend to adopt an analytic style of cognitive processing. This style of processing can be characterized as a bias to treat stimuli items in the environment as individual and distinctive objects composed on a set of features. Likewise, East Asians are embedded in a culture of collectivism that is associated with a holistic style of cognitive processing, which is reflected as a bias to regard items in the environment as related to one another, and more tightly bound to the context.

This section considers the evidence for the existence of these culture-related differences in analytic and holistic processing styles between Westerners and East Asians and their neural correlates. While many of these studies have been previously reviewed (Goh & Park, 2009b; Han & Northoff, 2008; Nisbett & Masuda, 2003; Nisbett & Miyamoto, 2005; Nisbett et al., 2001), we highlight important and novel aspects of these findings here as they pertain to the overall question on the interaction between age and culture. As will be seen, many of these studies show culture-related differences in the way Westerners and East Asians perceive and attend to items in the visual environment. Critically, both behavioral and neuroimaging studies report findings that are remarkably consistent with the analytic and holistic biases in Westerners and East Asians, respectively.

3.1 Cultural differences in perception and attention: Behavioral foundations
3.1.1 Face stimuli
In a study that used visual aesthetics as an approach to characterizing object-context perception in Westerners and East Asians, Masuda et al. (2008a) evaluated differences in the content of portrait photographs taken by American and Japanese participants. They found that American participants took portrait photographs in which the face, the object of the portrait, occupied a larger ratio of the frame than the background. In contrast, photographs taken by Japanese participants consisted of a much larger portion of the background relative to the face. Thus, Japanese may have considered the background context as more important to the portrait than Americans did. In another study on the degree to which Americans and Japanese incorporate contextual social information, Masuda et al. (2008b) asked participants

to judge the emotion of a facial expression that was presented amidst other emotional facial expressions that were either congruent or conflicting with the target expression. The results of that study suggested that Japanese were more likely to modulate their judgment of the target face emotion based on the other faces whereas Americans were less sensitive to contextual face emotions in their behavioral responses.

Eye movements to face stimuli also show distinctions between Westerners and East Asians. In Masuda et al. (2008b) study above, eye-movements of participants were also measured as they judged the emotional content of a target face amidst other faces in the background. They found that Japanese devoted less time fixating on the target face than Americans, and thus, Japanese were looking more at the contextual faces than the Americans as well. Blais et al. (2008) recorded eye movements as Westerners and East Asians viewed single face stimuli across several different types of tasks to examine which components of the face participants tended to look at. It was found that, across all tasks, Westerners tended to fixate on the eyes and mouth of the faces whereas East Asians focused on central regions of the face, around the nose. Westerners may have attended to facial features that contain distinguishing information about the face, consistent with an analytic style of face processing. In contrast, East Asians may have treated faces more holistically and thus de-emphasized the distinctiveness of facial features. Taken together, these findings reflect the bias for a more analytic style in Westerners and a more holistic style in East Asians when processing aesthetics and social information involving face stimuli.

3.1.2 Objects and backgrounds

Culture-related differences in analytic-holistic processing is supported by evidence that shows that Westerners have a greater affinity for visuo-spatial judgments involving absolute quantities whereas East Asians are better at relative comparisons. In the Frame Line Test, participants are presented with a test stimulus consisting of a line embedded within a square box frame. The test stimulus is then removed and replaced with probe, which was an empty square frame that was either smaller or larger in size relative to the test square. During the absolute judgment task, participants were instructed to draw a line in the probe square that was of the same length as the original test line, regardless of the size of the square. During the relative judgments task, however, participants were to draw a line that was of the same length relative to the size of the square frame. Kitayama et al. (2003) found that Americans were more accurate for the absolute line drawing and Japanese were more accurate for the relative line drawing. Thus, Westerners may have attended more to the features of the line (length), in accordance with an analytic style of processing, whereas East Asians integrated the line and square frame as a whole, in according with a holistic processing style.

Differences between Westerners and East Asians have also been found in the sensitivity to changing visual elements of complex scenes. Change blindness refers to the phenomenon whereby participants take some time to detect relatively salient changes in rapidly alternating scenes (Simons & Ambinder, 2005; Simons & Levin, 1997). Boduroglu et al. (2009) found that East Asians were better at detecting color changes in the stimuli periphery than Westerners, but East Asians also showed poorer performance than Westerners when the color changes occurred in the central regions of the screen. Using the change blindness paradigm as well, Masuda & Nisbett (2006) presented Americans and Japanese with rapidly alternating pictures of scenes with objects. They found that whereas Americans were faster at detecting changes occurring in the central object, they were slower with background changes.

In contrast, Japanese were equally fast for changes occurring in both objects and backgrounds. Moreover, Americans detected more object changes whereas Japanese detected more background changes. Thus, the more analytic style of processing in Westerners was reflected as greater sensitivity to central object changes, and the more holistic processing style in East Asians manifested as greater sensitivity to the peripheral background.

Again, evidence from eye-tracking studies provides compelling evidence that Westerners and East Asians are attending in different ways to the same scene stimuli. Chua et al. (2005) recorded eye-movements while American and Chinese participants looked at naturalistic pictures that depicted a central object presented against a contextual background scene. Compared to American participants, Chinese participants made more fixations to the background and had slower onsets of the first fixation to central objects. In addition, Chinese participants generally showed a greater proportion of background relative to object fixations throughout the time course of the stimulus viewing, whereas Westerners had greater proportions of object fixations over the time course with very brief periods of increased proportions of background fixations. Goh et al. (2009c) further evaluated whether these cultural differences in eye-movements were robust to visual stimuli that captured participants' attention against their own cultural preferences, using an experimental design adapted from Goh et al. (2007). It was found that, as expected, Westerners were more sensitive to object changes than East Asians, and East Asians alternated more between the objects and backgrounds. Moreover, these cultural differences in eye-movements were relatively robust to the attention capturing manipulation of changing objects and backgrounds. Critically, Westerners' eye-movements were characterized by fewer fixations with longer dwell times whereas East Asians had fewer but shorter fixations that covered a greater area of the visual stimuli (Figure 5).

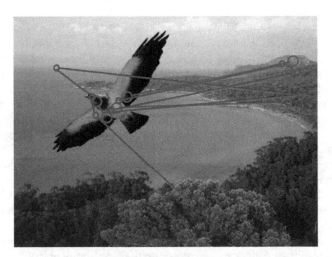

Fig. 5. A schematic of eye-movements during scene viewing in Westerners (blue) and East Asians (red). Circles represent fixations and size of circles represent fixation dwell times, with larger circles indicating longer times adapted from Goh et al. (2009c).

Some eye-tracking studies did not find cultural difference in eye-movements when Westerners and East Asians viewed scenes (Caldara et al., 2010; Miellet et al., 2010; Rayner et al., 2009). For example, Rayner et al. (2009) found that when visual scenes depicted a bizarre or impossible circumstance (e.g. a boy with an extra leg), there were no differences in the way Westerners and East Asians fixated on the scene. It is possible that in such cases, basic universal attentional processes take precedence over cultural differences in visual attention. It is also certainly possible that these results reflect how cultural biases are amenable to change since Westerners are capable of focusing on scenes and East Asians are capable of focusing on objects (see studies on cultural priming; Chiao et al., 2010; Miyamoto et al., 2006).

Overall, these findings show that there are culture-related differences in perception and attention between Westerners and East Asians. These differences are such that Westerners have a more analytic processing style, focusing on object features, and East Asians have a more holistic processing style, focusing on contextual information. With this in mind, we now consider the neural correlates of these visual processing behavioral patterns.

3.2 Cultural differences in perception and attention: Functional brain studies
3.2.1 Face, object, and scene processing in the ventral visual cortex

As mentioned previously, one of the most consistent observations related to visual processing in the brain is that specific regions within the ventral visual cortex show heightened sensitivity to specific categories of visual stimuli. It should also be noted that greater attention to the stimulus tends to increase the selectivity of the ventral visual region involved in processing that stimulus (Murray & Wojciulik, 2004; Yi et al., 2006). The following studies show that there are culture-related differences in the way the selective regions of the ventral visual cortex respond to faces, objects, and scenes in Westerners and East Asians, and that the analytic-holistic dichotomy operates in visual perception and attentional neural processes as well.

In a simple blocked-design fMRI experiment, Goh et al. (2010b) presented Americans (Westerners) and Singaporeans (East Asians) with face and house stimuli and compared the selectivity of their fusiform regions for faces relative to houses, and lingual regions for houses relative to faces. It was found that Americans showed greater face selectivity than Singaporeans in the left fusiform region, and face selectivity in the right fusiform regions was equivalent in both groups (Figure 6). Right fusiform engagement has been associated with more holistic processing of face stimuli as a whole; however, left fusiform activity has been associated with more analytic face processing of specific facial features (Rossion et al., 2000). Thus, the finding that Americans engaged greater left fusiform responses than Singaporeans to faces, and the findings on cultural differences in behavioral and eye-movement responses to faces reviewed above, provide a compelling basis for a greater bias to attend to facial features in Westerners than East Asians, consistent with a more analytic face processing style in Westerners. In addition, Goh et al. (2010c) found that Singaporeans showed some evidence for greater house selectivity than Americans in bilateral lingual regions. Taken together with the behavioral findings again, this suggests that Singaporeans were attending more than Americans to the contextual environment, consistent with a more holistic processing style for scenes in East Asians.

With respect to objects and scenes, fMRI studies have also found that Westerners engage more object-related processing in the ventral visual regions compared to East Asians. In Gutchess et al. (2006), Westerners and East Asians performed an incidental encoding task on stimuli consisting of objects and scenes. Whereas they did not find any group differences in

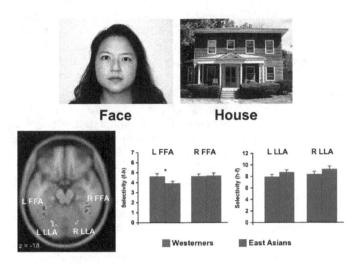

Fig. 6. Neural selectivity to face and house stimuli in the fusiform face areas (FFA) and lingual landmark areas (LLA) of Westerners and East Asians, adapted from Goh et al. (2010b), Culture differences in neural processing of faces and houses in the ventral visual cortex, *Social Cognitive and Affective Neuroscience*, 5(2-3), 227-235, with permission from Oxford University Press. Sample stimuli used in the blocked-design fMRI experiment are on top. The bottom left panel illustrates peak voxel locations of the FFA and LLA from a sample of individual participants. The bottom right panel shows greater selectivity for faces (f-h) in the left FFA in Westerners compared to East Asians (* p < .05), and marginally greater selectivity for houses (h-f) in bilateral LLA in East Asians compared to Westerners.

background-related processing regions, Westerners showed greater recruitment of object processing regions than East Asians in the middle temporal, supramarginal, and parietal regions. In Goh et al.'s (2007) fMRI adaptation study mentioned in the section on aging, brain imaging data from both Westerners and East Asians were also acquired to investigate cultural differences in ventral visual responses to objects and background scenes (see Figure 2). They found that although there were no group differences in scene processing regions, East Asians showed less object-related responses in the lateral occipital regions compared to Westerners. Interestingly, this culture-related difference in object processing was more evident in older adults than in younger adults, implying an age dependency, which is further discussed below.

Apart from cultural differences in the processing of objects and scenes as separate items, studies have also found evidence for cultural differences in sensitivity to the relationship between objects and scenes in the stimuli. Jenkins et al. (2010) used a similar fMRI adaptation experiment as in Goh et al. (2007), and presented participants pictures with selectively repeated objects and scenes. Critically in that study, some of the object-scene pairings were congruent (e.g. a plane in the sky) whereas some objects were incongruent with the scenes (e.g. an elephant in a kitchen), but not impossible. They found that whereas Westerners were relatively insensitive to object-scene congruity, East Asians showed greater responses to incongruent relative to congruent pairings, suggesting that they attended more to objects when the pairing with the scene was incongruent (see Goto et al., 2010, for a similar study using event-related potentials). Taken together, these findings are consistent with the analytic-holistic dichotomy, and suggest that Westerners treat each visual element in a picture more as separate objects, whereas East Asians regard the picture elements as more tightly bound together into the whole context.

3.2.2 Visual attention processing

Using the Frame Line Test from Kitayama et al. (2003), Hedden et al. (2008) acquired fMRI data as Westerners and East Asians made absolute and relative line judgments in the scanner. They found that Westerners showed greater brain responses during relative compared to absolute line judgments in frontal and parietal regions, brain areas typically associated with attentional processing. In contrast, East Asians showed greater brain responses during absolute compared to relative judgments in the same regions (Figure 7). These findings suggest that participants required greater effort when engaging non-preferred visual processing styles, which is associated with cultural differences in attention-related responses in fronto-parietal regions. Importantly, the finding that Westerners required greater effort for relative judgments and East Asians for absolute judgments is again consistent with the analytic-holistic dichotomy in these two groups.

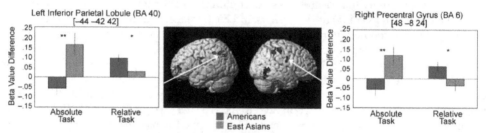

Fig. 7. Functional brain responses during the Frame Line Test in Americans and East Asians, adapted from Hedden et al. (2008), Cultural influences on neural substrates of attentional control, *Psychological Science*, 19(1), 53-81, copyright © 2008, with permission from Sage Publications. Americans showed greater responses in fronto-parietal regions during the relative compared to the absolute task. East Asians showed greater responses during the absolute compared to the relative task.

In a yet unpublished study, Goh et al. (submitted) acquired fMRI data as Westerners and East Asians made judgments on the distance between a dot and a horizontal line, relative to the length of a vertical line. In that study, while accuracy was equivalent in both groups, East Asians responded significantly faster than Westerners, suggesting that the task was easier for East Asians and harder for Westerners. In line with this interpretation, during task performance, Westerners showed greater activation of the frontal and parietal regions compared to East Asians. Importantly, they also found that Westerners showed greater suppression of responses compared to East Asians in the default-network regions that included the medial frontal and supramarginal regions. Suppression of these default-network regions has been linked to a greater need to attend to external stimuli (Anticevic et al., 2010; Benjamin et al., 2010; Greicius et al., 2003; Hayden et al., 2010; Mayer et al., 2010; Raichle et al., 2001). Thus, Westerners may have required greater attention than East Asians to perform the relative spatial judgment task, and correspondingly suppressed default-network activity more in the process.

In Goh et al. (2007), it was also suggested that the lack of object-processing responses in the lateral occipital regions in older adult East Asians was related to a reduction in attentional resources. Interestingly, Chee et al. (2006) investigated this by repeating the fMRI adaptation experiment on the same older East Asians but with the instruction to attend to the object while ignoring the scenes. Under those circumstances, the older East Asians showed a reinstatement of object-related processing in the lateral occipital region, suggesting that the lack of responses in the initial study was indeed due to attentional mechanisms. This finding suggests that under reduced attentional resources, the older East Asians maintained their focus on the background scenes but devoted less attention to objects, in line with a bias for holistic processing in East Asians.

Thus, culture-related functional brain differences are observed in perceptual regions as well as in regions involved in attention. It is possible that such chronic differential functional engagement may result in structural brain differences. And, while there are fewer studies on cultural differences in brain structure, there have been several studies on how different external experiences and expertise do bear on regional brain size and integrity.

3.3 Culture, experience, and brain structure

At present, only four studies have directly compared brain structural differences between Westerners and East Asians. Zilles et al. (2001) only examine gross brain size and shape differences and found that Japanese brains were shorter and wider, i.e. more circular in shape, compared to European brains, which were more elongated or oval. Green et al. (2007) and Kochunov et al. (2003) examined structural differences related to differences in the usage of the Chinese and English language. These latter two studies generally found that Chinese-speaking East Asians have more brain tissue than English-speaking Westerners in the left inferior frontal, middle temporal, and right superior temporal regions. The fourth study by Chee et al. (2011) examined a much larger sample of structural brain images of Americans and Singaporeans, which is critical since there is a large amount of variability in structural MRI data. Using various data analysis methods, including cortical thickness

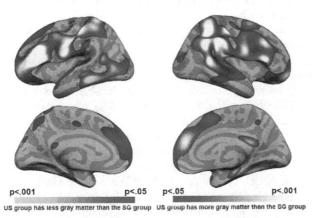

p<.001   p<.05   p<.05   p<.001

US group has less gray matter than the SG group   US group has more gray matter than the SG group

Fig. 8. Cortical thickness differences between Americans (US) and Singaporeans (SG). Adapted from Chee et al. (2011), Brain structure in young and old East Asians and Westerners: comparisons of structural volume and cortical thickness, *Journal of Cognitive Neuroscience*, 23(5), 1065-1079, copyright © 2011, with permission from MIT Press.

measures, voxel-based morphometry and pattern classification approaches, they found that Americans had thicker cortical gray matter than Singaporean in frontal, parietal, and temporal polymodal association areas, whereas Singaporeans had thicker left inferior temporal regions (Figure 8).

While more studies are required to relate these culture group differences in cortical thickness, it is clear from other non-culture studies that external experiences do have a modulatory influence on brain structure. For example, Maguire et al. (2000) showed London taxi-cab drivers have larger hippocampal volumes than control participants possibly due to the their expertise in navigating around the city streets. This finding was consistent with the important role that hippocampus has in spatial navigation as well as memory (Cohen et al., 1999). In addition, Draganski et al. (2004) showed that novices who acquired juggling skills longitudinally developed more gray matter in the middle temporal gyrus and intra-parietal sulcus, regions important for visuo-spatial coordination. It is therefore no surprise that cultural differences in functional engagement of specific brain regions would also result in the regional differences in brain structure described above, and future studies will establish more mechanistic links between cultural experience and brain structure.

4. Cultural differences across age

Having established that there are culture-related differences in brain structure and function, we now evaluate how these brain differences interact with the neural changes associated with aging described above. Studies that integrate age and culture are sparse at present. Nevertheless, the few studies that do consider this aspect of neural structure and function over the lifespan provides some initial guidance as to the nature of culture-related neural differences in older adulthood.

It is useful to first consider when culture-related neural differences start in the course of the human lifespan. As yet, we are not aware of any neuroimaging studies that have directly examined culture-related brain differences in children or adolescents. A few developmental studies, however, provide some clues as to when cultural experience may begin to have an influence on neurocognitive processes. For example, a linguistic study involving Western and East Asian infants developing in different language environments (English vs. Japanese) show language-specific perceptual biases as early as 7 months (Yoshida et al., 2010). In addition, Wang & Leichtman (2000) examined narratives of 6-year-old children and found that compared to Western children, East Asian children described stories and memories with a greater emphasis on social relationships and contextual information, characteristic of a collectivistic culture. Wang (2008) also examined autobiographical memory in Western and East Asian children as young as 3 years old. It was found that Western children tended to recall memories with greater specificity whereas East Asian children recalled memories in a more general manner, consisting of less specific details. In an fMRI study, Golarai et al. (2007) managed to examine the selectivity of the ventral visual cortex of young children, albeit just in a sample of Westerners. They showed that by 7 years of age, children had developed selective responses for faces in the FFA and scenes in the PPA to the level observed in mature adults. This imaging finding and the behavioral comparisons above suggest that the culture-related neural differences observed in young adults at approximately 20-30 years of age may begin in quite early in childhood.

With respect to culture-related differences in older adults, only one published functional neuroimaging study thus far has directly examined the interaction between age and culture.

As mentioned, Goh et al. (2007) used the fMRI adaptation paradigm to investigate ventral visual selectivity for objects and scenes in young and older, Westerners and East Asians (Figure 2). The main finding in that study was that older East Asians (aged 65 and above) showed reduced object-related processing compared to the other three groups. This finding was interpreted as an accentuation of the bias for contextual processing in older East Asians due to a reduction in attentional resources with age. In addition, Chee et al.'s (2011) structural brain study also compared young and older, Westerners and East Asians. It was found in that study that whereas the cultural differences in cortical thickness seen in younger adults was not present in older adults as a whole group, cultural differences emerged when older adults were split into high and low cognitive performance. This result suggests that in older adult individuals who show greater susceptibility to neurobiological decline with aging and thus poorer cognition, culture-related experiential influences on the brain become diminished with age. However, in older adults who remain relatively cognitively intact, cultural differences in brain structure are maintained throughout the lifespan.

Distinct from the more global effect of aging on the brain, the effect of cultural experience on the brain seems more localized and specific. That is, whereas aging is associated with a general decline in brain structure and function, culture and other experiential factors modulate neural structure and activity only in regions that are involved in a given cognitive process (e.g. the FFA for processing faces). While more studies are required to evaluate the extent and robustness of these effects, it appears that neurobiological declines associated with aging do not completely overwhelm the influence of experiential factors, at least those related to culture. Thus, the effect of culture-related experiences is likely to have an enduring impact on neural structure and function from adulthood to advanced age.

5. Methodological issues

Interpreting age-related differences in cognitive performance between age groups has proven to be a unique challenge, and exploring the effects of age and culture compounds these difficulties. Here we evaluate some important methodological issues that may limit the extent to which current data can be interpreted and applied to other samples, and suggest recommendations for future studies.

5.1 Cohort, age, and culture considerations

At all times, it should be noted that there is much heterogeneity in the cultural makeup of Westerners and East Asians and the attribution of cultural characteristics is always at the group level. In addition, while culture is defined in terms of value systems, many studies operationalize culture based on geopolitical boundaries, i.e. countries and nationalities. For example, Westerners are predominantly Americans and East Asians are typically Japanese, Chinese, or other Chinese Asian individuals (e.g., Hong Kong Chinese, Singaporean Chinese, Taiwanese Chinese, etc.). Moreover, people within these different cultural affiliations demonstrate varying degrees of individualism and collectivism. For example, Oyserman et al. (2002) documented that native Japanese are not necessarily more collectivistic relative to Caucasian Americans, and cultural differences in individualism and collectivism are not static over time between groups (Oyserman & S. W. S. Lee, 2008). Moreover, in an fMRI study involving native Japanese and Americans, Chiao et al. (2009) reported that neural activity within the ventral medial frontal regions predicted how individualistic or collectivistic a person is across cultures, regardless of the participants' cultural affiliation. These findings suggest that although some aspects of cultural groups remain stable across time, neural representations of self in Americans and East Asians are not inherently different, but instead reflect different cultural values that are endorsed by the individual.

Given the cost of conducting imaging studies and relatively low reliability of physiological signals, it is also particularly difficult to acquire neuroimaging data from participant samples that are saturated with culture- and/or age-specific experience, yet equated on other factors such as education, cohort-specific experiences and other demographics (Manly, 2008; Park et al., 1999; Whitfield & Morgan, 2008). Thus far, a variety of approaches to explore group differences across several neuroimaging studies have been utilized to deal with these sampling issues. The majority of cross-cultural studies involve East Asian and Western participants studying at the same institution (usually undergraduate/graduate students) as well as neuroimaging data from one MRI scanner (Gutchess et al., 2006; Hedden et al., 2008; Jenkins et al., 2010). However, there are two limitations to such an approach. First, immigrant participants from another culture (e.g., Chinese students in the United States) may already have had some biasing experiences in the host culture, even if they have not been exposed to the new environment for that long. This potentially results in an underestimation of cultural differences in behavioral performance and neural activation. Second, immigrant participants are often a select group of individuals (e.g. international students) who have been qualified to study or work overseas according to their conspicuous achievement, leading to a more high-performing, homogenous sample compared to native individuals. In such cases, conclusions of cultural variation may in fact be associated with sample differences in cognitive capabilities. To reduce these sampling biases described above, it is necessary to select samples based on equivalent levels of education, similar demographics and matched cognitive abilities between groups (Park & Huang, 2010).

Cohort-related effects within a cultural group may also influence the individual's value system, self-perceptions, cognitive processing, and even neural processing, over and above the cultural environment. For instance, in China, only older adults lived through the Cultural Revolution (~1970s), which had tremendous impact on their lifestyle and thinking, whereas younger adults in China had no such experience. A similarly situation applies to the Great Depression (~1930s) for young and older adults in America, and on a worldwide level, World War II. The effects of such socio-historical events on neuropsychological differences between age and culture groups are substantial and should be considered when recruiting participants in future studies.

The careful development of hypotheses and clear predictions of differentiated patterns of activation in older and young adults across cultures is also critical (Park et al., 1999; Park & Gutchess, 2006). Because of the distal nature of culture-related effects on the brain, combined with effects of education, diet, genetics and many other variables (Chee et al., 2011), it is difficult to simply theorize and test that differences observed in neural activation are directly linked to cultural experiences and behavioral practices. As an example, both well-established knowledge from the analytic-holistic framework (Nisbett & Masuda, 2003; Nisbett et al., 2001) and empirical findings from cross-cultural eye-movement studies (Chua et al., 2005) were used to guide Goh et al. (2007) and Goh et al.'s (2010) studies on neural correlates of age and culture in ventral visual processing. Using the existing knowledge base that prescribed specific expectations about the data facilitated the interpretation of the complex patterns of neuroimaging findings from different age and cultural groups in those studies.

5.2 Measurement and instrument comparability

Prior to cross-group comparisons in studies on cognitive neuroscience of aging and culture, it is first important to evaluate whether the experiment stimuli are equally familiar to both age and culture groups. Stimuli that are less familiar or evoke specific types of processing in one group during scanning would confound patterns of neural activation due to the stimuli familiarity differences rather than cognitive processes. Indeed, studies have found culture- and age-related variations in norms associated with how individuals from these groups name pictures of everyday objects (Yoon, et al., 2004a) and categorize words (Yoon et al., 2004b). Hedden et al. (2002) also found that Chinese had better performance than Americans in numerical cognitive tests such as digit comparison (a measure of speed of processing) and backward digit span (a measure of working memory). They suggested that such group differences could be due to differences in the number system and representation in the Chinese and English languages, rather than actual cognitive differences in speed or working memory. Thus, future studies should be aware of such differences in the stimuli used to ensure comparability of cognitive processing across cultural and age groups.

In studies that involved data from two different MRI scanner machines from different sites, it is possible that differences in the blood oxygen level dependent (BOLD) signal between cultural groups could occur as a result of differing properties between hardware rather than actual neural differences between cultures (Park, 2008; Park & Gutchess, 2002). Cases in point are Goh et al. (2007) and Goh et al. (2010), who acquired imaging data from Singapore and the United States, with both sites having identical imaging hardware and software.

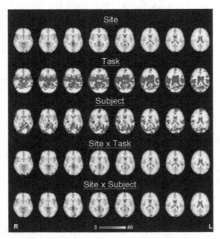

Fig. 9. Between-site comparison of functional MRI signal from Singapore and the United States equipped with identical imaging hardware and software. The same participants performed the same tasks at two magnet sites over several sessions. The statistical brain maps of a three-way Analysis of variance (ANOVA) are shown with the main effects and interactions of site, subject, and task, colored with increasing red intensities ($P < 0.001$ uncorrected). There were extensive regions showing significant main effects and interactions of subject and task, but the effects associated with magnet site were negligible. Adapted from Sutton et al. (2008), Investigation and validation of intersite fMRI studies using the same imaging hardware, *Journal of Magnetic Resonance Imaging*, 28(1), 21-28, copyright © 2008, with permission from John Wiley and Sons..

Prior to conducting these studies, the authors examined functional imaging data with a visual and motor task from four participants who were repeatedly imaged in both machines in Singapore and the United States (Sutton et al., 2008). They found that there was minimal variance in BOLD as a function of site, between-subject differences accounted for 10 times more variance than site of data collection, and task differences (motor versus visual) also accounted for a significant proportion of the variance (Figure 9). Phantom scans were also routinely acquired before testing participants in order to evaluate signal noise and stability of the two scanners as further checks that the two magnets were similarly calibrated. Given the careful evaluation of BOLD signal properties of the two different magnets, the results suggest that obtaining neuroimaging data from two geographically different sites with the identical systems used in those studies was feasible and had sufficient reliability.

6. Conclusion

In this review, we have covered imaging findings related to neurocognitive changes associated with aging and culture, and some findings pertaining to their interaction. Studies on neurocognitive aging show a general reduction in the distinctiveness of neural responses to different stimuli in the posterior brain regions that may be related to neurobiological declines. In the midst of such neurobiological declines, there is also consistent evidence showing increases in frontal responses that may be part of a compensatory response, in particular for the declines associated with posterior brain regions. In contrast to the more global effect of aging, studies on cultural differences in values, perception and attention have also shown specific and more localized differences in neural function that are consistently associated with the analytic-holistic dichotomy in Westerners and East Asians respectively. Specifically, Westerners show functional brain responses that reflect their bias for analytic processing styles that is associated with increased responses in object-processing regions probably related to greater attention to object features. In contrast, East Asians show brain responses that reflect a more holistic processing style associated with attention to contextual information in regions like the lingual landmark area. Some differences in brain structure have also been observed in these cultural groups, although a clear mechanism between cultural experience and brain structure has yet to be established. A few studies have shown that the impact of culture-related experiences on neural structure and function may be acquired at a very young age, and importantly, endures through to advanced aging with even some cases of accentuation.

In sum, the findings covered in this review suggest that there is a reliable and consistent effect of cultural experiences on neural structure and function. While more studies are required to strengthen the findings, initial studies have shown also that at least some of these culture-related effects present in young adults are maintained even in the face of neurobiological changes associated with aging. Importantly, these findings also suggest that neurobiological aging does not always lead to neurocognitive decline in a uniform manner, and that external experiences can modulate and perhaps alleviate some of the neural effects of aging in the brain.

7. Acknowledgement

We thank Dr. Wayne Chan and Dr. May Baydoun for their helpful comments. This research was supported in part by the Intramural Research Program of the NIH, National Institute on Aging, USA.

8. References

Aguirre, G. K., Zarahn, E., & D'Esposito, M. (1998a). An area within human ventral cortex sensitive to "building" stimuli: evidence and implications. *Neuron, 21*(2), 373-383.

Aguirre, G. K., Zarahn, E., & D'Esposito, M. (1998b). Neural components of topographical representation. *Proceedings of the National Academy of Sciences of the United States of America, 95*(3), 839-846.

Anticevic, A., Repovs, G., Shulman, Gordon L, & Barch, D. M. (2010). When less is more: TPJ and default network deactivation during encoding predicts working memory performance. *NeuroImage, 49*(3), 2638-2648.

Baltes, P. B., & Lindenberger, U. (1997). Emergence of a powerful connection between sensory and cognitive functions across the adult life span: a new window to the study of cognitive aging? *Psychology and Aging, 12*(1), 12-21.

Bartlett, J. C., & Leslie, J. E. (1986). Aging and memory for faces versus single views of faces. *Memory & cognition, 14*(5), 371-381.

Benjamin, C., Lieberman, D. A., Chang, M., Ofen, N., Whitfield-Gabrieli, S., Gabrieli, J. D. E., & Gaab, N. (2010). The influence of rest period instructions on the default mode network. *Frontiers in Human Neuroscience, 4*, 218.

Betts, L. R., Sekuler, A. B., & Bennett, P. J. (2007). The effects of aging on orientation discrimination. *Vision Research, 47*(13), 1769-1780.

Blais, C., Jack, R. E., Scheepers, C., Fiset, D., & Caldara, R. (2008). Culture shapes how we look at faces. *Public Library of Science ONE, 3*(8), e3022.

Boduroglu, A., Shah, P., & Nisbett, R. E. (2009). Cultural differences in allocation of attention in visual information processing. *Journal of Cross-Cultural Psychology, 40*(3), 349-360.

Burke, S. N., & Barnes, C. A. (2006). Neural plasticity in the ageing brain. *Nature Reviews Neuroscience, 7*(1), 30-40.

Burke, Sara N, & Barnes, Carol A. (2010). Senescent synapses and hippocampal circuit dynamics. *Trends in Neurosciences, 33*(3), 153-161.

Cabeza, R. (2002). Hemispheric asymmetry reduction in older adults: the HAROLD model. *Psychology and aging, 17*(1), 85–100.

Cabeza, R., Anderson, N. D., Locantore, J. K., & McIntosh, A. R. (2002). Aging gracefully: compensatory brain activity in high-performing older adults. *NeuroImage, 17*(3), 1394-1402.

Cabeza, R., Daselaar, S. M., Dolcos, F., Prince, S. E., Budde, M., & Nyberg, L. (2004). Task-independent and task-specific age effects on brain activity during working memory, visual attention and episodic retrieval. *Cerebral Cortex, 14*(4), 364-375.

Cabeza, R., Grady, C. L., Nyberg, L., McIntosh, A. R., Tulving, E., Kapur, S., Jennings, J. M., et al. (1997). Age-related differences in neural activity during memory encoding and retrieval: a positron emission tomography study. *Journal of Neuroscience, 17*(1), 391-400.

Caldara, R., Zhou, X., & Miellet, S. (2010). Putting culture under the "spotlight" reveals universal information use for face recognition. *PLoS One, 5*(3), e9708.

Carp, J., Park, J., Polk, T. A., & Park, D. C. (2010). Age differences in neural distinctiveness revealed by multi-voxel pattern analysis. *NeuroImage*. Epub ahead of print. doi:10.1016/j.neuroimage.2010.04.267

de Chastelaine, M., Wang, T. H., Minton, B., Muftuler, L. T., & Rugg, M. D. (2011). The Effects of Age, Memory Performance, and Callosal Integrity on the Neural Correlates of Successful Associative Encoding. *Cerebral Cortex*. Epub ahead of print. doi:10.1093/cercor/bhq294

Chee, M. W. L., Goh, J. O. S., Venkatraman, V., Chow Tan, J., Gutchess, A., Sutton, B., Hebrank, A., et al. (2006a). Age-related changes in object processing and contextual binding revealed using fMR-Adaptation. *Journal of Cognitive Neuroscience, 18*(4), 495-507.

Chee, M. W. L., Zheng, H., Goh, J. O. S., Park, D., & Sutton, B. P. (2011). Brain structure in young and old East Asians and Westerners: comparisons of structural volume and cortical thickness. *Journal of Cognitive Neuroscience, 23*(5), 1065-1079.

Chiao, J. Y., Harada, T., Komeda, H., Li, Z., Mano, Y., Saito, D., Parrish, T. B., et al. (2009). Neural basis of individualistic and collectivistic views of self. *Human Brain Mapping, 30*(9), 2813-2820.

Chiao, J. Y., Harada, T., Komeda, H., Li, Z., Mano, Y., Saito, D., Parrish, T. B., et al. (2010). Dynamic cultural influences on neural representations of the self. *Journal of Cognitive Neuroscience, 22*(1), 1-11.

Chua, H. F., Boland, J. E., & Nisbett, R. E. (2005). Cultural variation in eye movements during scene perception. *Proceedings of the National Academy of Sciences USA, 102*(35), 12629-12633.

Cohen, N., Ryan, J., Hunt, C., Romine, L., Wszalek, T., & Nash, C. (1999). The Hippocampal System and Declarative (Relational) Memory: Evidence from Functional Neuroimaging Studies. *Hippocampus, 9*, 83-98.

Daselaar, S. M., Veltman, D. J., Rombouts, S. A. R. B., Raaijmakers, J. G. W., & Jonker, C. (2003). Neuroanatomical correlates of episodic encoding and retrieval in young and elderly subjects. *Brain, 126*(1), 43-56.

Davis, S. W., Dennis, N. A., Daselaar, S. M., Fleck, M. S., & Cabeza, R. (2008). Que PASA? The Posterior Anterior Shift in Aging. *Cerebral Cortex, 18*(5), 1201-1209.

Davis, S. W., Dennis, N. A., Buchler, N. G., White, L. E., Madden, D. J., & Cabeza, R. (2009). Assessing the effects of age on long white matter tracts using diffusion tensor tractography. *NeuroImage, 46*(2), 530-541.

Dennis, N. A., & Cabeza, R. (2008). Neuroimaging of healthy cognitive aging. *Handbook of Aging and Cognition* (Vol. 3, pp. 1-54). New York, USA: Psychology Press.

Draganski, B., Gaser, C., Busch, V., Schuierer, G., Bogdahn, U., & May, A. (2004). Neuroplasticity: changes in grey matter induced by training. *Nature, 427*(6972), 311-2.

Duverne, S., Motamedinia, S., & Rugg, M. D. (2009). The relationship between aging, performance, and the neural correlates of successful memory encoding. *Cerebral Cortex, 19*(3), 733-744.

Epstein, R., & Kanwisher, N. (1998). A cortical representation of the local visual environment. *Nature, 392*(6676), 598-601.

Fjell, A. M., Westlye, L. T., Amlien, I., Espeseth, T., Reinvang, I., Raz, N., Agartz, I., et al. (2009). High consistency of regional cortical thinning in aging across multiple samples. *Cerebral Cortex, 19*(9), 2001-2012.

Goh, J. O. S., Leshikar, E. D., Sutton, B. P., Tan, J. C., Sim, S. K. Y., Hebrank, A. C., & Park, D. C. (2010b). Culture differences in neural processing of faces and houses in the ventral visual cortex. *Social Cognitive and Affective Neuroscience, 5*(2-3), 227-235.

Goh, J. O., Chee, M. W., Tan, J. C., Venkatraman, V., Hebrank, A., Leshikar, E. D., Jenkins, L., et al. (2007). Age and culture modulate object processing and object-scene binding in the ventral visual area. *Cognitive, Affective & Behavioral Neuroscience, 7*(1), 44-52.

Goh, J. O., Siong, S. C., Park, D., Gutchess, A., Hebrank, A., & Chee, M. W. (2004). Cortical areas involved in object, background, and object-background processing revealed with functional magnetic resonance adaptation. *Journal of Neuroscience, 24*(45), 10223-10228.

Goh, J. O. S. (2011). Functional Dedifferentiation and Altered Connectivity in Older Adults: Neural Accounts of Cognitive Aging. *Aging and Disease, 2*(1), 30-48.

Goh, J. O., & Park, D. C. (2009a). Neuroplasticity and cognitive aging: The scaffolding theory of aging and cognition. *Restorative Neurology and Neuroscience, 27*(5), 391-403.

Goh, J. O., & Park, D. C. (2009b). Culture sculpts the perceptual brain. *Progress in Brain Research, 178,* 95-111.

Goh, J. O., Suzuki, A., & Park, D. C. (2010a). Reduced neural selectivity increases fMRI adaptation with age during face discrimination. *NeuroImage, 51*(1), 336-344.

Goh, J. O., Tan, J. C., & Park, D. C. (2009c). Culture modulates eye-movements to visual novelty. *PloS One, 4*(12), e8238.

Golarai, G., Ghahremani, D. G., Whitfield-Gabrieli, S., Reiss, A., Eberhardt, J. L., Gabrieli, J. D. E., & Grill-Spector, Kalanit. (2007). Differential development of high-level visual cortex correlates with category-specific recognition memory. *Nature Neuroscience, 10*(4), 512-522.

Goto, S. G., Ando, Y., Huang, C., Yee, A., & Lewis, R. S. (2010). Cultural differences in the visual processing of meaning: Detecting incongruities between background and foreground objects using the N400. *Social Cognitive and Affective Neuroscience, 5*(2-3), 242 -253.

Grady, C L, McIntosh, A R, Horwitz, B., Maisog, J. M., Ungerleider, L. G., Mentis, M. J., Pietrini, P., et al. (1995). Age-related reductions in human recognition memory due to impaired encoding. *Science, 269*(5221), 218-221.

Grady, Cheryl L. (2008). Cognitive neuroscience of aging. *Annals of the New York Academy of Sciences, 1124,* 127-144.

Green, D. W., Crinion, J., & Price, C. J. (2007). Exploring cross-linguistic vocabulary effects on brain structures using voxel-based morphometry. *Bilingualism: Language and Cognition, 10*(02), 189-199.

Greenwood, P. M. (2007). Functional Plasticity in Cognitive Aging: Review and Hypothesis. *Neuropsychology, 21*(6), 657.

Greicius, M. D., Krasnow, B., Reiss, A. L., & Menon, V. (2003). Functional connectivity in the resting brain: a network analysis of the default mode hypothesis. *Proceedings of the National Academy of Sciences of the United States of America, 100*(1), 253-258.

Grill-Spector, K., Kourtzi, Z., & Kanwisher, N. (2001). The lateral occipital complex and its role in object recognition. *Vision Res, 41*(10-11), 1409-1422.

Grill-Spector, K., Kushnir, T., Hendler, T., Edelman, S., Itzchak, Y., & Malach, R. (1998). A sequence of object-processing stages revealed by fMRI in the human occipital lobe. *Human Brain Mapping, 6*(4), 316-328.

Grill-Spector, K., & Malach, R. (2001). fMR-adaptation: A tool for studying the functional properties of human cortical neurons. *Acta Psychologica, 107*(1-3), 293-321.

Grill-Spector, K., & Malach, R. (2004). The human visual cortex. *Annual Review of Neuroscience, 27*, 649-677.

Grill-Spector, K., Golarai, G., & Gabrieli, J. (2008). Developmental neuroimaging of the human ventral visual cortex. *Trends in Cognitive Sciences, 12*(4), 152-162.

Gutchess, A. H., Welsh, R. C., Hedden, T., Bangert, A., Minear, M., Liu, L. L., & Park, D. C. (2005). Aging and the neural correlates of successful picture encoding: frontal activations compensate for decreased medial-temporal activity. *Journal of Cognitive Neuroscience, 17*(1), 84-96.

Gutchess, A. H., Welsh, R. C., Boduroglu, A., & Park, D. C. (2006). Cultural differences in neural function associated with object processing. *Cognitive, Affective & Behavioral Neuroscience, 6*(2), 102-109.

Han, S., & Northoff, G. (2008). Culture-sensitive neural substrates of human cognition: a transcultural neuroimaging approach. *Nature Reviews.Neuroscience, 9*(8), 646-54.

Hasher, L., & Zacks, R. T. (1988). Working memory, comprehension, and aging: A review and a new view. In G. H. Bower (Ed.), *The Psychology of Learning and Motivation* (Vol. 22, p. 193–225). San Diego, CA: Academic Press.

Haxby, J. V., Gobbini, M. I., Furey, M. L., Ishai, A., Schouten, J. L., & Pietrini, P. (2001). Distributed and overlapping representations of faces and objects in ventral temporal cortex. *Science, 293*(5539), 2425-2430.

Haxby, J. V., Hoffman, E. A., & Gobbini, M. I. (2000). The distributed human neural system for face perception. *Trends in cognitive sciences, 4*(6), 223-233.

Hayden, B. Y., Smith, D. V., & Platt, M. L. (2010). Cognitive control signals in posterior cingulate cortex. *Frontiers in Human Neuroscience, 4*, 223.

Head, D., Buckner, R. L., Shimony, J. S., Williams, L. E., Akbudak, E., Conturo, T. E., McAvoy, M., et al. (2004). Differential vulnerability of anterior white matter in nondemented aging with minimal acceleration in dementia of the Alzheimer type: evidence from diffusion tensor imaging. *Cerebral Cortex, 14*(4), 410-423.

Hedden, T., Park, D. C., Nisbett, R., Ji, L. J., Jing, Q., & Jiao, S. (2002). Cultural variation in verbal versus spatial neuropsychological function across the life span. *Neuropsychology, 16*(1), 65-73.

Hedden, Trey, Ketay, S., Aron, A., Markus, Hazel Rose, & Gabrieli, J. D. E. (2008). Cultural influences on neural substrates of attentional control. *Psychological Science, 19*(1), 12-7.

Henson, R. N. (2003). Neuroimaging studies of priming. *Progress in neurobiology, 70*(1), 53-81.

Heuninckx, S., Wenderoth, N., & Swinnen, S. P. (2008). Systems neuroplasticity in the aging brain: recruiting additional neural resources for successful motor performance in elderly persons. *Journal of Neuroscience, 28*(1), 91-9.

Hofstede, G. (1980). Culture and organizations. *International Studies of Management & Organization, 10*(4), 15–41.

Hofstede, G. (2001). *Culture's Consequences: Comparing Values, Behaviors, Institutions, and Organizations Across Nations.* Thousand Oaks, CA: Sage Publications.

Jenkins, L. J., Yang, Y. J., Goh, Joshua, Hong, Y. Y., & Park, Denise C. (2010). Cultural differences in the lateral occipital complex while viewing incongruent scenes. *Social Cognitive and Affective Neuroscience, 5*(2-3), 236-241.

Jimura, K., & Braver, T. S. (2010). Age-related shifts in brain activity dynamics during task switching. *Cerebral Cortex, 20*(6), 1420-1431.

Kaasinen, V., Vilkman, H., Hietala, J., Nagren, K., Helenius, H., Olsson, H., Farde, L., et al. (2000). Age-related dopamine D2/D3 receptor loss in extrastriatal regions of the human brain. *Neurobiology of Aging, 21*(5), 683-8.

Kanwisher, N., McDermott, J., & Chun, M. M. (1997). The fusiform face area: a module in human extrastriate cortex specialized for face perception. *Journal of Neuroscience, 17,* 4302-4311.

Kempermann, G., & Gage, F. H. (1999). Experience-dependent regulation of adult hippocampal neurogenesis: effects of long-term stimulation and stimulus withdrawal. *Hippocampus, 9*(3), 321-32.

Kempermann, G., Gast, D., & Gage, F. H. (2002). Neuroplasticity in old age: Sustained fivefold induction of hippocampal neurogenesis by long-term environmental enrichment. *Annals of Neurology, 52*(2), 135-143.

Kempermann, G., Kuhn, H. G., & Gage, F. H. (1998). Experience-induced neurogenesis in the senescent dentate gyrus. *Journal of Neuroscience, 18*(9), 3206-3212.

Kennedy, K. M., & Raz, N. (2009a). Aging white matter and cognition: differential effects of regional variations in diffusion properties on memory, executive functions, and speed. *Neuropsychologia, 47*(3), 916-927.

Kennedy, K. M., & Raz, N. (2009b). Pattern of normal age-related regional differences in white matter microstructure is modified by vascular risk. *Brain Research, 1297,* 41-56.

Kitayama, S., Duffy, S., Kawamura, T., & Larsen, J. T. (2003). Perceiving an object and its context in different cultures: a cultural look at new look. *Psychological Science, 14*(3), 201-206.

Kitayama, S., Markus, H. R, Matsumoto, H., & Norasakkunkit, V. (1997). Individual and collective processes in the construction of the self: Self-enhancement in the United States and self-criticism in Japan. *Journal of personality and social psychology, 72,* 1245–1267.

Kochunov, P., Fox, P., Lancaster, J., Tan, L. H., Amunts, K., Zilles, K., Mazziotta, J., et al. (2003). Localized morphological brain differences between English-speaking Caucasians and Chinese-speaking Asians: new evidence of anatomical plasticity. *Neuroreport, 14*(7), 961.

Leshikar, E. D., Gutchess, A. H., Hebrank, A. C., Sutton, B. P., & Park, D. C. (2010). The impact of increased relational encoding demands on frontal and hippocampal function in older adults. *Cortex, 46*(4), 507-521.

Leventhal, A. G., Wang, Y., Pu, M., Zhou, Y., & Ma, Y. (2003). GABA and its agonists improved visual cortical function in senescent monkeys. *Science, 300*(5620), 812-815.

Li, S. C. (2003). Biocultural orchestration of developmental plasticity across levels: the interplay of biology and culture in shaping the mind and behavior across the life span. *Psychological Bulletin, 129*(2), 171-194.

Li, S. C., & Sikström, S. (2002b). Integrative neurocomputational perspectives on cognitive aging, neuromodulation, and representation. *Neuroscience and Biobehavioral Reviews*, 26(7), 795-808.

Lindenberger, U., & Baltes, P. B. (1994). Sensory functioning and intelligence in old age: a strong connection. *Psychology and Aging*, 9(3), 339-355.

Logan, J. M., Sanders, A. L., Snyder, A. Z., Morris, J. C., & Buckner, R. L. (2002). Under-recruitment and nonselective recruitment dissociable neural mechanisms associated with aging. *Neuron*, 33(5), 827-840.

Madden, D. J., Turkington, T. G., Provenzale, J. M., Denny, L. L., Hawk, T. C., Gottlob, L. R., & Coleman, R. E. (1999). Adult age differences in the functional neuroanatomy of verbal recognition memory. *Human brain mapping*, 7(2), 115-35.

Maguire, E. A., Gadian, D. G., Johnsrude, I. S., Good, C D, Ashburner, J., Frackowiak, R. S., & Frith, C. D. (2000). Navigation-related structural change in the hippocampi of taxi drivers. *Proceedings of the National Academy of Sciences of the United States of America*, 97(8), 4398-4403.

Malach, R., Reppas, J. B., Benson, R. R., Kwong, K. K., Jiang, H., Kennedy, W. A., Ledden, P. J., et al. (1995). Object-related activity revealed by functional magnetic resonance imaging in human occipital cortex. *Proceedings of the National Academy of Sciences of the United States of America*, 92(18), 8135-8139.

Manly, J. J. (2008). Critical issues in cultural neuropsychology: profit from diversity. *Neuropsychology review*, 18(3), 179-83.

Masuda, T., Gonzalez, R., Kwan, L., & Nisbett, R. E. (2008a). Culture and aesthetic preference: Comparing the attention to context of East Asians and Americans. *Personality and Social Psychology Bulletin*, 34(9), 1260.

Masuda, T., & Nisbett, R. E. (2006). Culture and change blindness. *Cognitive Science*, 30, 1-19.

Masuda, T., Ellsworth, P. C., Mesquita, B., Leu, J., Tanida, S., & Van de Veerdonk, E. (2008b). Placing the face in context: cultural differences in the perception of facial emotion. *Journal of Personality and Social Psychology*, 94(3), 365-381.

Mayer, J. S., Roebroeck, A., Maurer, K., & Linden, D. E. J. (2010). Specialization in the default mode: Task-induced brain deactivations dissociate between visual working memory and attention. *Human Brain Mapping*, 31(1), 126-139.

Miellet, S., Zhou, X., He, L., Rodger, H., & Caldara, R. (2010). Investigating cultural diversity for extrafoveal information use in visual scenes. *Journal of Vision*, 10(6), 21.

Mishkin, M., Ungerleider, L. G., & Macko, K. A. (1983). Object vision and spatial vision: Two cortical pathways. *Trends in Neurosciences*, 6(10), 414-417.

Miyamoto, Y., Nisbett, R. E., & Masuda, T. (2006). Culture and the physical environment: Holistic versus analytic perceptual affordances. *Psychological Science*, 17(2), 113-119.

Morcom, A. M., Good, Catriona D, Frackowiak, R. S. J., & Rugg, M. D. (2003). Age effects on the neural correlates of successful memory encoding. *Brain*, 126(1), 213-229.

Murray, S. O., & Wojciulik, E. (2004). Attention increases neural selectivity in the human lateral occipital complex. *Nature Neuroscience*, 7(1), 70-74.

Nisbett, R. E. (2003). *The geography of thought: How Asians and Westerners think differently - And why*. New York: Free Press.

Nisbett, R. E., & Masuda, T. (2003). Culture and point of view. *Proceedings of the National Academy of Sciences*, 100(19), 11163-11170.

Nisbett, R. E., & Miyamoto, Y. (2005). The influence of culture: holistic versus analytic perception. *Trends in Cognitive Sciences, 9*(10), 467-473.

Nisbett, R. E., Peng, K., Choi, I., & Norenzayan, A. (2001). Culture and systems of thought: Holistic versus analytic cognition. *Psychological review, 108*(2), 291-310.

Oyserman, D., Coon, H. M., & Kemmelmeier, M. (2002). Rethinking individualism and collectivism: evaluation of theoretical assumptions and meta-analyses. *Psychological bulletin, 128*(1), 3-72.

Oyserman, D., & Lee, S. W. S. (2008). Does culture influence what and how we think? Effects of priming individualism and collectivism. *Psychological Bulletin, 134*(2), 311-342.

Park, D. C. (2008). Developing a cultural cognitive neuroscience of aging. *Handbook of Cognitive Aging* (pp. 352-367). Thousand Oaks, CA, USA: Sage Publications.

Park, D. C., & Goh, J. O. S. (2009). Successful aging. In J. Cacioppo & G. Berntson (Eds.), *Handbook of Neuroscience for the Behavioral Sciences* (pp. 1203-1219). Hoboken, NJ: John Wiley & Sons.

Park, D. C., & Gutchess, A. H. (2002). Aging, cognition, and culture: a neuroscientific perspective. *Neuroscience and Biobehavioral Reviews, 26*(7), 859-867.

Park, D. C., & Gutchess, A. H. (2005). Long-Term Memory and Aging: A Cognitive Neuroscience Perspective. *Cognitive Neuroscience of Aging: Linking Cognitive and Cerebral Aging* (pp. 218-245). New York, USA: Oxford University Press.

Park, D. C., & Huang, C. M. (2010). Culture Wires the Brain: A Cognitive Neuroscience Perspective. *Perspectives on Psychological Science, 5*, 391–400.

Park, D. C., Nisbett, R., & Hedden, T. (1999). Aging, culture, and cognition. *The Journals of Gerontology.Series B, Psychological Sciences and Social Sciences, 54*(2), P75-84; P75-84.

Park, D. C., Polk, T. A., Park, R., Minear, M., Savage, A., & Smith, M. R. (2004). Aging reduces neural specialization in ventral visual cortex. *Proceedings of the National Academy of Sciences of the United States of America, 101*(35), 13091-13095.

Park, D. C., & Reuter-Lorenz, P. (2009). The adaptive brain: aging and neurocognitive scaffolding. *Annual Review of Psychology, 60*(1), 173-196.

Park, D. C., Smith, A. D., Lautenschlager, G., Earles, J. L., Frieske, D., Zwahr, M., & Gaines, C. L. (1996). Mediators of long-term memory performance across the life span. *Psychology and aging, 11*(4), 621-637.

Park, D. C., Welsh, R. C., Marshuetz, C., Gutchess, A. H., Mikels, J., Polk, T. A., Noll, D. C., et al. (2003). Working memory for complex scenes: age differences in frontal and hippocampal activations. *Journal of cognitive neuroscience, 15*(8), 1122-1134.

Park, D., & Gutchess, A. (2006). The cognitive neuroscience of aging and culture. *Current Directions in Psychological Science, 15*(3), 105-108.

Park, D. C., Lautenschlager, G., Hedden, T., Davidson, N. S., Smith, A. D., & Smith, P. K. (2002). Models of visuospatial and verbal memory across the adult life span. *Psychology and Aging, 17*(2), 299-320.

Park, D. C., Polk, T. A., Hebrank, A. C., & Jenkins, L. J. (2010). Age differences in default mode activity on easy and difficult spatial judgment tasks. *Frontiers in Human Neuroscience, 3*, 75.

Park, J., Carp, J., Hebrank, A., Park, D. C., & Polk, T. A. (2010). Neural specificity predicts fluid processing ability in older adults. *Journal of Neuroscience, 30*(27), 9253-9259.

Polk, T. A., Stallcup, M., Aguirre, G. K., Alsop, D. C., D'Esposito, M., Detre, J. A., & Farah, M. J. (2002). Neural Specialization for Letter Recognition. *Journal of Cognitive Neuroscience, 14*(2), 145-159.

Raichle, M. E., MacLeod, A. M., Snyder, A. Z., Powers, W. J., Gusnard, D. A., & Shulman, G. L. (2001). A default mode of brain function. *Proceedings of the National Academy of Sciences of the United States of America, 98*(2), 676-682.

Rayner, K., Castelhano, M. S., & Yang, J. (2009). Eye movements when looking at unusual/weird scenes: Are there cultural differences? *Journal of Experimental Psychology.Learning, Memory, and Cognition, 35*(1), 254-9.

Raz, N., Lindenberger, Ulman, Rodrigue, K. M., Kennedy, K. M., Head, Denise, Williamson, A., Dahle, C., et al. (2005). Regional brain changes in aging healthy adults: general trends, individual differences and modifiers. *Cerebral Cortex, 15*(11), 1676-1689.

Raz, N., & Rodrigue, K. M. (2006). Differential aging of the brain: patterns, cognitive correlates and modifiers. *Neuroscience and Biobehavioral Reviews, 30*(6), 730-748.

Reuter-Lorenz, P. A., & Cappell, K. A. (2008). Neurocognitive aging and the compensation hypothesis. *Current Directions in Psychological Science, 17*(3), 177-182.

Reuter-Lorenz, P. A., Jonides, J., Smith, E. E., Hartley, A., Miller, A., Marshuetz, C., & Koeppe, R. A. (2000). Age differences in the frontal lateralization of verbal and spatial working memory revealed by PET. *Journal of Cognitive Neuroscience, 12*(1), 174-187.

Reuter-Lorenz, P. A., & Park, D. C. (2010). Human neuroscience and the aging mind: a new look at old problems. *Journal of Gerontology Series B: Psychological Sciences and Social Sciences, 65*(4), 405-415.

Rossi, S., Miniussi, C., Pasqualetti, P., Babiloni, C., Rossini, P. M., & Cappa, S. F. (2004). Age-related functional changes of prefrontal cortex in long-term memory: a repetitive transcranial magnetic stimulation study. *Journal of Neuroscience, 24*(36), 7939-44.

Rossion, B., Dricot, L., Devolder, A., Bodart, J. M., Crommelinck, M., De Gelder, B., & Zoontjes, R. (2000). Hemispheric asymmetries for whole-based and part-based face processing in the human fusiform gyrus. *Journal of Cognitive Neuroscience, 12*(5), 793-802.

Salat, D. H., Buckner, R. L., Snyder, A. Z., Greve, D. N., Desikan, R. S. R., Busa, E., Morris, J. C., et al. (2004). Thinning of the cerebral cortex in aging. *Cerebral Cortex, 14*(7), 721-730.

Salthouse, T. (1996). The processing-speed theory of adult age differences in cognition. *Psychol Rev, 103*(3), 403-428.

Schmolesky, M. T., Wang, Y., Pu, M., & Leventhal, A. G. (2000). Degradation of stimulus selectivity of visual cortical cells in senescent rhesus monkeys. *Nature Neuroscience, 3*(4), 384-390.

Schneider-Garces, N. J., Gordon, B. A., Brumback-Peltz, C. R., Shin, E., Lee, Y., Sutton, Bradley P, Maclin, E. L., et al. (2010). Span, CRUNCH, and beyond: working memory capacity and the aging brain. *Journal of Cognitive Neuroscience, 22*(4), 655-669.

Simons, D. J., & Ambinder, M. S. (2005). Change blindness. Theory and consequences. *Current Directions in Psychological Science, 14*(1), 44.

Simons, D. J., & Levin, D. T. (1997). Change blindness. *Trends in cognitive sciences*, *1*(7), 261-267.

Spiridon, M., & Kanwisher, N. (2002). How distributed is visual category information in human occipito-temporal cortex? An fMRI study. *Neuron*, *35*(6), 1157-1165.

Stark, S. M., Yassa, M. A., & Stark, C. E. L. (2010). Individual differences in spatial pattern separation performance associated with healthy aging in humans. *Learning & Memory*, *17*(6), 284-288.

Sutton, B. P., Goh, J., Hebrank, A., Welsh, R. C., Chee, M. W. L., & Park, D. C. (2008). Investigation and validation of intersite fMRI studies using the same imaging hardware. *Journal of Magnetic Resonance Imaging*, *28*(1), 21-28.

Triandis, H. C., Bontempo, R., Villareal, M. J., Asai, M., & Lucca, N. (1988). Individualism and collectivism: Cross-cultural perspectives on self-ingroup relationships. *Journal of personality and Social Psychology*, *54*(2), 323–338.

Triandis, H. C. (1995). *Individualism and Collectivism*. Boulder, CO, USA: Westview.

Vallesi, A., McIntosh, Anthony R, & Stuss, D. T. (2011). Overrecruitment in the aging brain as a function of task demands: evidence for a compensatory view. *Journal of Cognitive Neuroscience*, *23*(4), 801-815.

Voss, M. W., Erickson, K. I., Chaddock, L., Prakash, R. S., Colcombe, S. J., Morris, K. S., Doerksen, S., et al. (2008). Dedifferentiation in the visual cortex: an fMRI investigation of individual differences in older adults. *Brain Research*, *1244*, 121-31.

Wang, Q., & Leichtman, M. D. (2000). Same beginnings, different stories: a comparison of American and Chinese children's narratives. *Child Development*, *71*(5), 1329-1346.

Wang, Q. (2008). Emotion knowledge and autobiographical memory across the preschool years: a cross-cultural longitudinal investigation. *Cognition*, *108*(1), 117-135.

Wang, Y., Zhou, Y., Ma, Y., & Leventhal, A. G. (2005). Degradation of signal timing in cortical areas V1 and V2 of senescent monkeys. *Cerebral Cortex*, *15*(4), 403-408.

Whitfield, K., & Morgan, A. A. (2008). Minority populations and cognitive aging. *Handbook of Cognitive Aging* (pp. 384-397). Thousand Oaks, CA, USA: Sage.

Wlotko, E. W., Lee, C. L., & Federmeier, K. D. (2010). Language of the aging brain: Event-related potential studies of comprehension in older adults. *Language and Linguistics Compass*, *4*(8), 623-638.

Yi, D. J., Kelley, T. A., Marois, R., & Chun, M. M. (2006). Attentional modulation of repetition attenuation is anatomically dissociable for scenes and faces. *Brain Research*, *1080*(1), 53-62.

Yoon, C., Feinberg, F., Hu, P., Gutchess, A. H., Hedden, T., Chen, H. Y., Jing, Q., et al. (2004b). Category norms as a function of culture and age: comparisons of item responses to 105 categories by american and chinese adults. *Psychology and aging*, *19*(3), 379-393.

Yoon, C., Feinberg, F., Luo, T., Hedden, T., Gutchess, A. H., Chen, H. Y., Mikels, J. A., et al. (2004a). A cross-culturally standardized set of pictures for younger and older adults: American and Chinese norms for name agreement, concept agreement, and familiarity. *Behavior research methods, instruments, & computers : a journal of the Psychonomic Society, Inc*, *36*(4), 639-649.

Yoshida, K. A., Iversen, J. R., Patel, A. D., Mazuka, R., Nito, H., Gervain, J., & Werker, J. F. (2010). The development of perceptual grouping biases in infancy: a Japanese-English cross-linguistic study. *Cognition, 115*(2), 356-361.

Yu, S., Wang, Y., Li, X., Zhou, Y., & Leventhal, A. G. (2006). Functional degradation of extrastriate visual cortex in senescent rhesus monkeys. *Neuroscience, 140*(3), 1023-1029.

Zilles, K., Kawashima, R., Dabringhaus, A., Fukuda, H., & Schormann, T. (2001). Hemispheric shape of European and Japanese brains: 3-D MRI analysis of intersubject variability, ethnical, and gender differences. *NeuroImage, 13*(2), 262-271.

7

Resting State Blood Flow and Glucose Metabolism in Psychiatric Disorders

Nobuhisa Kanahara, Eiji Shimizu, Yoshimoto Sekine and Masaomi Iyo
Chiba University
Japan

1. Introduction

Over the last 20 years, SPECT and PET, along with CT and MRI have been the main methodologies used in studies investigating psychiatric disorders. The structural alterations in patients' brains found by CT and MRI are usually quite subtle, while those found by the nuclear imaging modalities (PET and SPECT) are more pronounced. Partly for this reason, the latter methods have led to discoveries in a wide range of psychiatric disorders. In the 90s, region of interest (ROI) method provided only sketchy results due to the low spatial resolution of the nuclear imaging, but rapid progression in analytic and statistical methods in the 2000s had led to more detailed and accurate determinations of the differences in regional cerebral blood flow (rCBF) and glucose metabolic ratios (rGMR) between patients and comparison subjects. On the other hand, whereas an improved understanding of the etiology of psychiatric disorders has led to significant progress in multiple research areas, SPECT and PET studies measuring only the rCBF/rGMR distribution at rest have come to face some limitations for elucidation of the disease pathophysiology. Accordingly, at resting studies using SPECT/PET have tended to focus on certain kinds of clinical information, such as symptomatology and treatment. This review summarizes the history of at rest SPECT and PET studies, and provides a comprehensive survey in psychiatric disorders including schizophrenia, major depressive disorder, bipolar disorder and obsessive-compulsive disorder.

2. Schizophrenia

Functional neuroimaging has been used to elucidate patterns of increased or decreased activity within the brains of schizophrenic and normal subjects during rest and various assigned tasks, revealing that the affected parts of the central nervous system are not contained within a single brain region, but rather lie within neural networks over several brain regions. Numerous structural brain researches studies employing CT and MRI have demonstrated significant volume reductions in key brain regions such as the lateral prefrontal cortex, anterior cingulate cortex (ACC), superior temporal cortex, hippocampus/parahippocampus, striatum and thalamus in patients with schizophrenia relative to normal subjects (Shenton et al., 2001). In support of these structural alterations, functional neuroimaging studies have produced representations of abnormalities in and across these regions. Taking these results together, a variety of symptoms, including hallucination/delusion and negative symptoms, have been attributed not to abnormalities in a single brain region but to abnormalities in a distributed network of spatially distinct regions. Furthermore, functional neuroimaging studies have demonstrated that antipsychotics have substantial effects on brain functions, and have helped to elucidate the differences in action mechanisms among them.

2.1 Hypofrontality and negative symptoms in schizophrenia

Ingvar and Franzen (1974) reported that patients with chronic schizophrenia showed significant reduction in the rCBF ratio of the frontal to occipital region compared to normal subjects and subjects with first-episode schizophrenia measured with ^{133}Xe. This was the first study to report an abnormality in rCBF in schizophrenia. Following this work, several other studies examined the resting state blood flow and metabolism (Buchsbaum et al., 1982; Wolkin et al., 1985; Tamminga et al., 1992; Sachdev et al., 1997) and repeatedly reported significant decreases in patients with schizophrenia relative to normal participants. On the other hand, there have been studies showing no difference in this parameter between patients and normal controls (Gur et al., 1995; Sabri et al., 1997, Scottish Schizophrenia Research Group, 1998), or even an increase in rCBF/rGMR in patients compared to normal controls (Cleghorn et al., 1989; Ebmeier et al., 1993).

Early studies on this issue have presented very disparate results with respect to not only the presence or absence of hypoperfusion/hypomtabolism, but also, in cases in which it was present, the degree, relevant regions and correlation with symptoms of hypoperfusion/hypometabolism. The reason for these differences is presumed to be the large number of confounding factors, such as disease heterogeneity, treatment with antipsychotics, imcompleteness of results derived from the ROI method, measured value of absolute or relative data, different reference regions for relative data, measurement conditions under varied physiological states, and so on. Therefore, additional explorations with a more sophisticated study design for the drug-naïve subjects group, the same scanning conditions and reliable analytic methods are needed to reach a definitive conclusion on this issue.

As for the effects of antipsychotic medications, several studies on drug-naïve patients with first-episode schizophrenia demonstrated a significant reduction in blood flow and metabolism in the frontal cortex relative to age-matched normal controls under a resting condition (Buchsbaum et al., 1992a; Steinberg et al., 1995; Vita et al., 1995; Erkwoh et al., 1997) and task-related activation (Andreasen et al., 1992, 1997; Ashton et al., 2000) and suggested that the abnormal reduction in the prefrontal region occurs from a very early stage of the disease. With respect to the problem of analytic methods, ROI methods have been a mainstream from the 80s to late 90s, but voxel-wise methods representative of Statistic Parametric Mapping (SPM) have prevailed from the mid-90s and are the standard modality at present. This voxel-wise methods have successfully addressed two important problems in brain analyses: individual structural differences between the brains of participants and examiners' arbitress on target brain regions depending on *a priori* hypothesis. Numerical researches based on these methods have demonstrated a significant reduction in particularly the lateral, medial and orbital phases of the prefrontal cortex relative to normal controls (Andreasen et al., 1997; Ashton et al., 2000; Kim et al., 2000; Potkin et al., 2002; Lehrer et al., 2005; Molina et al., 2005a, 2005b, 2009), and these findings have shown that areas with hypoperfusion and hypometabolism were pervasive and further accompanied by other areas with hyperperfusion/hypermetabolism within the frontal cortex (Andreasen et al., 1997; Kim et al., 2000). The measurement conditions used under rest or the performance of a given task should also be taken into consideration. Whereas most of the studies with SPECT have been conducted under a resting state, many studies using FDG-PET have performed the comparison under a cognitive task such as continuous performance task (CPT) or California verbal learning task (CVLT). This is because of the possibility that a spontaneous fluctuation of mental state under a resting condition during scanning could result in varied distribution of rGMR in the participant group as a whole. Indeed, several PET studies using CPT (Potkin et al., 2002; Molina et al., 2005a, 2005b, 2009) or a visual attention task (Lehrer et al., 2005) showed a significant reduction of rGMR in the prefrontal cortex in patients compared to normal controls, very similar to the results obtained in almost all studies under a resting state. Then, reduction of rCBF/rGMR in the prefrontal cortex in patients relative to normal controls under a static state during the performance of cognitive tasks and under a resting state collectively indicates hypofrontality.

Although earlier studies have dealt this issue with dichotomous problem; presence or absence of hypofrontality, afterward, improvements in research design and analytic methods provide more detailed information such as distributed patterns within the frontal lobe within patients' brains or the degree of difference of the finding between patients and controls. In this context, in some meta-analysis studies (Davidson and Heinrichs, 2003; Hill et al., 2004), the finding of hypofrontality has been supported and thus established as a more convictive finding in the disease.

The hypoperfusion and hypometabolism in the frontal lobe have been presumed to be closely linked with negative symptoms and cognitive impairments in schizophrenia. These notions were demonstrated by the negative relationship between negative symptoms and blood flow/metabolism (Liddle et al., 1992; Wolkin et al., 1992; Ebmeier et al., 1993; Schröder et al., 1996; Andreasen et al., 1997; Erkwoh et al., 1997; Sabri et al., 1997; Ashton et al., 2000) and the significant reductions of blood flow/metabolism in the patients group with profound negative symptoms (Potkin et al., 2002; Gonul et al., 2003a), although several negative studies have existed (Vita et al., 1995; Min et al., 1999). On the other hand, whereas the cognitive dysfunctions that have recently received so much attention are closely related with negative symptoms, the reports exploring the relationship between the impairments and at rest blood flow/metabolism are very restricted (Penadés et al., 2002; Molina et al., 2009). A hypodopaminergic state in the prefrontal cortex is presumed to underlie the negative symptoms and cognitive impairments (Lynch, 1992; Remington et al., 2011) and thus, in this context, it is noted that hypofrontality strongly suggests an important part of core pathophysiology in schizophrenia.

2.2 rCBF/rGMR patterns in key regions other than the frontal lobe

As for brain regions other than the frontal lobe, a number of previous studies have demonstrated substantial variations between the patients with schizophrenia and normal controls, with some reports observing increases in various activities and other reports documenting decreases, and thus no convincing consensus has been reached.

Both the lateral and medial phases in the temporal cortex have been closely related with positive symptoms, particularly hallucination and delusion. Based on accumulating evidence from fMRI studies, for example, the primary auditory cortex located in the superior temporal cortex has been demonstrated to be closely related to auditory hallucination (Dierks et al., 1999; Lennox et al., 2000). Indeed, the first-episode and drug-naïve patients with auditory hallucinations presented higher (Horga et al., 2011) and lower metabolism (Cleghorn et al., 1992; Vita et al., 1995) compared with normal controls. Further, activity in this region was reported to be negatively associated with disorganization as a form of thought disorders (Ebmeier et al., 1993; Erkwoh et al., 1997; Sabri et al., 1997). The hippocampal and/or parahippocampal gyrus are also related with hallucination/delusion and disorganization. PET studies have shown an increase (Gur et al., 1995; Molina et al., 2005b) and decrease (Tamminga et al., 1992; Kim et al., 2000; Horga et al., 2011) in rCBF/rGMR of the regions in schizophrenia compared with normal controls, and positive (Liddle et al., 1992) and negative correlations (Schröder et al., 1996) between metabolism in the regions and hallucinations. Although these reports have very conflicting results and do not reach a definitive conclusion, they do suggest that both the lateral and medial parts of the temporal lobe are closely related with the positive symptoms.

The findings of activity within other key brain regions in schizophrenia have been very controversial. As for the striatum, several reports on drug-naïve patients have shown a significant reduction relative to normal controls (Buchsbaum et al., 1987, 1992a; Shihabuddin et al., 1998), suggesting a relation with putative neurological soft signs in the very early stage (Dazzan et al., 2004). The thalamus has a function of filtering all sensory signals from input to the cortex, and is known to play a primary role in the etiology of schizophrenia- namely, dysfunction in the correct perception of information- from the external world. The activity in the thalamus has been alternatively reported to increase (Andreasen et al., 1997; Jacobsen et al., 1997; Kim et al., 2000; Clark et al., 2001) or decrease (Vita et al., 1995; Hazlett et al., 1999, 2004; Buchsbaum et al., 1996; Lehrer et al., 2005). Moreover, increases of rCBF/rGMR in the cerebellum (Andreasen et al., 1997; Kim et al., 2000; Desco et al., 2003) and the subcortical regions (Buchsbaum et al., 1998, 2007a; Desco et al., 2003) have been observed. As described above, attempts to clarify the pathophysiology of schizophrenia have focused on brain regions from the frontal and temporal cortex to the subcortical regions including the striatum, thalamus, hippocampus and cerebellum. It appears that the approach of elucidating the pathophysiology requires an integrative interpretation based on the putative aberrant networks and their correlation with symptoms. Taken together, these findings suggest that resting blood flow and metabolism studies contribute to the elucidation of the disease pathophysiology by macroscopic investigation over the whole brain and microscopic investigation focusing on key regions.

2.3 Impacts of antipsychotics on blood flow and metabolism

Antipsychotics have some significant effects on brain blood flow and metabolism, and are presumed to be closely related to the potency of neuroleptics. All antipsychotics commonly induce dopamine (DA) D2 receptor antagonistic actions, resulting in the most direct action for improvement of delusions and hallucinations. Traditionally, typical antipsychotics such as haloperidol, an almost pure DA D2 blocker, had been widely used. But more recently, atypical antipsychotics have become the mainstay in the clinical practice. These atypical antipsychotics can reduce the extra-pyramidal symptoms and improve the negative symptoms and cognitive impairments by an antagonistic action on the 5-HT 2A receptors. Functional neuroimaging studies have provided important insights about the differences in pharmacological action and treatment effect among a diverse range of antipsychotics, and the subsequent functional changes in the central nervous system.

A number of previous studies have shown that typical neuroleptics such as haloperidol reduce blood flow and metabolism in the frontal lobe. These effects were repeatedly replicated in studies of both acute (Bartlett et al., 1998; Lahti et al., 2005) and chronic administration (Bartlett et al., 1991; Buchsbaum et al., 1992b; Miller et al., 1997, 2001; Lahti et al., 2003). Further, whereas haloperidol was reported to be related with hypoperfusion and hypometabolism in the hippocampus in terms of amelioration of positive symptoms (Lahti et al., 2003), increases of rCBF/rGMR in the motor cortex induced by haloperidol were presumed to be related with extra-pyramidal symptoms (Molina et al., 2003; Buchsbaum et al., 2007), and the decrease in activity in the occipital cortex following haloperidol treatment might be related with sedative effects (Bartlett et al., 1991; Desco et al., 2003; Lahti et al., 2003).

An increase in rCBF/rGMR in the basal ganglia in patients with schizophrenia by neuroleptics, in particular haloperidol, is the most consistent finding among numerous reports on antipsychotics. This has been replicated very well in the acute effect (Lahti et al., 2005) as well as the chronic effect (Buchsbaum et al., 1987, 1992a, 2007a; Miller et al., 1997, 2001; Scottish Schizophrenia Research Group, 1998; Corson et al., 2002; Desco et al., 2003; Lahti et al., 2003). The increase of blood flow and metabolism in this area is presumed to be due to increases of activity in the post synapses through upregulation of DA D2 receptors induced by a potent blocking action of the receptor by haloperidol (Miller et al., 1997; Corson et al., 2002). This notion is in line with the increase of volume in this area following haloperidol treatment in structural MRI studies (Shenton et al., 2001).

Studies on the effects of atypical antipsychotics on brain perfusion/metabolism have become to be examined based on more detailed neuronal substrates than studies on typical antipsychotics by appearance of voxel wise analysis. Although risperidone has less effect on the reduction of blood flow in the frontal lobe than haloperidol (Miller et al., 2001), the drug induces a significant reduction in the prefrontal cortex relative to baseline (Berman et al., 1996; Liddle et al., 2000; Ngan et al., 2002; Molina et al., 2008). In the basal ganglia, the degree of increase in blood flow/metabolism by risperidone is likely smaller than that by haloperidol (Liddle et al., 2000; Miller et al., 2001). Liddle et al. (2000) demonstrated that treatment with risperidone for 6 weeks showed a significant positive relation between decrease in the hippocampus and decrease in reality distortion, suggesting that the hippocampus is an important target area of risperidone.

Olanzapine is likely that its effect of blood flow/metabolism in the frontal lobe is lesser than that by risperidone (Gonul et al., 2003b; Molina et al., 2005c; Buchsbaum et al., 2007b).

Clozapine, the gold standard among the atypical neuroleptics, has a pharmacological profile with weaker blockade of DA D2 receptors and broader actions for multiple receptors than other atypical antipsychotics, and these characteristics are presumed to be related to its superior clinical efficacy relative to other neuroleptics. Interestingly, several previous studies have reported that clozapine induced a significant reduction in blood flow/metabolism in the prefrontal cortex (Potkin et al., 1994, 2003; Cohen et al., 1997; Lahti et al., 2003; Molina et al., 2005d, 2008). On the other hand, increases in several parts of the prefrontal cortex, including the ACC (Lahti et al., 2003) and decreases in the hippocampus (Lahti et al., 2003; Potkin et al., 2003) have been shown by some studies, supporting the drug's clinical actions such as ameliorations of delusions/hallucinations and cognitive impairments. Indeed, responders to clozapine exhibited more prominent changes in blood flow/metabolism above mentioned rather than non-responders (Potkin et al., 2003; Molina et al., 2008). These complex patterns induced by clozapine have been suggested to be strongly related to the drug's superior clinical characteristics.

2.4 Conclusion

Functional neuroimaging studies performed in schizophrenic subjects under a resting state have made progress in the accumulation of findings on hypoperfusion/hypometabolism in the frontal lobe. It is noted that the hypofrontality is closely related with negative symptoms. On the other hand, the brain regions relevant to positive symptoms are still clearly unknown. The studies performed thus far have well explored the effects of various antipsychotics on the brain blood flow and metabolism, but neuroleptic-induced reductions in blood flow/metabolism in the prefrontal cortex have been obscure in terms of their relationship with the improvement of positive symptoms or secondary negative symptoms. By contrast, alteration in the limbic regions or the medial phase of the temporal cortex, such as the hippocampus, has been shown to be related with positive symptoms, and functional neuroimaging studies have contributed to detection of the origin of positive symptoms.

3. Major Depressive Disorder

Functional neuroimaging studies measuring at-rest brain perfusion and metabolism in patients with major depressive disorder (MDD) have demonstrated that the etiology of the disease is closely linked with multiple components of the frontal lobe, temporal lobe, parietal lobe, limbic/paralimbic regions, and basal ganglia. Recent knowledge on affection and perception acquired from multiple human and animal research fields strongly support the findings that have been observed within depressive patients' brains in neuroimaging studies. Although a number of functional neuroimaging studies for MDD have been conducted to date, the results were varied widely among the studies. However, a sequence of inconsistent findings on MDD has demonstrated that depressive patient groups consist of highly heterogeneous subtypes, and that the etiology of depression contains multiple symptoms.

Studies on the effects of antidepressants on brain perfusion and metabolism have reported the relatively consistent finding that abnormal activity in the key brain regions relevant to depression could be normalized by successful treatment. However, no reliable markers on response prediction have been available to date in the imaging studies. On the other hand, studies of electroconvulsive therapy (ECT), an established treatment modality for refractory depression, have suggested that its effective mechanism is involved in the inhibitory process within subjects' brains that occurred immediately following the ECT course.

3.1 Abnormalities in multiple prefrontal cortex and limbic regions in MDD

Earlier functional neuroimaging studies on depression have reported significant reduction in rCBF/rGMR in the frontal lobe or prefrontal cortex in patients with depression relative to normal subjects (Baxter et al., 1989; Martinot et al., 1990; Bench et al., 1992). However, several subsequent studies with the voxel based analyses have failed to confirm this finding (Skaf et al., 2002; Videbach et al., 2002; Bonne et al., 2003). Great progression made in research on human and animal emotion and perception has elucidated that the frontal lobe and limbic/paralimbic systems are tightly involved in affective and perceptive controls, including   mood,   attention,   decision-making,   anxiety,   behaviors   dependent   on reward/punishment, and so on. It is, therefore, very reasonable that hypoactivity in the frontal lobe is observed in subjects with depression relative to normal subjects. Inconsistent results among the previous studies mentioned above, suggest great heterogeneity of patients with the disease. Therefore, a number of confounding factors, such as age, sex, brain organic condition (ischemia and atrophy), pharmacotherapy (drug class, dose and duration), and disease stage (acute or remit), could easily affect brain activity, leading to a varied distribution of rCBF/rGMR in the patient group as a whole.

Studies with careful sample selection, in which subjects who were, for example, in a drug-naïve state or in withdrawal from antidepressants for several weeks, were careful selected in order to reduce the heterogeneity have reported significant hypoperfusion and hypometabolism in the dorsolateral prefrontal cortex in subjects with depression relative to normal controls (Kimbrell et al., 2002; Gonul et al., 2004). The reduction in activity in this region was the most consistent finding among those in the frontal lobe as a whole. Additionally, rCBF and rGMR in the dorsolateral prefrontal cortex were negatively correlated with the severity of depression (Baxter et al., 1989; Martinot et al., 1990; Hurwitz et al., 1990; Bonne et al., 1996; Kimbrell et al., 2002; Gonul et al., 2004). Subanalyses of each symptom have shown the degree of psycho-motor retardation and the activity in the prefrontal cortex to be negative correlated (Bench et al., 1993; Dolan et al., 1993; Videbach et al., 2002). Although increased activities in the ventrolateral prefrontal cortex and OFC have been suggested by a sequence of studies by Drevets (Drevets et al., 1992, 1997; Drevets, 1999, 2000), other studies did not sufficiently examine these areas. With respect to the medial prefrontal cortex and ACC, although most studies with relatively large ROIs in this area, observed hypoperfusion and hypometabolism (Hurwitz et al., 1990; Bench et al., 1992, 1993; Bonne et al., 1996; Mayberg et al., 1997; Videbach et al., 2002; Gonul et al., 2004), several detailed studies on these regions demonstrated decreased activities in the dorsal medial prefrontal and dorsal ACC (Kimbrell et al., 2002; Fitzgerald et al., 2008) and increased activities in the rostral ACC (Drevets, 1999; Konarski et al., 2007). In particular, the latter region was suggested that the greater perfusion and metabolism was, the better clinical response to antidepressant treatment was predicted (Mayberg et al., 1997).

As for the limbic region, increases in rCBF/rGMR in the amygdala (Drevets et al., 1992; Abercrombie et al., 1998; Videbach et al., 2002) and caudate (Gonul et al., 2004; Périco et al., 2005) were observed in patients with depression relative to normal subjects. The subgenual ACC, a component within the paralimbic system, was hypoactive in patients with unipolar depression (Drevets et al., 1997; Skaf et al., 2002; Fitzgerald et al., 2008), but also in patients with bipolar depression (Drevets et al., 1997). The caudate was also reported to show hypometabolism (Baxter et al., 1985; Drevets et al., 1992). These reductions in activity in anatomically small areas, such as the subgenual ACC and caudate, might be due to the partial volume effects (Krishnan et al., 1992; Drevets, 2000). The ventrolateral prefrontal cortex, including the subgenual ACC, has closely reciprocal connectivities with the amygdala, hypotharamus and brain stem, and disturbances of these networks could lead to the hypersensitivity to failure, pathological guilt and exaggeration of self-esteem shown in patients with MDD.

3.2 Change of rCBF/rGMR induced by antidepressants and ECT

Antidepressant agents are shown to be effective for 50-60% patients with MDD (Hirschfeld et al., 2002), and only 20-35% of patients reach remission (Mann, 2005). While diverse classes of antidepressants are available in clinical practice at present, studies on the effect of specific antidepressants on brain perfusion or metabolism and the studies on the relationship between clinical improvement and the brain activity induced by antidepressants have been very restricted, and, further, the few such studies that exist usually have very small sample sizes. According to previous studies on these issues, aberrant regions at baseline prior to initial treatment in subjects with MDD appear to be normalized, particularly in responders to the agent. However, it is very uncertain whether the abnormalities can be recovered to a level similar to that in normal subjects (Baxter et al., 1985, 1989; Tutus et al., 1998; Ishizaki et al., 2008) or remain to a certain degree (Hurwitz et al., 1990; Martinoti et al., 1990). The discrepancies among these studies might be due to differences in class, dose of antidepressant, diverse treatment durations, different definitions of effectiveness or recovery of symptoms, or small sample sizes. Several selective serotonin reuptake inhibitors (SSRIs; paroxetine and citalopram) and serotonin and noradrenaline reuptake inhibitors (SNRIs; venlafaxine) in some well-designed studies have been examined most extensively in terms of their effects on brain perfusion/metabolism in patients with MDD. However, although several key regions, such as the frontal, temporal, parietal, and limbic regions and the basal ganglia, have been widely found to be relevant areas affected by the depressants studied, consistent findings on the combination of the relevant areas or their change directions have been very scarce. With respect to the prediction of the response to antidepressants, the greater the perfusion in the ACC (Mayberg et al., 1997), rectul gyrus (Buchsbaum et al., 1997), and lateral prefrontal cortex (Joe et al., 2006; Brockmann et al., 2009) prior to treatment was, the better the expected response. On the other hand, a decrease in rCBF/rGMR prior to treatment in the ACC (Brody et al., 1999; Konarski et al., 2009), lateral prefrontal cortex (Navarro et al., 2004) and hippocampus/basal ganglia/thalamus (Milak et al., 2009) led to a good treatment response. Therefore, the studies on this issue to date have failed to confirm conclusions.

ECT is usually indicated the patients with MDD who have been treatment-resistant to antidepressants. While this modality provides a relatively high rate of response for these patients, the understanding of its mechanism of action remains very poor. During seizures induced by ECT, evident reductions in rCBF/rGMR occurred over large brain areas (Takano et al., 2007). Afterwards, hypoperfusion and hypometabolism, to a lesser degree than during the seizure, in several brain regions, including the prefrontal region, have continued for a maximum of several months. This findings is presumed to be related to clinical responsiveness (Prohovnik et al., 1986; Rosenberg et al., 1988; Guze et al., 1991). However, some studies have demonstrated significant increases in rCBF in several brains (Bonne et al., 1996; Kohn et al., 2007). These discrepancies might be due to several confounding factors, such as procedural-related factors including anesthetics and electrode replacements, or to varying durations between the termination of the ECT course and imaging scanning.

3.3 Conclusion
The etiology of depression is strongly suggested to be related to the frontal lobe and limbic/paralimbic regions. However, the highly heterogeneity of patients with depression could lead to inconsistent results observed among studies. In addition, assessing the results in anatomically small areas or components with obscure boundaries, such as the subgenual ACC, amygdala, and OFC, is very difficult, and this serious problem in the interpretations of these regions stems from the effects of volume reduction in these regions in patients with

depression relative to normal. With respect to antidepressants and ECT, their mechanisms have been under examination.

4. Bipolar Disorder

Bipolar Disorder is characterized by distinctive affective labile episodes of manic/hypomanic state and/or depressive state. Concurrently, cognitive dysfunctions such as impairments of attention, working memory and executive function usually accompany the disease. Based on recent careful clinical observations, lifetime prevalence, including all bipolar II disorder, subthreshold bipolar disorder and drug-induced manic/hypomanic episode, is up to 5% (Merikangas et al., 2007). About 60% of patients with bipolar disorder are misdiagnosed as having MDD, and further, one-third of patients experience any psychiatric symptoms for more than 10 years before a correct diagnosis is made (Hirschfeld et al., 2003). Therefore, understanding the pathophysiology of bipolar disorder is very important for exact diagnosis and effective treatment. In neuroimaging studies on bipolar disorder, however, there have been a number of difficulties with the research, such as difficulty in recruiting patients with mania into the study and with safely scanning them, and the large heterogeneity within such patient groups in terms of affective state and disease subtype. Therefore, neuroimaging studies conducted to date have tended to have small sample sizes. Also, almost all studies on bipolar disorder have employed depressive patient groups combining cases of bipolar and unipolar depression, and the data acquired to date in manic and euthymic patients have been relatively restricted compared to the findings in depressive patients. In this context, resting state rCBF/rGMR studies on bipolar disorder have appeared to be inconsistent (Stoll et al., 2000; Strakowski et al., 2000). Still, recent resting state studies are providing a cortical-anterior subcortical dysfunction model of the disease pathology through several kinds of examination, including studies on mania and comparative studies between bipolar and unipolar depression (Keener and Phillips, 2007; Pan et al., 2009).

4.1 Bipolar mania

There have been few studies on manic patients, and those that have been performed have been largely biased by very small sample size, patients with manic level that can cooperate with study, and continuous pharmacotherapy consisting of a mixture of mood stabilizers, antidepressants and antipsychotics. In these studies, rCBF/rGMR reduction in the prefrontal cortice, particularly the ventral prefrontal cortex and increase in the subcortical areas compared to normal controls have been relatively consistent, providing cortical-subcortical or cortical–limbic/paralimbic regions impairment as a disease model in bipolar disorder. Decrease in brain perfusion/metabolism in the frontal cortex has been reported in the lateral prefrontal cortex at rest (al-Mousawi et al., 1996; Bhardwaj et al., 2010; Brooks III et al., 2010) and during cognitive tasks (Blumberg et al., 1999; Rubinsztein et al., 2001) and in the orbitofrontal cortex at rest (Blumberg et al., 1999) and during cognitive tasks (Blumberg et al., 1999; Rubinsztein et al., 2001). On the other hand, increases of rCBF/rGMR have been reported in the dorsal ACC (Rubinsztein et al., 2001), caudal ACC (Blumberg et al., 2000) and ventral/subgenual ACC (Drevets et al., 1997; Blumberg et al., 2000; Brooks III et al., 2010) and the head of the caudate (Blumberg et al., 2000; Brooks III et al., 2010). Goodwin et al. (1997) reported that in patients with relapsed manic episodes following withdrawal of lithium, increase of rCBF in the ACC was positively correlated with manic symptoms. These findings lead to and partly support the anatomical-functional hypothesis that while the orbitofrontal and lateral prefrontal impairments are related with affective/impulsive dysregulation and cognitive dysfunction, respectively, compensatory functional hyperactivity reflects the findings of increase in the ACC and limbic/paralimbic regions observed in resting-state studies (Keener and Phillips, 2007; Pan et al., 2009).

4.2 Bipolar depression

Although there have been more reports on bipolar depression than on mania, the findings from this body of work are rather confusing. This may be due, at least in part, to the design of these studies. That is, earlier studies have frequently used a disease group combining cases of unipolar and bipolar depression, and when they have compared bipolar depression with other conditions, they have alternatively used normal healthy subjects, patients with unipolar depression and subjects with mania/euthymia as the comparison group. Moreover, the different studies have different target regions (ACC, subgenual prefrontal cortex and amygdala). With respect to the cortex, although few reports demonstrated any regions with hyperperfusion and hypermetabolism in bipolar depression relative to normal controls, areas with hypoperfusion/hypometabolosm in the patients compared to normal controls spread very broader in the lateral prefrontal (Baxter et al., 1985, 1989; Ketter et al., 2001; Brooks III et al., 2009a), medial prefrontal (Baxter et al., 1985; Bauer et al., 2005; Brooks III et al., 2009a), subgenual ACC (Drevets et al., 1997; Brooks III et al., 2009a), temporal lobe (Baxter et al., 1985; Ketter et al., 2001; Bhardwaj et al., 2010), occipital lobe (Baxter et al., 1985; Ketter et al., 2001) and parietal lobe (Baxter et al., 1985; Ketter et al., 2001). On the other hand, hyperperfusion/hypermetabolism have also been observed in the subcortical or limbic/paralimbic areas, including the amygdala (Ketter et al., 2001; Drevets et al., 2002; Bauer et al., 2005; Mah et al., 2007), subgenual ACC (Drevets et al., 1997; Bauer et al., 2005; Mah et al., 2007), ventral striatum (Bauer et al., 2005), caudate nucleus (Ketter et al., 2001; Mah et al., 2007), and putamen (Ketter et al., 2001; Mah et al., 2007), nucleus accumbens (Ketter et al., 2001; Mah et al., 2007), thalamus (Ketter et al., 2001; Bauer et al., 2005) and cerebellum (Bauer et al., 2005).

There have been a few reports comparing patients with bipolar depression and bipolar mania within the same study. Examination of the subgenual ACC (Brodmann area 25) by Drevets et al. (1997) demonstrated clear distinction of increased activity when mania and decreased activity when depression, and growing attention has been paid to this area as a mood-state marker in bipolar disorder. However, some subsequent studies showed higher metabolism in the depressive state (Bauer et al., 2005; Mah et al., 2007), indicating a failure to conform. The inconsistency among studies on small anatomical area such as the subgenual ACC may be related to shortcomings in the characteristics of nuclear imaging, such as insufficient spatial resolution of the scanner or inaccurate normalization to the standard brain (Drevets et al., 2002).

4.3 Euthymia

Although manic state and depressive state represent clinically extreme and opposite symptoms, neuroimaging findings on the two states are relatively similar. Thus, a cortical-subcortical model raises some questions as to whether this model means trait marker in the disease, or whether reliable mood-state markers in the disease exist. In this context, studies on euthymia will be more and more important for addressing these issues.

Some studies on patients with euthymic state compared to normal controls have reported a decrease of rCBF/rGMR in the lateral prefrontal (Culha et al., 2008; Brooks III et al., 2009b) and ACC (Culha et al., 2008) at rest, and the lateral prefrontal (Krüger et al., 2003) and OFC (Blumberg et al., 1999; Krüger et al., 2003) during cognitive tasks or symptom-provocation. On the other hand, regions with increased perfusion/metabolism were observed in the subcortical areas such as the amygdala (Brooks III et al., 2009b) and parahippocampus (Brooks III et al., 2009b) at rest. Krüger et al (2003, 2006) in symptom-provocation studies demonstrated that although increased rCBF in the subgenual ACC seen in normal controls was deficit in euthymic patients, increased perfusion in the dorsal ACC was observed only in the patients. Though there have been very few studies conducted on euthymia, patients with euthymia appear to show a decrease of rCBF/rGMR in the prefrontal cortex and an increase in rCBF/rGMR in the subcortical areas, according to previous reports. These notions are comparable to recent clinical observations that patients in a euthymic state show significant cognitive impairments identical to the distinctive pathological states of mania and depression (Kessing, 1998; Elshahawi et al., 2011), and they are in preparatory stage to relapse fragile to stress (Swann, 2010), but not asymptomatic state not meeting manic and depression.

4.4 Conclusion

Functional neuroimaging studies on bipolar disorder have demonstrated hypoactivity in the cortex, particularly the ventral prefrontal cortex, and concurrent hyperactivity in the subcortical or limbic/paralimbic regions. To data, however, this knowledge has not reflected the clinical bipolarity of mania and depression and thus remains a trait marker. Furthermore, these findings cannot be distinguished from those of other psychiatric disorders, including unipolar depression. Studies with more sophisticated designed and larger sample size will be needed in the future.

5. Obsessive-Compulsive Disorder

Obsessive-compulsive disorder (OCD) has a lifetime prevalence of 2-3% (Weissman et al., 1994). OCD is characterized by persistent and recurrent thoughts that invade conscious awareness against a patient's will (obsessions) and is further usually accompanied by ego-dystonic, ritualistic behaviors that the patient is obliged to perform in order to prevent overwhelming anxiety (compulsions). Patients with OCD form a more homogeneous group than those with other psychiatric disorders, and this perhaps accounts for the fact that previous functional neuroimaging studies have provided relatively consistent findings on aberrant brain regions in this disorder, which include the OFC, ACC, caudate nuclei, thalamus and so on. That is, the etiology of OCD has been presumed to follow a cortico-subcortical model. Functional neuroimaging techniques have contributed substantially to the exploration of these areas relevant to the disorder. Furthermore, recent reports on treatment intervention for OCD have strongly suggested that selective serotonin reuptake inhibitors (SSRI) and cognitive behavior therapy (CBT), both established treatment approaches, raise some effects on patients' brain blood flow and metabolism, and further normalize aberrant regional perfusion and metabolism within these networks in treatment responders.

5.1 Dysfunction of the orbitofrontal-subcortical circuit in OCD

The basal ganglia is a candidate abnormal area in OCD to which great attention was initially paid. The reason for this is a high rate of patients with obsessive symptoms were found to have certain diseases, such as Von Economo encephalitis (Schilder, 1938), Sydenham's chorea (Swedo et al., 1989) and Tourette's syndrome (Nee et al., 1980), which have presumed to be impaired in the basal ganglia. Afterwards, functional neuroimaging studies on OCD have focused on the striatum, in particular caudate nucleus as aberrant region within patients' brains and concurrently have successively detected some abnormal brain areas such as the OFC, ACC and thalamus in patients with OCD, when compare them with normal healthy subjects. In this context, researchers have proposed a dysfunction of cortico-striatum-thalamus-cortical network as an etiological model of OCD (Modell et al., 1989; Baxter et al., 1996; Saxena et al., 1998).

It has been classically recognized that the cortico-subcortical network consists of direct and indirect pathways. The thalamus in the network has a gating function which filters all stimuli from the outer world and receives two main inputs from the striatum. The one is the direct pathway where signals from the striatum input to the thalamus via the globus pallidus internal/substantial nigra and the other is the indirect pathway where signals from the striatum input to the globus pallidus internal/substantial nigra through the globus pallidus external or subthalamic nucleus, and are further sent to the thalamus. Afterwards, feedback signals from the thalamus are sent to the cortex. These pathways consist of neurotransmissions combined with excitatory signals by glutamate and inhibitory signals by GABA. The direct pathway inputting to the thalamus disinhibits the thalamus (reinforcement of positive feedback) and the indirect pathway inhibits the thalamus (negative feedback), thereby helping to maintain the balance of the system (Alexander and Crutcher, 1990). In patients with OCD, it is presumed that this circuit represents an imbalance of hyperactivity. In the dysfunctional network, impairment in the striatum leads to an insufficient gating function of the thalamus, resulting in cortical hyperactivities. In this context, the direct pathway in the patients with OCD predominates over the indirect pathway. In terms of symptom-relations, the striatum is essentially involved in unconscious acquisition of the initial process of action or behavior, and hypermobilization of the impaired striatum could lead to compulsive symptoms in the manner of ritual behaviors, in order to normalize the undesirable thoughts or anxieties occurring via the dysfunctional thalamus. On the other hand, these invasive thoughts and excess anxieties would relate with hyperactivity in the OFC and ACC, respectively.

Previous functional neuroimaging studies in subjects at rest or undergoing symptom-provocation have implicated an increase in rCBF/rGMR in the OFC (Baxter et al., 1987, 1988; Benkelfat et al., 1990; Horwitz et al., 1991; Rubin et al., 1992, 1995; McGuire et al., 1994; Alptekin et al., 2001), ACC (Swedo et al., 1989; Horwitz et al., 1991; Perani et al., 1995), caudate nucleus (Baxter et al., 1987, 1988; Diler et al., 2004; Saxena et al., 2004), putamen (Benkelfat et al., 1990; Perani et al., 1995) and thalamus (McGuire et al., 1994; Perani et al., 1995; Alptekin et al., 2001; Saxena et al., 2001, 2004), strongly suggesting hyperactivities in the cortico-subcortical loop in patients with OCD. However, other studies have demonstrated inverse results, i.e., decreases in the OFC (Crespo-Faccoro et al., 1999; Busatto et al., 2000), ACC (Busatto et al., 2000), caudate nucleus (Rubin et al., 1992, 1995; Edmonstone et al., 1994; Lucey et al., 1995, 1997), putamen (Edmonstone et al.,

1994) and thalamus (Martinot et al., 1990; Lucey et al., 1995). These discrepancies were presumed to be due to varied treatment duration of serotonin reuptake inhibitors (SRIs) (Rubin et al., 1995), or to childhood- or adult-onset of the disease (Geller et al., 1995), presence or absence of comorbidity disorders such as MDD or tic disorder (Crespo-Faccoro et al., 1999; Hoehn-Saric et al., 2001) and the measurement of different parameters (brain blood flow or metabolism). Interestingly, whereas SPECT studies tended to indicate a decrease in rCBF, FDG-PET studies tended to show an increase in rGMR in the key regions in the disease, suggesting a possibility of uncoupling between brain blood flow and glucose utilization (Whiteside et al., 2004). At the very least, these regions are closely involved in the pathophysiology of OCD.

Studies on the relation between the symptom severity and the degree of abnormality in these areas have presented very varied results and failed to provide consistent findings.

5.2 Change following intervention by SRIs and cognitive-behavior therapy

Previous studies have replicated well that aberrant findings of rCBF/rGMR relevant to OCD-related regions could be normalized by pharmacological intervention of SRIs. Treatment of clomipramine, a tricyclic antidepressant, over several months could normalize regional blood flow or metabolism in the OFC and/or caudate nucleus from significant increase level prior to intervention compared to normal controls (Benkelfat et al., 1990; Swedo et al., 1992; Rubin et al., 1995). Also, intervention by two SSRIs, paroxetine and fluoxetine, provided similar results to clomipramine; increased rCBF/rGMR in the OFC and/or caudate nucleus at baseline were reduced significantly following treatment with paroxetine (Saxena et al., 1999, 2002; Hansen et al., 2002; Diler et al., 2004) and increased rCBF/rGMR in the ACC/caudate nucleus/thalamus at baseline decreased significantly after fluoxetine treatment (Hoehn-Saric et al., 1991; Baxter et al., 1992). Furthermore, in most of these studies, responders in clinical symptoms to pharmacological intervention tended to show a significant decrease relative to baseline, whereas non-responders showed no change by the treatment (Benkelfat et al., 1990; Baxter et al., 1992; Swedo et al., 1992; Saxena et al., 1999; Hoehn-Saric et al., 2001; Diler et al., 2004; Ho Pian et al., 2005). With respect to response prediction, several studies have found that the lower the brain blood flow or metabolism in relevant regions prior to treatment was, the greater was the reduction in OCD symptoms (Benkelfat et al., 1990; Saxena et al., 1999). In addition, there were significant correlations between decrease of metabolism at baseline in the OFC or caudate nucleus and improvement of OCD symptoms (Benkelfat et al., 1990; Swedo et al., 1992; Baxter et al., 1992). However, studies on significant response predictors have been very restricted and reliable parameters on response prediction have never been explored to date.

CBT, interestingly, also appears to normalize increased rCBF/rGMR in some relevant areas, including the caudate nucleus (Baxter et al., 1992; Schwartz et al., 1996; Nakatani et al., 2003) and thalamus (Saxena et al., 2009). Additionally, responders to CBT exhibited greater reduction in the caudate nucleus from baseline to CBT intervention than did non-responders (Schwartz et al., 1996). Although there have been few studies up to now on the alteration of brain function before and after CBT, growing notions on the effects of CBT on brain functions within subjects would address some important issues on whether the functional brain change induced by SRIs is a direct consequence of their pharmacological actions, or a state consequence occurring regardless of treatment approaches.

5.3 Depression as a comorbidity with OCD

Although most studies have been directed to the patients with OCD without MDD, in clinical practice OCD patients frequently have major depression as a comorbidity; approximately one-third of OCD patients also have MDD (Rasmussen and Eisen, 1992; Weismann et al., 1994), whereas 22-38% of patients with MDD have obsessive-compulsive symptoms (Kendell and DiScipio, 1970). Thus, notions acquired from studies performed on pure OCD patients without depression might deviate from the actual pathophysiology of OCD. Further, since SRIs and CBT are commonly effective for improvement of both OCD and MDD, exploration of the neuronal substrates shared by the two diseases might provide very valuable information for understanding the etiology.

Saxena et al. (1999) demonstrated that patients with concurrent OCD and MDD showed a significant reduction in metabolism in the hippocampus similar to that of patients with MDD alone. Furthermore, treatment with paroxetine for patients with concurrent OCD and MDD induced a reduction of rGMR in the ventral lateral prefrontal cortex, which was similar to the findings in patients with MDD alone, but did not show a decrease in the OFC and caudate nucleus like that seen in the patients with OCD alone (Saxena et al., 2002). These findings suggested that patients with concurrent OCD and MDD had the pathophysiology of MDD, and thus may constitute a distinctive subtype within OCD, such that both the etiologies of OCD and MDD should be considered carefully when devising a treatment strategy.

5.4 Conclusion

Functional neuroimaging studies on OCD have provided much more consistent findings than structural MRI studies. That is, in patients with OCD, some important regions in the cortical and subcortical areas present with hyperactivity and are normalized by pharmacotherapy. Since improvements by SRIs and CBT occur in only about half of patients (responders), further neuroimaging studies controlled by treatment intervention are strongly needed.

6. References

Abercrombie HC, Schaefer SM, Larson CL, Oakes TR, Lindgren KA, Holden JE, Perlman SB, Turski PA, Krahn DD, Benca RM, Davidson RJ. (1998). Metabolic rate in the right amygdala predicts negative affect in depressed patients. *Neuroreport*, 5. 9(14), 3301-3307.

Alexander GE, Crutcher MD. (1990). Functional architecture of basal ganglia circuits: neural substrates of parallel processing. *Trends Neurosci*, 13(7), 266-271.

al-Mousawi AH, Evans N, Ebmeier KP, Roeda D, Chaloner F, Ashcroft GW. (1996). Limbic dysfunction in schizophrenia and mania. A study using 18F-labelled fluorodeoxyglucose and positron emission tomography. *Br J Psychiatry*, 169(4), 509-516.

Alptekin K, Degirmenci B, Kivircik B, Durak H, Yemez B, Derebek E, Tunca Z. (2001). Tc-99m HMPAO brain perfusion SPECT in drug-free obsessive-compulsive patients without depression. *Psychiatry Res*, 1. 107(1), 51-56.

Andreasen NC, Rezai K, Alliger R, Swayze VW 2nd, Flaum M, Kirchner P, Cohen G, O'Leary DS. (1992). Hypofrontality in neuroleptic-naive patients and in patients with chronic schizophrenia. Assessment with xenon 133 single-photon emission computed tomography and the Tower of London. *Arch Gen Psychiatry*, 49(12), 943-958.

Andreasen NC, O'Leary DS, Flaum M, Nopoulos P, Watkins GL, Boles Ponto LL, Hichwa RD. (1997). Hypofrontality in schizophrenia: distributed dysfunctional circuits in neuroleptic-naïve patients. *Lancet*, 14. 349(9067), 1730-1734.

Ashton L, Barnes A, Livingston M, Wyper D; Scottish Schizophrenia Research Group. (2000). Cingulate abnormalities associated with PANSS negative scores in first episode schizophrenia. *Behav Neurol*, 12(1-2), 93-101.

Bartlett EJ, Wolkin A, Brodie JD, Laska EM, Wolf AP, Sanfilipo M. (1991). Importance of pharmacologic control in PET studies: effects of thiothixene and haloperidol on cerebral glucose utilization in chronic schizophrenia. *Psychiatry Res*, 40(2), 115-124.

Bartlett EJ, Brodie JD, Simkowitz P, Schlösser R, Dewey SL, Lindenmayer JP, Rusinek H, Wolkin A, Cancro R, Schiffer W. (1998). Effect of a haloperidol challenge on regional brain metabolism in neuroleptic-responsive and nonresponsive schizophrenic patients. *Am J Psychiatry*, 155(3), 337-343.

Bauer M, London ED, Rasgon N, Berman SM, Frye MA, Altshuler LL, Mandelkern MA, Bramen J, Voytek B, Woods R, Mazziotta JC, Whybrow PC. (2005). Supraphysiological doses of levothyroxine alter regional cerebral metabolism and improve mood in bipolar depression. *Mol Psychiatry*, 10(5), 456-469.

Baxter LR Jr, Phelps ME, Mazziotta JC, Schwartz JM, Gerner RH, Selin CE, Sumida RM. (1985). Cerebral metabolic rates for glucose in mood disorders. Studies with positron emission tomography and fluorodeoxyglucose F 18. *Arch Gen Psychiatry*, 42(5), 441-447.

Baxter LR Jr, Phelps ME, Mazziotta JC, Guze BH, Schwartz JM, Selin CE. (1987). Local cerebral glucose metabolic rates in obsessive-compulsive disorder. A comparison with rates in unipolar depression and in normal controls. *Arch Gen Psychiatry*, 44(3), 211-218.

Baxter LR Jr, Schwartz JM, Mazziotta JC, Phelps ME, Pahl JJ, Guze BH, Fairbanks L. (1988). Cerebral glucose metabolic rates in nondepressed patients with obsessive-compulsive disorder. *Am J Psychiatry*, 145(12), 1560-1563.

Baxter LR Jr, Schwartz JM, Phelps ME, Mazziotta JC, Guze BH, Selin CE, Gerner RH, Sumida RM. (1989). Reduction of prefrontal cortex glucose metabolism common to three types of depression. *Arch Gen Psychiatry*, 46(3), 243-250.

Baxter LR Jr, Schwartz JM, Bergman KS, Szuba MP, Guze BH, Mazziotta JC, Alazraki A, Selin CE, Ferng HK, Munford P, et al. (1992). Caudate glucose metabolic rate changes with both drug and behavior therapy for obsessive-compulsive disorder. *Arch Gen Psychiatry*, 49(9), 681-689.

Baxter LR Jr, Saxena S, Brody AL, Ackermann RF, Colgan M, Schwartz JM, Allen-Martinez Z, Fuster JM, Phelps ME. (1996). Brain Mediation of Obsessive-Compulsive Disorder Symptoms: Evidence From Functional Brain Imaging Studies in the Human and Nonhuman Primate. *Semin Clin Neuropsychiatry*, 1(1), 32-47.

Benkelfat C, Nordahl TE, Semple WE, King AC, Murphy DL, Cohen RM. (1990). Local cerebral glucose metabolic rates in obsessive-compulsive disorder. Patients treated with clomipramine. *Arch Gen Psychiatry*, 47(9), 840-848.

Berman I, Merson A, Sison C, Allan E, Schaefer C, Loberboym M, Losonczy MF. (1996). Regional cerebral blood flow changes associated with risperidone treatment in elderly schizophrenia patients: a pilot study. *Psychopharmacol Bull*, 32(1), 95-100.

Bench CJ, Friston KJ, Brown RG, Scott LC, Frackowiak RS, Dolan RJ. (1992). The anatomy of melancholia--focal abnormalities of cerebral blood flow in major depression. *Psychol Med,* 22(3), 607-615.

Bench CJ, Friston KJ, Brown RG, Frackowiak RS, Dolan RJ. (1993). Regional cerebral blood flow in depression measured by positron emission tomography: the relationship with clinical dimensions. *Psychol Med,* 23(3), 579-590.

Bhardwaj R, Chakrabarti S, Mittal BR, Sharan P. (2010). A single photon emission computerized tomography (SPECT) study of regional cerebral blood flow in bipolar disorder. *World J Biol Psychiatry,* 11(2 Pt 2), 334-343.

Biver F, Goldman S, Delvenne V, Luxen A, De Maertelaer V, Hubain P, Mendlewicz J, Lotstra F. (1994). Frontal and parietal metabolic disturbances in unipolar depression. *Biol Psychiatry,* 15. 36(6), 381-388.

Blumberg HP, Stern E, Ricketts S, Martinez D, de Asis J, White T, Epstein J, Isenberg N, McBride PA, Kemperman I, Emmerich S, Dhawan V, Eidelberg D, Kocsis JH, Silbersweig DA. (1999). Rostral and orbital prefrontal cortex dysfunction in the manic state of bipolar disorder. *Am J Psychiatry,* 156(12), 1986-1988.

Blumberg HP, Stern E, Martinez D, Ricketts S, de Asis J, White T, Epstein J, McBride PA, Eidelberg D, Kocsis JH, Silbersweig DA. (2000). Increased anterior cingulate and caudate activity in bipolar mania. *Biol Psychiatry,* 1. 48(11), 1045-1052.

Bonne O, Krausz Y, Gorfine M, Karger H, Gelfin Y, Shapira B, Chisin R, Lerer B. (1996). Cerebral hypoperfusion in medication resistant, depressed patients assessed by Tc99m HMPAO SPECT. *J Affect Disord,* 16. 41(3), 163-171.

Bonne O, Louzoun Y, Aharon I, Krausz Y, Karger H, Lerer B, Bocher M, Freedman N, Chisin R. (2003). Cerebral blood flow in depressed patients: a methodological comparison of statistical parametric mapping and region of interest analyses. *Psychiatry Res,* 20. 122(1), 49-57.

Brockmann H, Zobel A, Joe A, Biermann K, Scheef L, Schuhmacher A, von Widdern O, Metten M, Biersack HJ, Maier W, Boecker H. (2009). The value of HMPAO SPECT in predicting treatment response to citalopram in patients with major depression. *Psychiatry Res,* 30. 173(2), 107-112.

Brody AL, Saxena S, Silverman DH, Alborzian S, Fairbanks LA, Phelps ME, Huang SC, Wu HM, Maidment K, Baxter LR Jr. (1999). Brain metabolic changes in major depressive disorder from pre- to post-treatment with paroxetine. *Psychiatry Res,* 11. 91(3), 127-139.

Brooks JO 3rd, Bonner JC, Rosen AC, Wang PW, Hoblyn JC, Hill SJ, Ketter TA. (2009a). Dorsolateral and dorsomedial prefrontal gray matter density changes associated with bipolar depression. *Psychiatry Res,* 30. 172(3), 200-204.

Brooks JO 3rd, Hoblyn JC, Woodard SA, Rosen AC, Ketter TA. (2009b). Corticolimbic metabolic dysregulation in euthymic older adults with bipolar disorder. *J Psychiatr Res.* 43(5), 497-502.

Brooks JO 3rd, Hoblyn JC, Ketter TA. (2010). Metabolic evidence of corticolimbic dysregulation in bipolar mania. *Psychiatry Res,* 28. 181(2), 136-140.

Buchsbaum MS, Ingvar DH, Kessler R, Waters RN, Cappelletti J, van Kammen DP, King AC, Johnson JL, Manning RG, Flynn RW, Mann LS, Bunney WE Jr, Sokoloff L. (1982). Cerebral glucography with positron tomography. Use in normal subjects and in patients with schizophrenia. *Arch Gen Psychiatry,* 39(3), 251-259.

Buchsbaum MS, Wu JC, DeLisi LE, Holcomb HH, Hazlett E, Cooper-Langston K, Kessler R. (1987). Positron emission tomography studies of basal ganglia and somatosensory cortex neuroleptic drug effects: differences between normal controls and schizophrenic patients. *Biol Psychiatry*, 22(4), 479-494.

Buchsbaum MS, Haier RJ, Potkin SG, Nuechterlein K, Bracha HS, Katz M, Lohr J, Wu J, Lottenberg S, Jerabek PA, et al. (1992a). Frontostriatal disorder of cerebral metabolism in never-medicated schizophrenics. *Arch Gen Psychiatry*, 49(12), 935-942.

Buchsbaum MS, Potkin SG, Siegel BV Jr, Lohr J, Katz M, Gottschalk LA, Gulasekaram B, Marshall JF, Lottenberg S, Teng CY, et al. (1992b). Striatal metabolic rate and clinical response to neuroleptics in schizophrenia. *Arch Gen Psychiatry*, 49(12), 966-974.

Buchsbaum MS, Someya T, Teng CY, Abel L, Chin S, Najafi A, Haier RJ, Wu J, Bunney WE Jr. (1996). PET and MRI of the thalamus in never-medicated patients with schizophrenia. *Am J Psychiatry*, 153(2), 191-199.

Buchsbaum MS, Wu J, Siegel BV, Hackett E, Trenary M, Abel L, Reynolds C. (1997). Effect of sertraline on regional metabolic rate in patients with affective disorder. *Biol Psychiatry*, 1. 41(1), 15-22.

Buchsbaum MS, Tang CY, Peled S, Gudbjartsson H, Lu D, Hazlett EA, Downhill J, Haznedar M, Fallon JH, Atlas SW. (1998). MRI white matter diffusion anisotropy and PET metabolic rate in schizophrenia. *Neuroreport*, 16. 9(3), 425-430.

Buchsbaum MS, Buchsbaum BR, Hazlett EA, Haznedar MM, Newmark R, Tang CY, Hof PR. (2007a). Relative glucose metabolic rate higher in white matter in patients with schizophrenia. *Am J Psychiatry*, 164(7), 1072-1081.

Buchsbaum MS, Haznedar MM, Aronowitz J, Brickman AM, Newmark RE, Bloom R, Brand J, Goldstein KE, Heath D, Starson M, Hazlett EA. (2007b). FDG-PET in never-previously medicated psychotic adolescents treated with olanzapine or haloperidol. *Schizophr Res*, 94(1-3), 293-305.

Busatto GF, Zamignani DR, Buchpiguel CA, Garrido GE, Glabus MF, Rocha ET, Maia AF, Rosario-Campos MC, Campi Castro C, Furuie SS, Gutierrez MA, McGuire PK, Miguel EC. (2000). A voxel-based investigation of regional cerebral blood flow abnormalities in obsessive-compulsive disorder using single photon emission computed tomography (SPECT). *Psychiatry Res*, 10. 99(1), 15-27.

Clark C, Kopala L, Li DK, Hurwitz T. (2001). Regional cerebral glucose metabolism in never-medicated patients with schizophrenia. *Can J Psychiatry*, 46(4), 340-345.

Cleghorn JM, Garnett ES, Nahmias C, Firnau G, Brown GM, Kaplan R, Szechtman H, Szechtman B. (1989). Increased frontal and reduced parietal glucose metabolism in acute untreated schizophrenia. *Psychiatry Res*, 28(2), 119-133.

Cleghorn JM, Franco S, Szechtman B, Kaplan RD, Szechtman H, Brown GM, Nahmias C, Garnett ES. (1992). Toward a brain map of auditory hallucinations. *Am J Psychiatry*, 149(8), 1062-1069.

Cohen RM, Gross M, Nordahl TE, Semple WE, Oren DA, Rosenthal N. (1992). Preliminary data on the metabolic brain pattern of patients with winter seasonal affective disorder. *Arch Gen Psychiatry*, 49(7), 545-552.

Cohen RM, Nordahl TE, Semple WE, Andreason P, Litman RE, Pickar D. (1997). The brain metabolic patterns of clozapine- and fluphenazine-treated patients with schizophrenia during a continuous performance task. *Arch Gen Psychiatry*, 54(5), 481-486.

Corson PW, O'Leary DS, Miller DD, Andreasen NC. (2002). The effects of neuroleptic medications on basal ganglia blood flow in schizophreniform disorders: a comparison between the neuroleptic-naïve and medicated states. *Biol Psychiatry*, 1. 52(9), 855-962.

Crespo-Facorro B, Cabranes JA, López-Ibor Alcocer MI, Payá B, Fernández Pérez C, Encinas M, Ayuso Mateos JL, López-Ibor JJ Jr. (1999). Regional cerebral blood flow in obsessive-compulsive patients with and without a chronic tic disorder. A SPECT study. *Eur Arch Psychiatry Clin Neurosci*, 249(3), 156-161.

Culha AF, Osman O, Dogangün Y, Filiz K, Suna K, Kalkan ON, Gulfizar V, Beyza A. (2008). Changes in regional cerebral blood flow demonstrated by 99mTc-HMPAO SPECT in euthymic bipolar patients. *Eur Arch Psychiatry Clin Neurosci*, 258(3), 144-151.

Davidson LL, Heinrichs RW. (2003). Quantification of frontal and temporal lobe brain-imaging findings in schizophrenia: a meta-analysis. *Psychiatry Res*, 15. 122(2), 69-87.

Dazzan P, Morgan KD, Orr KG, Hutchinson G, Chitnis X, Suckling J, Fearon P, Salvo J, McGuire PK, Mallett RM, Jones PB, Leff J, Murray RM. (2004). The structural brain correlates of neurological soft signs in AESOP first-episode psychoses study. *Brain*, 127(Pt 1), 143-153.

Desco M, Gispert JD, Reig S, Sanz J, Pascau J, Sarramea F, Benito C, Santos A, Palomo T, Molina V. (2003). Cerebral metabolic patterns in chronic and recent-onset schizophrenia. *Psychiatry Res*, 15. 122(2), 125-135.

Dierks T, Linden DE, Jandl M, Formisano E, Goebel R, Lanfermann H, Singer W. (1999). Activation of Heschl's gyrus during auditory hallucinations. *Neuron*, 22(3), 615-621.

Diler RS, Kibar M, Avci A. (2004). Pharmacotherapy and regional cerebral blood flow in children with obsessive compulsive disorder. *Yonsei Med J*, 29. 45(1), 90-99.

Dolan RJ, Bench CJ, Liddle PF, Friston KJ, Frith CD, Grasby PM, Frackowiak RS. (1993). Dorsolateral prefrontal cortex dysfunction in the major psychoses; symptom or disease specificity? *J Neurol Neurosurg Psychiatry*, 56(12), 1290-1294.

Drevets WC, Videen TO, Price JL, Preskorn SH, Carmichael ST, Raichle ME. (1992). A functional anatomical study of unipolar depression. *J Neurosci*, 12(9), 3628-3641.

Drevets WC, Price JL, Simpson JR Jr, Todd RD, Reich T, Vannier M, Raichle ME. (1997). Subgenual prefrontal cortex abnormalities in mood disorders. *Nature*, 24. 386(6627), 824-827.

Drevets WC. (1999). Prefrontal cortical-amygdalar metabolism in major depression. *Ann N Y Acad Sci*, 29. 877, 614-637.

Drevets WC. (2000). Neuroimaging studies of mood disorders. *Biol Psychiatry*, 15. 48(8), 813-829.

Drevets WC, Price JL, Bardgett ME, Reich T, Todd RD, Raichle ME. (2002). Glucose metabolism in the amygdala in depression: relationship to diagnostic subtype and plasma cortisol levels. *Pharmacol Biochem Behav*, 71(3), 431-447.

Ebmeier KP, Blackwood DH, Murray C, Souza V, Walker M, Dougall N, Moffoot AP, O'Carroll RE, Goodwin GM. (1993). Single-photon emission computed tomography with 99mTc-exametazime in unmedicated schizophrenic patients. *Biol Psychiatry*, 1. 33(7), 487-495.

Edmonstone Y, Austin MP, Prentice N, Dougall N, Freeman CP, Ebmeier KP, Goodwin GM. (1994). Uptake of 99mTc-exametazime shown by single photon emission computerized tomography in obsessive-compulsive disorder compared with major depression and normal controls. *Acta Psychiatr Scand*, 90(4), 298-303.

Elshahawi HH, Essawi H, Rabie MA, Mansour M, Beshry ZA, Mansour AN. (2011). Cognitive functions among euthymic bipolar I patients after a single manic episode versus recurrent episodes. *J Affect Disord*, 130(1-2), 180-191.

Erkwoh R, Sabri O, Steinmeyer EM, Bull U, Sass H. (1997). Psychopathological and SPECT findings in never-treated schizophrenia. *Acta Psychiatr Scand*, 96(1), 51-57.

Fitzgerald PB, Laird AR, Maller J, Daskalakis ZJ. (2008). A meta-analytic study of changes in brain activation in depression. *Hum Brain Mapp*, 29(6), 683-695.

Geller DA, Biederman J, Reed ED, Spencer T, Wilens TE. (1995). Similarities in response to fluoxetine in the treatment of children and adolescents with obsessive-compulsive disorder. *J Am Acad Child Adolesc Psychiatry*, 34(1), 36-44.

Gonul AS, Kula M, Eşel E, Tutuş A, Sofuoglu S. (2003a). A Tc-99m HMPAO SPECT study of regional cerebral blood flow in drug-free schizophrenic patients with deficit and non-deficit syndrome. *Psychiatry Res*, 30. 123(3), 199-205.

Gonul AS, Kula M, Sofuoglu S, Tutus A, Esel E. (2003b). Tc-99 HMPAO SPECT study of regional cerebral blood flow in olanzapine-treated schizophrenic patients. *Eur Arch Psychiatry Clin Neurosci*, 253(1), 29-33.

Gonul AS, Kula M, Bilgin AG, Tutus A, Oguz A. (2004). The regional cerebral blood flow changes in major depressive disorder with and without psychotic features. *Prog Neuropsychopharmacol Biol Psychiatry*, 28(6), 1015-1021.

Goodwin GM, Cavanagh JT, Glabus MF, Kehoe RF, O'Carroll RE, Ebmeier KP. (1997). Uptake of 99mTc-exametazime shown by single photon emission computed tomography before and after lithium withdrawal in bipolar patients: associations with mania. *Br J Psychiatry*, 170, 426-430.

Gur RC, Gur RE. (1995). Hypofrontality in schizophrenia: RIP. *Lancet*, 3. 345(8962), 1383-1384.

Guze BH, Baxter LR Jr, Schwartz JM, Szuba MP, Liston EH. (1991). Electroconvulsive Therapy and Brain Glucose Metabolism. *Convuls Ther*, 7(1), 15-19.

Hansen ES, Hasselbalch S, Law I, Bolwig TG. (2002). The caudate nucleus in obsessive-compulsive disorder. Reduced metabolism following treatment with paroxetine: a PET study. *Int J Neuropsychopharmacol*, 5(1), 1-10.

Hazlett EA, Buchsbaum MS, Byne W, Wei TC, Spiegel-Cohen J, Geneve C, Kinderlehrer R, Haznedar MM, Shihabuddin L, Siever LJ. (1999). Three-dimensional analysis with MRI and PET of the size, shape, and function of the thalamus in the schizophrenia spectrum. *Am J Psychiatry*, 156(8), 1190-1199.

Hazlett EA, Buchsbaum MS, Kemether E, Bloom R, Platholi J, Brickman AM, Shihabuddin L, Tang C, Byne W. (2004). Abnormal glucose metabolism in the mediodorsal nucleus of the thalamus in schizophrenia. *Am J Psychiatry*, 161(2), 305-314.

Hill K, Mann L, Laws KR, Stephenson CM, Nimmo-Smith I, McKenna PJ. (2004). Hypofrontality in schizophrenia: a meta-analysis of functional imaging studies. *Acta Psychiatr Scand*, 110(4), 243-256.

Hirschfeld RM, Montgomery SA, Aguglia E, Amore M, Delgado PL, Gastpar M, Hawley C, Kasper S, Linden M, Massana J, Mendlewicz J, Möller HJ, Nemeroff CB, Saiz J, Such P, Torta R, Versiani M.(2002). Partial response and nonresponse to antidepressant therapy: current approaches and treatment options. *J Clin Psychiatry*, 63(9), 826-837.

Hirschfeld RM, Lewis L, Vornik LA. (2003). Perceptions and impact of bipolar disorder: how far have we really come? Results of the national depressive and manic-depressive association 2000 survey of individuals with bipolar disorder. *J Clin Psychiatry*, 64(2), 161-174.

Hoehn-Saric R, Pearlson GD, Harris GJ, Machlin SR, Camargo EE. (1991). Effects of fluoxetine on regional cerebral blood flow in obsessive-compulsive patients. *Am J Psychiatry*, 148(9), 1243-1245.

Hoehn-Saric R, Schlaepfer TE, Greenberg BD, McLeod DR, Pearlson GD, Wong SH. (2001). Cerebral blood flow in obsessive-compulsive patients with major depression: effect of treatment with sertraline or desipramine on treatment responders and non-responders. *Psychiatry Res*, 30. 108(2), 89-100.

Ho Pian KL, van Megen HJ, Ramsey NF, Mandl R, van Rijk PP, Wynne HJ, Westenberg HG. (2005). Decreased thalamic blood flow in obsessive-compulsive disorder patients responding to fluvoxamine. *Psychiatry Res*, 28. 138(2), 89-97.

Horga G, Parellada E, Lomeña F, Fernández-Egea E, Mané A, Font M, Falcón C, Konova AB, Pavia J, Ros D, Bernardo M. (2011). Differential brain glucose metabolic patterns in antipsychotic-naïve first-episode schizophrenia with and without auditory verbal hallucinations. *J Psychiatry Neurosci*, 1. 36(5), 312-321.

Horwitz B, Swedo SE, Grady CL, Pietrini P, Schapiro MB, Rapoport JL, Rapoport SI. (1991). Cerebral metabolic pattern in obsessive-compulsive disorder: altered intercorrelations between regional rates of glucose utilization. *Psychiatry Res*, 40(4), 221-237.

Hurwitz TA, Clark C, Murphy E, Klonoff H, Martin WR, Pate BD (1990). Regional cerebral glucose metabolism in major depressive disorder. *Can J Psychiatry*, 35(8), 684-688.

Ingvar DH, Franzén G. (1974). Abnormalities of cerebral blood flow distribution in patients with chronic schizophrenia. *Acta Psychiatr Scand*, 50(4), 425-462.

Ishizaki J, Yamamoto H, Takahashi T, Takeda M, Yano M, Mimura M. (2008). Changes in regional cerebral blood flow following antidepressant treatment in late-life depression. *Int J Geriatr Psychiatry*, 23(8), 805-811.

Jacobsen LK, Hamburger SD, Van Horn JD, Vaituzis AC, McKenna K, Frazier JA, Gordon CT, Lenane MC, Rapoport JL, Zametkin AJ. (1997). Cerebral glucose metabolism in childhood onset schizophrenia. *Psychiatry Res*, 31. 75(3), 131-144.

Joe AY, Tielmann T, Bucerius J, Reinhardt MJ, Palmedo H, Maier W, Biersack HJ, Zobel A. (2006). Response-dependent differences in regional cerebral blood flow changes with citalopram in treatment of major depression. *J Nucl Med*, 47(8), 1319-1325.

Keener MT, Phillips ML. (2007). Neuroimaging in bipolar disorder: a critical review of current findings. *Curr Psychiatry Rep*, 9(6), 512-520.

Kendell RE, Discipio WJ. (1970). Obsessional symptoms and obsessional personality traits in patients with depressive illnesses. *Psychol Med*, 1(1), 65-72.

Kessing LV. (1998). Cognitive impairment in the euthymic phase of affective disorder. *Psychol Med*, 28(5), 1027-1038.

Ketter TA, Kimbrell TA, George MS, Dunn RT, Speer AM, Benson BE, Willis MW, Danielson A, Frye MA, Herscovitch P, Post RM. (2001). Effects of mood and subtype on cerebral glucose metabolism in treatment-resistant bipolar disorder. *Biol Psychiatry*, 15. 49(2), 97-109.

Kim JJ, Mohamed S, Andreasen NC, O'Leary DS, Watkins GL, Boles Ponto LL, Hichwa RD. (2000). Regional neural dysfunctions in chronic schizophrenia studied with positron emission tomography. *Am J Psychiatry*, 157(4), 542-548.

Kimbrell TA, Ketter TA, George MS, Little JT, Benson BE, Willis MW, Herscovitch P, Post RM. (2002). Regional cerebral glucose utilization in patients with a range of severities of unipolar depression. *Biol Psychiatry*, 1. 51(3), 237-252.

Kohn Y, Freedman N, Lester H, Krausz Y, Chisin R, Lerer B, Bonne O. (2007). 99mTc-HMPAO SPECT study of cerebral perfusion after treatment with medication and electroconvulsive therapy in major depression. *J Nucl Med*, 48(8), 1273-1278.

Konarski JZ, Kennedy SH, McIntyre RS, Rafi-Tari S, Soczynska JK, Mayberg HS. (2007). Relationship between regional brain metabolism, illness severity and age in depressed subjects. *Psychiatry Res*, 15. 155(3), 203-210.

Konarski JZ, Kennedy SH, Segal ZV, Lau MA, Bieling PJ, McIntyre RS, Mayberg HS. (2009). Predictors of nonresponse to cognitive behavioural therapy or venlafaxine using glucose metabolism in major depressive disorder. *J Psychiatry Neurosci*, 34(3), 175-180.

Krishnan KR, McDonald WM, Escalona PR, Doraiswamy PM, Na C, Husain MM, Figiel GS, Boyko OB, Ellinwood EH, Nemeroff CB. (1992). Magnetic resonance imaging of the caudate nuclei in depression. Preliminary observations. *Arch Gen Psychiatry*, 49(7), 553-557.

Krüger S, Seminowicz D, Goldapple K, Kennedy SH, Mayberg HS. (2003). State and trait influences on mood regulation in bipolar disorder: blood flow differences with an acute mood challenge. *Biol Psychiatry*, 1. 54(11), 1274-1283.

Krüger S, Alda M, Young LT, Goldapple K, Parikh S, Mayberg HS. (2006). Risk and resilience markers in bipolar disorder: brain responses to emotional challenge in bipolar patients and their healthy siblings. *Am J Psychiatry*, 163(2), 257-264.

Lahti AC, Holcomb HH, Weiler MA, Medoff DR, Tamminga CA. (2003). Functional effects of antipsychotic drugs: comparing clozapine with haloperidol. *Biol Psychiatry*, 1. 53(7), 601-608.

Lahti AC, Weiler MA, Medoff DR, Tamminga CA, Holcomb HH. (2005). Functional effects of single dose first- and second-generation antipsychotic administration in subjects with schizophrenia. *Psychiatry Res*, 30. 139(1), 19-30.

Lehrer DS, Christian BT, Mantil J, Murray AC, Buchsbaum BR, Oakes TR, Byne W, Kemether EM, Buchsbaum MS. (2005). Thalamic and prefrontal FDG uptake in never medicated patients with schizophrenia. *Am J Psychiatry*, 162(5), 931-938.

Lennox BR, Park SB, Medley I, Morris PG, Jones PB. (2000). The functional anatomy of auditory hallucinations in schizophrenia. *Psychiatry Res*, 20. 100(1), 13-20.

Liddle PF, Friston KJ, Frith CD, Hirsch SR, Jones T, Frackowiak RS. (1992). Patterns of cerebral blood flow in schizophrenia. *Br J Psychiatry*, 160, 179-186.

Liddle PF, Lane CJ, Ngan ET. (2000). Immediate effects of risperidone on cortico-striato-thalamic loops and the hippocampus. *Br J Psychiatry*, 177, 402-407.

Lucey JV, Costa DC, Blanes T, Busatto GF, Pilowsky LS, Takei N, Marks IM, Ell PJ, Kerwin RW. (1995). Regional cerebral blood flow in obsessive-compulsive disordered patients at rest. Differential correlates with obsessive-compulsive and anxious-avoidant dimensions. *Br J Psychiatry*, 167(5), 629-634.

Lucey JV, Costa DC, Busatto G, Pilowsky LS, Marks IM, Ell PJ, Kerwin RW. (1997). Caudate regional cerebral blood flow in obsessive-compulsive disorder, panic disorder and healthy controls on single photon emission computerised tomography. *Psychiatry Res*, 14. 74(1), 25-33.

Lynch MR. (1992). Schizophrenia and the D1 receptor: focus on negative symptoms. *Prog Neuropsychopharmacol Biol Psychiatry*, 16(6), 797-832.

Mah L, Zarate CA Jr, Singh J, Duan YF, Luckenbaugh DA, Manji HK, Drevets WC. (2007). Regional cerebral glucose metabolic abnormalities in bipolar II depression. *Biol Psychiatry*, 15. 61(6), 765-775.

Mann JJ. (2005). The medical management of depression. *N Engl J Med*, 27, 353(17), 1819-1834.

Martinot JL, Hardy P, Feline A, Huret JD, Mazoyer B, Attar-Levy D, Pappata S, Syrota A. (1990). Left prefrontal glucose hypometabolism in the depressed state: a confirmation. *Am J Psychiatry*, 147(10), 1313-1317.

Mayberg HS, Brannan SK, Mahurin RK, Jerabek PA, Brickman JS, Tekell JL, Silva JA, McGinnis S, Glass TG, Martin CC, Fox PT. (1997). Cingulate function in depression: a potential predictor of treatment response. *Neuroreport*, 3. 8(4), 1057-1061.

McGuire PK, Bench CJ, Frith CD, Marks IM, Frackowiak RS, Dolan RJ. (1994). Functional anatomy of obsessive-compulsive phenomena. *Br J Psychiatry*, 164(4), 459-468.

Merikangas KR, Ames M, Cui L, Stang PE, Ustun TB, Von Korff M, Kessler RC. (2007). The impact of comorbidity of mental and physical conditions on role disability in the US adult household population. *Arch Gen Psychiatry*, 64(10), 1180-1188.

Milak MS, Parsey RV, Lee L, Oquendo MA, Olvet DM, Eipper F, Malone K, Mann JJ. (2009). Pretreatment regional brain glucose uptake in the midbrain on PET may predict remission from a major depressive episode after three months of treatment. *Psychiatry Res*, 15, 173(1), 63-70.

Miller DD, Rezai K, Alliger R, Andreasen NC. (1997). The effect of antipsychotic medication on relative cerebral blood perfusion in schizophrenia: assessment with technetium-99m hexamethyl-propyleneamine oxime single photon emission computed tomography. *Biol Psychiatry*. 1. 41(5), 550-559.

Miller DD, Andreasen NC, O'Leary DS, Watkins GL, Boles Ponto LL, Hichwa RD. (2001).Comparison of the effects of risperidone and haloperidol on regional cerebral blood flow in schizophrenia. *Biol Psychiatry*, 15. 49(8), 704-715.

Min SK, An SK, Jon DI, Lee JD. (1999). Positive and negative symptoms and regional cerebral perfusion in antipsychotic-naive schizophrenic patients: a high-resolution SPECT study. *Psychiatry Res*, 30. 90(3), 159-168.

Modell JG, Mountz JM, Curtis GC, Greden JF. (1989). Neurophysiologic dysfunction in basal ganglia/limbic striatal and thalamocortical circuits as a pathogenetic mechanism of obsessive-compulsive disorder. *J Neuropsychiatry Clin Neurosci*, 1(1), 27-36.

Molina V, Sanz J, Reig S, Martínez R, Sarramea F, Luque R, Benito C, Gispert JD, Pascau J, Desco M. (2005a). Hypofrontality in men with first-episode psychosis. *Br J Psychiatry*, 186, 203-208.

Molina V, Sanz J, Sarramea F, Benito C, Palomo T. (2005b). Prefrontal atrophy in first episodes of schizophrenia associated with limbic metabolic hyperactivity. *J Psychiatr Res*, 39(2), 117-127.

Molina V, Gispert JD, Reig S, Pascau J, Martínez R, Sanz J, Palomo T, Desco M. (2005c). Olanzapine-induced cerebral metabolic changes related to symptom improvement in schizophrenia. *Int Clin Psychopharmacol*, 20(1), 13-18.

Molina V, Gispert JD, Reig S, Sanz J, Pascau J, Santos A, Desco M, Palomo T. (2005d). Cerebral metabolic changes induced by clozapine in schizophrenia and related to clinical improvement. *Psychopharmacology (Berl)*, 178(1), 17-26.

Molina V, Tamayo P, Montes C, De Luxán A, Martin C, Rivas N, Sancho C, Domínguez-Gil A. (2008). Clozapine may partially compensate for task-related brain perfusion abnormalities in risperidone-resistant schizophrenia patients. *Prog Neuropsychopharmacol Biol Psychiatry*, 15. 32(4), 948-954.

Molina V, Solera S, Sanz J, Sarramea F, Luque R, Rodríguez R, Jiménez-Arriero MA, Palomo T. (2009). Association between cerebral metabolic and structural abnormalities and cognitive performance in schizophrenia. *Psychiatry Res*, 30. 173(2), 88-93.

Nakatani E, Nakgawa A, Ohara Y, Goto S, Uozumi N, Iwakiri M, Yamamoto Y, Motomura K, Iikura Y, Yamagami T. (2003). Effects of behavior therapy on regional cerebral blood flow in obsessive-compulsive disorder. *Psychiatry Res*, 30. 124(2), 113-120.

Navarro V, Gastó C, Lomeña F, Torres X, Mateos JJ, Portella MJ, Masana G, Marcos T. (2004). Prognostic value of frontal functional neuroimaging in late-onset severe major depression. *Br J Psychiatry*, 184, 306-311.

Ngan ET, Lane CJ, Ruth TJ, Liddle PF. (2002). Immediate and delayed effects of risperidone on cerebral metabolism in neuroleptic naïve schizophrenic patients: correlations with symptom change. *J Neurol Neurosurg Psychiatry*, 72(1), 106-110.

Nee LE, Caine ED, Polinsky RJ, Eldridge R, Ebert MH (1980). Gilles de la Tourette syndrome: clinical and family study of 50 cases. *Ann Neurol*, 7(1), 41-49.

Pan L, Keener MT, Hassel S, Phillips ML. (2009). Functional neuroimaging studies of bipolar disorder: examining the wide clinical spectrum in the search for disease endophenotypes. *Int Rev Psychiatry*, 21(4), 368-379.

Penadés R, Boget T, Lomeña F, Mateos JJ, Catalán R, Gastó C, Salamero M. (2002). Could the hypofrontality pattern in schizophrenia be modified through neuropsychological rehabilitation? *Acta Psychiatr Scand*, 105(3), 202-208.

Perani D, Colombo C, Bressi S, Bonfanti A, Grassi F, Scarone S, Bellodi L, Smeraldi E, Fazio F. (1995). [18F]FDG PET study in obsessive-compulsive disorder. A clinical/metabolic correlation study after treatment. *Br J Psychiatry*, 166(2), 244-250.

Périco CA, Skaf CR, Yamada A, Duran F, Buchpiguel CA, Castro CC, Soares JC, Busatto GF. (2005). Relationship between regional cerebral blood flow and separate symptom clusters of major depression: a single photon emission computed tomography study using statistical parametric mapping. *Neurosci Lett*, 26. 384(3), 265-270.

Potkin SG, Buchsbaum MS, Jin Y, Tang C, Telford J, Friedman G, Lottenberg S, Najafi A, Gulasekaram B, Costa J, et al. (1994). Clozapine effects on glucose metabolic rate in striatum and frontal cortex. *J Clin Psychiatry*, 55 Suppl B, 63-66.

Potkin SG, Alva G, Fleming K, Anand R, Keator D, Carreon D, Doo M, Jin Y, Wu JC, Fallon JH. (2002). A PET study of the pathophysiology of negative symptoms in schizophrenia. Positron emission tomography. *Am J Psychiatry*, 159(2), 227-237.

Potkin SG, Basile VS, Jin Y, Masellis M, Badri F, Keator D, Wu JC, Alva G, Carreon DT, Bunney WE Jr, Fallon JH, Kennedy JL. (2003). D1 receptor alleles predict PET metabolic correlates of clinical response to clozapine. *Mol Psychiatry*, 8(1), 109-113.

Prohovnik I, Sackeim HA, Decina P, Malitz S. (1986). Acute reductions of regional cerebral blood flow following electroconvulsive therapy. Interactions with modality and time. *Ann N Y Acad Sci*, 462, 249-262.

Rasmussen SA, Eisen JL. (1992). The epidemiology and differential diagnosis of obsessive compulsive disorder. *J Clin Psychiatry*, 53 Suppl, 4-10.

Remington G, Agid O, Foussias G. (2011). Schizophrenia as a disorder of too little dopamine: implications for symptoms and treatment. *Expert Rev Neurother*, 11(4), 589-607.

Rosenberg R, Vorstrup S, Andersen A, Bolwig TG. (1988). Effect of ECT on Cerebral Blood Flow in Melancholia Assessed with SPECT. *Convuls Ther*, 4(1), 62-73.

Rubin RT, Villanueva-Meyer J, Ananth J, Trajmar PG, Mena I. (1992). Regional xenon 133 cerebral blood flow and cerebral technetium 99m HMPAO uptake in unmedicated patients with obsessive-compulsive disorder and matched normal control subjects. Determination by high-resolution single-photon emission computed tomography. *Arch Gen Psychiatry*, 49(9), 695-702.

Rubin RT, Ananth J, Villanueva-Meyer J, Trajmar PG, Mena I. (1995). Regional 133xenon cerebral blood flow and cerebral 99mTc-HMPAO uptake in patients with obsessive-compulsive disorder before and during treatment. *Biol Psychiatry*, 1. 38(7), 429-437.

Rubinsztein JS, Fletcher PC, Rogers RD, Ho LW, Aigbirhio FI, Paykel ES, Robbins TW, Sahakian BJ. (2001). Decision-making in mania: a PET study. *Brain*, 124 (Pt 12), 2550-2563.

Sabri O, Erkwoh R, Schreckenberger M, Cremerius U, Schulz G, Dickmann C, Kaiser HJ, Steinmeyer EM, Sass H, Buell U. (1997). Regional cerebral blood flow and negative/positive symptoms in 24 drug-naive schizophrenics. *J Nucl Med*, 38(2), 181-188.

Sachdev P, Brodaty H, Rose N, Haindl W. (1997). Regional cerebral blood flow in late-onset schizophrenia: a SPECT study using 99mTc-HMPAO. *Schizophr Res*, 30. 27(2-3), 105-117.

Saxena S, Brody AL, Schwartz JM, Baxter LR. (1998). Neuroimaging and frontal-subcortical circuitry in obsessive-compulsive disorder. *Br J Psychiatry*, Suppl (35), 26-37.

Saxena S, Brody AL, Maidment KM, Dunkin JJ, Colgan M, Alborzian S, Phelps ME, Baxter LR Jr. (1999). Localized orbitofrontal and subcortical metabolic changes and predictors of response to paroxetine treatment in obsessive-compulsive disorder. *Neuropsychopharmacology*, 21(6), 683-693.

Saxena S, Brody AL, Ho ML, Alborzian S, Ho MK, Maidment KM, Huang SC, Wu HM, Au SC, Baxter LR Jr. (2001). Cerebral metabolism in major depression and obsessive-compulsive disorder occurring separately and concurrently. *Biol Psychiatry*, 1.50(3), 159-170.

Saxena S, Brody AL, Ho ML, Alborzian S, Maidment KM, Zohrabi N, Ho MK, Huang SC, Wu HM, Baxter LR Jr. (2002). Differential cerebral metabolic changes with paroxetine treatment of obsessive-compulsive disorder vs major depression. *Arch Gen Psychiatry*, 59(3), 250-261.

Saxena S, Brody AL, Maidment KM, Smith EC, Zohrabi N, Katz E, Baker SK, Baxter LR Jr. (2004). Cerebral glucose metabolism in obsessive-compulsive hoarding. *Am J Psychiatry*, 161(6), 1038-1048.

Saxena S, Gorbis E, O'Neill J, Baker SK, Mandelkern MA, Maidment KM, Chang S, Salamon N, Brody AL, Schwartz JM, London ED. (2009). Rapid effects of brief intensive cognitive-behavioral therapy on brain glucose metabolism in obsessive-compulsive disorder. *Mol Psychiatry*, 14(2), 197-205.

Schilder P. (1938). The organic background of obsessions and compulsions. Am J Psychiatry, 94, 1397-1414.Schlegel S, Aldenhoff JB, Eissner D, Lindner P, Nickel O. (1989). Regional cerebral blood flow in depression: associations with psychopathology. J Affect Disord, 17(3), 211-218.

Schroder J, Buchsbaum MS, Siegel BV, Geider FJ, Lohr J, Tang C, Wu J, Potkin SG. (1996). Cerebral metabolic activity correlates of subsyndromes in chronic schizophrenia. Schizophr Res, 19(1), 41-53.

Schwartz JM, Stoessel PW, Baxter LR Jr, Martin KM, Phelps ME. (1996). Systematic changes in cerebral glucose metabolic rate after successful behavior modification treatment of obsessive-compulsive disorder. Arch Gen Psychiatry, 53(2), 109-113.

Scottish Schizophrenia Research Group. (1998). Regional cerebral blood flow in first-episode schizophrenia patients before and after antipsychotic drug treatment. Acta Psychiatr Scand, 97(6), 440-449.

Shenton ME, Dickey CC, Frumin M, McCarley RW. (2001). A review of MRI findings in schizophrenia. Schizophr Res, 15. 49(1-2), 1-52.

Shihabuddin L, Buchsbaum MS, Hazlett EA, Haznedar MM, Harvey PD, Newman A, Schnur DB, Spiegel-Cohen J, Wei T, Machac J, Knesaurek K, Vallabhajosula S, Biren MA, Ciaravolo TM, Luu-Hsia C. (1998). Dorsal striatal size, shape, and metabolic rate in never-medicated and previously medicated schizophrenics performing a verbal learning task. Arch Gen Psychiatry, 55(3), 235-243.

Skaf CR, Yamada A, Garrido GE, Buchpiguel CA, Akamine S, Castro CC, Busatto GF. (2002). Psychotic symptoms in major depressive disorder are associated with reduced regional cerebral blood flow in the subgenual anterior cingulate cortex: a voxel-based single photon emission computed tomography (SPECT) study. J Affect Disord, 68(2-3), 295-305.

Steinberg JL, Devous MD SR, Paulman RG, Gregory RR. (1995). Regional cerebral blood flow in first break and chronic schizophrenic patients and normal controls. Schizophr Res, 17(3), 229-240.

Stoll AL, Renshaw PF, Yurgelun-Todd DA, Cohen BM. (2000). Neuroimaging in bipolar disorder: what have we learned? Biol Psychiatry, 15. 48(6), 505-517.

Strakowski SM, DelBello MP, Adler C, Cecil DM, Sax KW. (2000). Neuroimaging in bipolar disorder. Bipolar Disord, 2(3 Pt 1), 148-164.

Swann AC. (2010). Approaches to preventing relapse in bipolar disorder: addressing nonadherence and prodromal symptoms. J Clin Psychiatry, 71(12), e35.

Swedo SE, Rapoport JL, Cheslow DL, Leonard HL, Ayoub EM, Hosier DM, Wald ER. (1989). High prevalence of obsessive-compulsive symptoms in patients with Sydenham's chorea. Am J Psychiatry, 146(2), 246-249.

Swedo SE, Pietrini P, Leonard HL, Schapiro MB, Rettew DC, Goldberger EL, Rapoport SI, Rapoport JL, Grady CL. (1992). Cerebral glucose metabolism in childhood-onset obsessive-compulsive disorder. Revisualization during pharmacotherapy. Arch Gen Psychiatry, 49(9), 690-694.

Takano H, Motohashi N, Uema T, Ogawa K, Ohnishi T, Nishikawa M, Kashima H, Matsuda H. (2007). Changes in regional cerebral blood flow during acute electroconvulsive therapy in patients with depression: positron emission tomographic study. Br J Psychiatry, 190, 63-68.

Tamminga CA, Thaker GK, Buchanan R, Kirkpatrick B, Alphs LD, Chase TN, Carpenter WT. (1992). Limbic system abnormalities identified in schizophrenia using positron emission tomography with fluorodeoxyglucose and neocortical alterations with deficit syndrome. *Arch Gen Psychiatry*, 49(7), 522-530.

Tutus A, Simsek A, Sofuoglu S, Nardali M, Kugu N, Karaaslan F, Gönül AS. (1998). Changes in regional cerebral blood flow demonstrated by single photon emission computed tomography in depressive disorders: comparison of unipolar vs. bipolar subtypes. *Psychiatry Res*, 28. 83(3), 169-177.

Videbech P, Ravnkilde B, Pedersen TH, Hartvig H, Egander A, Clemmensen K, Rasmussen NA, Andersen F, Gjedde A, Rosenberg R. (2002). The Danish PET/depression project: clinical symptoms and cerebral blood flow. A regions-of-interest analysis. *Acta Psychiatr Scand*, 106(1), 35-44.

Vita A, Bressi S, Perani D, Invernizzi G, Giobbio GM, Dieci M, Garbarini M, Del Sole A, Fazio F. (1995). High-resolution SPECT study of regional cerebral blood flow in drug-free and drug-naive schizophrenic patients. *Am J Psychiatry*, 152(6), 876-882.

Weissman MM, Bland RC, Canino GJ, Greenwald S, Hwu HG, Lee CK, Newman SC, Oakley-Browne MA, Rubio-Stipec M, Wickramaratne PJ, et al. (1994). The cross national epidemiology of obsessive compulsive disorder. The Cross National Collaborative Group. *J Clin Psychiatry*, 55 Suppl, 5-10.

Whiteside SP, Port JD, Abramowitz JS. (2004). A meta-analysis of functional neuroimaging in obsessive-compulsive disorder. *Psychiatry Res*, 15. 132(1), 69-79.

Wolkin A, Jaeger J, Brodie JD, Wolf AP, Fowler J, Rotrosen J, Gomez-Mont F, Cancro R. (1985). Persistence of cerebral metabolic abnormalities in chronic schizophrenia as determined by positron emission tomography. *Am J Psychiatry*, 142(5), 564-571.

Wolkin A, Sanfilipo M, Wolf AP, Angrist B, Brodie JD, Rotrosen J. (1992). Negative symptoms and hypofrontality in chronic schizophrenia. *Arch Gen Psychiatry*, 49(12), 959-965.

8

The Memory, Cognitive and Psychological Functions of Sleep: Update from Electroencephalographic and Neuroimaging Studies

Roumen Kirov[1] and Serge Brand[2]
[1]*Institute of Neurobiology, Bulgarian Academy of Sciences*
[2]*Depression Research Unit, Psychiatric Hospital of the University of Basel*
[1]*Bulgaria*
[2]*Switzerland*

1. Introduction

Sleep is a universal biological feature in almost all, if not in all species, and represents a global state of immobility with greatly reduced responsiveness to environmental stimuli, which can be distinguished from coma or anaesthesia by its rapid reversibility (Cirelli & Tononi, 2008). It is by no means a dormant state. When it is prevented, the body tries to recover the lost amount. The existence of sleep rebound after deprivation reveals that sleep is not simply a period of reduced activity or alertness regulated by circadian or ultradian rhythms (Dinges et al., 2005). Notably, in most vertebrates and all mammal species, including man, sleep displays a specific architecture roughly described as a cyclic occurrence of rapid eye movement (REM) sleep and non-REM sleep. Further, dramatic changes in brain electrophysiology, neurochemistry and functional anatomy biologically distinguish the different sleep stages from one another (Hobson & Pace-Schott, 2002; Pace-Schott & Hobson, 2002). Also, human and animal neurophysiologic studies have shown that the magnitude of changes in brain metabolism and neuronal activity in many discrete brain structures during certain sleep stages exceeds that during most of the waking periods (Gottesmenn, 1999; Maquet et al., 1996; Nofzinger et al., 1997; Steriade & Timofeev, 2003).

Although the precise functions of sleep are still beyond comprehensive understanding (Cirelli & Tononi, 2008), many studies point to the critical role of sleep for physiological functioning and adaptation. Its vital importance is well documented by the fact that its deprivation in rodents and flies can cause death more quickly relative to food deprivation (Rechtschaffen, 1998). Thus, sleep is shown to serve many energetic and metabolic, immune, thermoregulatory, cardiovascular, and respiratory functions, all responsible for normal brain and body homeostasis (Siegel, 2009; Tononi & Cirelli, 2006). Notably, along with these functions, sleep is shown to play a key role for important cognitive and psychological processes, among which learning and memory have been most intensively studied (Diekelmann & Born, 2010; Rasch & Born, 2007; Stickgold, 2005; Walker, 2008; Walker & Stickgold, 2006; 2010). Accordingly, an extensive body of research has revealed a cruicial role for sleep in human cognitive abilities (Mander et al., 2008; Schabus et al., 2006; 2008; Yoo et al., 2007b), heuristic creativity and insightfulness (Cai et al., 2009; Stickgold et al., 1999; 2001; Wagner et al., 2004; Yordanova et al., 2008; 2009; 2010), constructive thinking and decision making (Durrant et al., 2011; Venkatraman et al., 2011), and emotional regulation (Walker, 2009; Walker & van der Helm, 2009). The latter engages consolidation of emotional memory (Nishida et al., 2009; Wagner et al., 2001; 2006; Walker, 2009) and emotional processing (Gujar et al., 2011a; 2011b; Yoo et al., 2007a). Collectively, these various associations suggest that sleep provides unique conditions for off-line memory consolidation, reconsolidation and information reprocessing to take place. However, it is still not precisely known whether these mechanisms are distinctly different from the restoring and energetic functions of sleep, whether the two types of functions are coupled, or whether the latter simply facilitate the cognitive functions of sleep.

Many electroencephalographic (EEG) and neuroimaging studies including functional magnetic resonance imaging (fMRI) have found that the structural and functional organization of the neural substrate undergoes changes during sleep in relation to human cognition. The entity of neural mechanisms underpinning cognitive and psychological functions of the brain is generally recognized as brain plasticity, i.e., as the capability of the neural substrate to reorganize over time as a result of previous experiences. In this chapter, studies demonstrating that sleep affects cognition by neural plasticity mechanisms in humans will be updated and overviewed to provide a converging framework for better understanding the role of sleep for memory, cognitive abilities and psychological functioning. Since mechanisms of brain plasticity are closely related to sleep physiology, architecture and neurobiological regulation, the reader will be first introduced to neurobiology of sleep.

2. Neurobiology of sleep

2.1 Sleep architecture and physiology

The heterogeneous nature of sleep can be seen in human and in most animal polysomnographic (PSG) records, which traditionally use electrophysiological techniques including electroencephalography (EEG), electromyography (EMG) and electro-oculography (EOG) to characterize sleep at system levels. In humans, overnight sleep is characterized by a cyclic occurrence of non-REM sleep and REM sleep. Non-REM sleep includes lighter sleep stages 1 and 2 and stages 3 and 4 of the deeper slow wave sleep (SWS) (Rechtschaffen & Kales, 1968). Whereas SWS dominates the first half of the night, REM sleep and stage 2 of non-REM sleep dominate the second half. This ultradian dynamics reflects the circadian regulation of sleep that is distinguishable from its homeostatic regulation seen after sleep deprivation or prolonged wakefulness (Borbély 1982; Borbély & Ackermann, 1999). Normally, sleep onset begins with a brief period of stage 1 of non-REM sleep, which is subsequently followed by sleep deepening marked by appearance of stage 2 of non-REM sleep and a further progressive transition to stages 3 and 4 of SWS. The latter is followed by a relatively short transient of stage 2 of non-REM sleep, after which a period of REM sleep appears. This progression of sleep stages, and in particular, the non-REM sleep - REM sleep alternation forms one sleep cycle with approximately 90 min duration. About 5 or more such sleep cycles are usually observed in the normal human overnight sleep (Broughton, 1987; Rechschaffen & Kales, 1968; Sinton & McCarley, 2000).

The Memory, Cognitive and Psychological Functions of Sleep: Update from Electroencephalographic
and Neuroimaging Studies

157

2.2 Electrophysiological signatures of sleep stages

The distinct sleep stages of either human overnight sleep or human daily naps can be determined by their specific "macroscopic" electrophysiological signatures, which are described by Rechschaffen & Kales (1968) and are commonly used for human sleep stages scoring. Unlike the desynchronized mode of EEG activity during wakefulness, the electrophysiological signatures of different sleep stages are more complex, which reflects a more heterogeneous nature of sleep than that of wake (Hobson & Pace-Schott, 2002). Basically, wakefulness is divided into active wake, characterized by desynchronized low-voltage fast EEG activity including beta (~ 15-30 Hz) and gamma (> 30 Hz) rhythms as well as by theta (~ 5 Hz) EEG activity with frontal-midline location, and quiet wake, characterized by posterior alpha (~ 10 Hz) and central sigma (~ 12-14 Hz) EEG rhythms that replace the desynchronized EEG mode of the active wake (Niedermeyer, 1993). The electrophysiological signatures of both active and quiet are show in Figure 1.

Sleep initiation is described as a replacement of waking EEG by theta or slower rhythms paralleled by an appearance of very slow circular eye movements, and both electrophysiological features form stage 1 of non-REM sleep (Broughton, 1987; Sinton & McCarley, 2000). Stage 2 of non-REM sleep is defined by presence of the classical EEG sleep spindles oscillating at ~ 12-15 Hz with central-parietal location, slower sleep spindles oscillating at ~ 9-13 Hz with frontal location and sporadic biphasic slow waves known as K-complexes (Anderer et al., 2001; De Gennaro & Ferrara, 2003). Sleep spindles are present also in the deeper SWS stages, but in less pronounced and discrete forms, among which spindle activity in the frequency range of ~ 8-12 Hz with frontal location is recognized to dominate SWS (Cantero et al., 2002; Salih et al., 2009). K-complexes are regarded as precursors of EEG components of the SWS (Amzica & Steriade, 1997; De Gennaro & Ferrara, 2003). These "macroscopic" human electrophysiological signatures of distinct sleep-wake stages are shown in Figure 1.

SWS is hallmarked by synchronous high-voltage (> 75 µV) EEG delta (~ 1-4 Hz) waves and slow (< 1 Hz) oscillations (SO) (Achrermann & Borbely, 1997; Crunelli & Hughes, 2010; Steriade et al., 1993), both recognized as slow wave activity (SWA) (Fig. 1). SO are also shown to occur in stage 2 of non-REM sleep (Crunelli & Hughes, 2010; Nir et al., 2011), and the SO during both stage 2 of non-REM sleep and SWS are shown to group and synchronize sleep spindles and delta waves (Mölle et al., 2002; Mölle et al., 2004; Steriade, 2001). Whereas sleep spindles originate form interactions between thalamo-cortical circuits involving γ-aminobutyric (GABA)-ergic thalamic neurons and glutamate-ergic cortical neurons (De Gennaro & Ferrara, 2003; Steriade, 2006), SO are shown to have a neocortical origin (Achrermann & Borbely, 1997; Nir et al., 2011; Steriade et al., 1993), although they are also proposed to emerge form the thalamus (Crunelli & Hughes, 2010). Another important EEG signature of SWS seen not only in animals but also in human intracranial EEG recordings, is reflected by hippocampal sharp-wave/ripple (SWR) bursts. Hippocampal sharp waves generated in the hippocampal CA3 region are fast depolarizing events, on which high-frequency oscillations (~ 80-200 Hz) originating from an interaction between inhibitory interneurons and pyramidal cells in CA1 (so-called ripples) are superimposed (Buzsáki, 2006; Csicsvari et al., 1999). Notably, SO have been shown to group also SWR in rodents (Battaglia et al., 2004; Sirota et al., 2003), and a temporal phase-coupling between SO, sleep spindles and SWR has been demonstrated in human depth EEG records during SWS (Clemens et al., 2007; 2011; Nir et al., 2011). The complex relationship between these sleep signatures is regarded as reflecting brain plasticity mechanisms at a system level, which is important for the memory consolidation and reconsolidation during SWS (Diekelmann & Born, 2010).

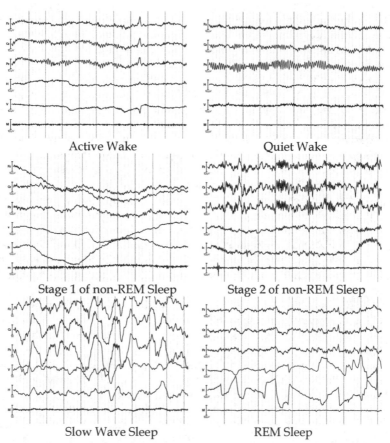

Fig. 1. Electrophysiological signatures of distinct sleep-wake stages: EEG recorded from Fz, Cz and Pz, vertical (v) and horizontal (h) eye movements, and electromyogram (m). Calibration marks are set-up at 100 μV, time (horizontal) marks are 1 s.

Unlike non-REM sleep electrophysiology, REM sleep EEG signatures (Fig. 1) include low-voltage desynchronized wake-like EEG activity comprising theta and fast (beta and gamma) rhythms accompanied by a swift occurrence of rapid eye movements (REM) upon lack of muscle tone (Aserinsky & Kleitman, 1953; Cantero et al., 2003; Clemens et al., 2009). Hippocampal theta rhythm is a prominent REM sleep EEG signature in rodents (Gottesmann, 1999; Kirov & Moyanova, 2002) and felines (Hobson & Pace Schott, 2002), while in human hippocampus and neocortex it is less coherent (Cantero et al., 2003). Further, REM sleep is hallmarked by ponto-geniculo-occipital (PGO) waves. PGO waves are driven by intense bursts of synchronized activity that propagate from the pontine brainstem mainly to the lateral geniculate nucleus and visual cortex (Callaway et al., 1987; Hobson & Pace-Schott, 2002; Pace-Schott & Hobson, 2002). They occur in temporal association with

The Memory, Cognitive and Psychological Functions of Sleep: Update from Electroencephalographic
and Neuroimaging Studies

159

REM in rats and felines (Callaway et al., 1987; Stickgold et al, 2001), as well as in humans (Lim et al, 2007; Miyauchi et al., 2009), and are suggested to reflect both dream mental states of REM sleep and cognitive processing during this sleep stage (Stickgold et al., 2001). REM sleep signatures are shown to reflect mechanisms of brain plasticity at synaptic and genetic levels (Ribeiro et al., 1999; 2002), which may promote not only REM sleep specific processes, but also a further transformation of consolidated memories (Walker & Stickgold, 2010).

2.3 Mechanisms of sleep regulation

The regulation of sleep is active in its own rights, and is closely related to sleep's physiology and functions (Hobson, 2005; Pace-Schott & Hobson, 2002). The respective neurobiological mechanisms are represented by complex reciprocal interactions between different neuronal populations and their chemical modulators and transmitters in distinct functional states across sleep-wake cycle leading to distinct functional states (Gottesmann, 1999; Hobson et al., 1975; Hobson & Peace-Schott, 2002; Peace-Schott & Hobson, 2002). Two major brain regions are mostly considered in sleep regulation, especially when functions of sleep are concerned (Pace-Schott & Hobson, 2002). The first engages neuronal populations located in the diencephalon, in particular, the hypothalamus, mostly involved in the circadian regulation of sleep. The second brain region engages brainstem or meso-pontine and basal forebrain nuclei spread in the reticular ascending system (RAS) and projecting noradrenaline (NA), serotonin (5-Hydroxytryptamine, 5-HT) and acetylcholine (Ach) neuromodulatory signals to upper brain structures including the basal ganglia and amygdala, thalamus, hippocampus, and cortex. These mechanisms are essential for the ultradian alternating expression of non-REM sleep-REM sleep periods (Gottesmann, 1999; Hobson et al., 1975; Pace-Schott & Hobson, 2002). Briefly, during wake, brainstem/meso-pontine NA, 5-HT, Ach, and hypothalamic histamine (HIS) neurons projecting to upper brain structures and cortex, are all active, thus sustaining functional brain states optimal to the environmental requirements (Gottesmann, 1999; Hobson & Pace-Schott, 2002; Pace-Schott & Hobson, 2002). As sleep deepens from stages 1 and 2 to SWS, all these neuromodulators progressively decrease their activities, with their lowest levels observed during SWS. This leads to strongly diminished or lacking RAS neuromodulation of upper brain structures and cortex, which in turn, is responsible for the appearance of non-REM sleep EEG signals represented by sleep spindles, K-complexes and SWA, all originating from thalamo-cortical and cortico-cortical interplay (McCormick & Bal, 1997; Pace-Schott & Hobson, 2002; Steriade & Timofeev, 2003). In REM sleep, all NA, 5-HT and HIS neurons cease their firing. In contrast, Ach excessive over-activity emerges projecting to the cortex and all sub-cortical structures, which produces the electrophysiological signatures of REM sleep (Gottesmann, 1999; Pace-Schott & Hobson, 2002).

2.4 Neuroimaging of sleep and wake

Several neuroimaging studies using either fMRI or positron-emission tomography (PET) have investigated the pattern of brain activation across wake, non-REM and REM sleep. These studies have demonstrated that anterior cingulate cortex, right and left amygdaloid complexes, pons, parahippocampal cortex, and extrastriate visual cortex are more active during REM sleep compared with wake and non-REM sleep, whereas the activation of other brain areas including right and left dorsolateral prefrontal cortices, right and left parietal cortices and precuneus, posterior cingulate cortex, and primary visual cortex, is suppressed in REM sleep compared with wake. All these brain regions have been shown to be the most suppressed during non-REM sleep (Broun et al., 1997; 1998; Maquet et al., 1996; Miyauchi et al., 2009; Nofzinger et al., 1997). Yet, other brain structures are shown to specifically increase their activation in relation to distinct non-REM sleep stages and their EEG signatures. For example, blood oxygen level-dependent (BOLD) signal from the thalamus is strongest during spindle activity in stage 2 of non-REM sleep (Schabus et al., 2007), whereas during SO in SWS, brain functional activation is strong in the medial temporal cortex, the parahippocampal cortex, and neocortical areas (Dang-Vu et al., 2005; 2008; Maquet et al., 1997).

2.5 Mental characteristics of the sleep-wake stages

Notably, from a cognitive point of view, the mental characteristics of sleep-wake stages well correspond to their brain activation patterns found in neuroimaging studies (Fosse et al., 2001; 2004; Hobson & Pace-Schott, 2002; Hobson et al., 2000; Stickgold et al., 2001). Thus, wake is characterized by strongest and most logic thoughts in the presence of sensory input, executive control and goal-directed behavior. Sleep onset is hallmarked by the so called hypnagogic hallucinations, and as sleep deepens from stage 2 of non-REM sleep to SWS, thinking becomes more and more scares, and almost absent during SWS. Yet, there are logic thoughts mostly associated with previous wake experiences (Fosse et al., 2004; Hobson, 2005; Hobson et al., 2000; Stickgold et al., 2001). During REM sleep, mental activity is likely hallucinatory, and is behaviorally expressed in vivid, bizarre and elusive dreams (Fosse et al., 2004; Hobson et al., 2000; Stickgold et al., 2001). Also, REM sleep mentality is characterized by a most salient emotional tone upon lack of sensory input (Hobson et al., 2000) and executive control, as evidenced by the neuroimaging data (suppression of the dorsolateral prefrontal cortex, e.g., Maquet et al., 1996).

3. Sleep and memory

Likewise the heterogeneous structure of sleep, memory categories believed to exist in human brain are distinctly different. Roughly, they can be divided into declarative and non-declarative or procedural memory, and the same categorization holds true for the processes of learning (Dienes & Perner 1999). Declarative memory is considered to comprise consciously accessible memories of fact-based information (i.e., knowing "what"). Several subcategories of the declarative system exist, including episodic memory (autobiographical memory for events of one's past) and semantic memory (memory for general knowledge, not tied to specific events, but rather tied to its verbal components) (Tulving 1985). Current neural models of declarative memory formation emphasize the critical importance of structures in the medial temporal lobe, especially the hippocampus, and thus, declarative memory is also known as hippocampus-dependent memory (Eichenbaum, 2000). In contrast, procedural or implicit memory is regarded as non-conscious, comprising memory of knowing "how", such as learning of actions, habits, and skills, as well as implicit learning (Dienes & Perner 1999). Procedural memory formation appears to be less dependent on medial temporal lobe structures, and to include sensori-motor cortices, basal ganglia and cerebellum (Forkstam & Petersson 2005).

3.1 Overview of human EEG data

Since the discovery of SO (< 1 Hz) in cats (Steriade et al., 1993) and (~ 0.7-0.8 Hz) in humans (Achrermann & Borbely, 1997), this hallmark of human non-REM sleep, and SWS in

The Memory, Cognitive and Psychological Functions of Sleep: Update from Electroencephalographic
and Neuroimaging Studies

161

particular, has been proposed as an essential mechanism underlying the consolidation of hippocampus-dependent memories (Buzsáki, 1989; Marshall & Born, 2007; Mölle et al., 2004; Steriade, 2001). In human SWS, "up" and "down" EEG states of SO are shown be dissimilarly associated with a number of electrophysiological events. Specifically, the "up" state of the SO is marked by increased occurrence of delta slow waves and sleep spindles, whereas during the 'down" state of SO, delta slow wave and sleep spindle activities markedly decrease (Mölle et al., 2002; 2004). Thus, human SO are demonstrated to group both slow waves and spindles. Further, a rapid increase of the underlying neuronal activity (depolarizing state) and a rapid decrease in it (hyperpolarizing state) have recently been shown to characterize human SO "up" and "down" wave forms, respectively (Nir et al., 2011). Finally, human studies have demonstrated time and phase coupling between SO, slow waves, sleep spindles, and hippocampal SWR bursts (Clemens et al., 2007; 2011; Nir et al., 2011). Collectively, these findings strongly indicate that non-REM sleep/SWS SO represent an EEG mechanism involved in plastic changes sub-serving the hippocampus-dependent memory consolidation.

Indeed, SO have been shown to be strongly associated with both procedural (Huber et al., 2004) and declarative (Mölle et al., 2004) memory consolidation taking place in human non-REM sleep/SWS. Later, to verify the specific role for SO in hippocampus-dependent memory consolidation, a series of studies, in which brain rhythms have been modulated using trans-cranial direct current stimulation (tDCS), has been conducted in humans. This method is now recognized as a reliable tool for modulating both the internally generated brain rhythms and the activity of underlying neuronal populations, depolarized under anodal tDCS and hyperpolarized under cathodal tDCS, respectively (Fröhlich & McCormick, 2010; Reis et al., 2008).

Initially, weak (not perceived by subjects) anodal tDCS oscillating at 0.75 Hz (slow oscillation stimulation, SOS) has been delivered during the transition from stage 2 of non-REM sleep to SWS after declarative and procedural learning before sleep. Compared with a sham condition, stimulation has selectively produced a gain in only declarative memory after sleep. Importantly, it has also produced a substantial increase in SO (~ 0.75 Hz) and frontal slow alpha spindle (8-12 Hz) activity, possibly by entraining these sleep EEG rhythms (Marshall et al., 2006). These findings have provided strong evidence for the role of SO and/or frontal slow spindle activity for the hippocampus-dependent memory consolidation. However, they have not addressed the question of whether SOS itself or whether endogenous SO boosted by the SOS have resulted in improvement of the consolidation of declarative memory found. This question was addressed in two later studies. In these studies, weak anodal tDCS oscillating at frequencies not common for the respective functional brain states was applied. In particular, SOS oscillating at 0.75 Hz was applied during quiet or resting wake retention period after learning declarative and procedural tasks. SOS did not affect either declarative or procedural memory consolidation, nor did it affect working memory and mood at retest. However, in contrast to its EEG effects during non-REM sleep (Marshall et al., 2006), it produced only a local (at the frontal sites of stimulation) increase in EEG power in SO (0.4-1.2 Hz) frequency band, accompanied by a widespread and strong increase in theta (4-8 Hz) EEG power. Further, when delivered in active wake state during encoding of a verbal learning memory task, the 0.75 Hz SOS produced virtually the same EEG effects as during quite wake (local increase in SO and widespread increase in theta power), but it significantly improved encoding of declarative verbal information (Kirov et al., 2009). Recently, tDCS oscillating at 5 Hz (wake and/or REM sleep EEG rhythm, theta stimulation) was applied in the first non-REM sleep cycle of overnight sleep, during the transition from stage 2 of non-REM sleep to SWS, after subjects have learned tasks of both declarative and procedural memory before sleep. Notably, theta stimulation disrupted the normal progression of SWS, SO (0.5-1 Hz) and SWA (1-4 Hz) EEG power in the course of the stimulation. Also, it significantly decreased slow spindle activity (8-12 Hz) only frontally. These EEG changes were associated with a strong impairment of only declarative memory consolidation at recall after sleep (Marshall et al., 2011). Collectively, these findings strongly indicate that SO, SWA and frontal slow spindle activity reflect specific EEG mechanisms of hippocampus-dependent memory consolidation, which do not act beyond non-REM sleep/SWS. Moreover, they provide one of the strongest evidence for the assumption that during active wake, encoding of memory is reflected by theta EEG oscillations, which possibly reflect a transfer of information from the cortex to the hippocampus (Sederberg et al., 2003). Essentially, they strongly support the notion that memories encoded during wake undergo off-line consolidation during non-REM sleep/SWS by mechanisms involving an interplay between the hippocampus and the cortex, as reflected by the SO and frontal slow alpha activity (Buzsáki, 2006; Mölle et al., 2002; 2004; Marshall et al., 2006). Another recent investigation clearly showed strong and positive correlations between SO and sleep spindle EEG activities during the earliest portion of overnight non-REM sleep/SWS and rates of off-line improvement of both declarative and non-declarative memories (Wilhelm et al., 2011). These sleep EEG rhythms correlated positively with gain of improvement of only memories that were expected to be of further relevance, and not with memories that were not, with the latter memories being not found affected by sleep. Notably, this study demonstrates that SO and sleep spindles during non-REM sleep/SWS, are important EEG patterns not only for memory consolidation but also for memory reprocessing or reconsolidation (Wilhelm et al., 2011).

Some of the observations in the studies of Marshall et al. (2006; 2011) and Wilhelm et al. (2011) deserve further mentioning. These studies clearly show associations of non-REM sleep/SWS EEG signatures with either memory consolidation or reconsolidation in the first non-REM sleep cycle (Marshall et al., 2006; 2011) and even before the occurrence of the first SWS period (Wilhelm et al., 2011). A more recent study demonstrates that during the first half of overnight sleep, SO and SWA represent a global electric brain event that can be reliably recorded from hippocampus, medial temporal lobe and neocortex, whereas during the second half, both SO and SWA are expressed rather like a local phenomenon without strong phase and time coupling (Nir et al., 2011). Thus, regarding the studies using oscillating tDCS during sleep (Marshall et al., 2006; 2011) together with these of Wilhelm et al. (2011) and Nir et al. (2011), it can be concluded that SO, frontal slow alpha activity and sleep spindles, all represent important sleep EEG signatures reflecting processes of hippocampus-dependent memory consolidation and reconsolidation, which processes take place in the earliest part of non-REM sleep.

Similarly, classical sleep spindles, the major EEG signature of stage 2 of non-REM sleep, have been proposed to reflect mechanisms of brain plasticity that take place during non-REM sleep (Sejnowski & Destexhe, 2000; Steriade, 2001). Many human studies have demonstrated that either number, density, or EEG power spectral activity of spindles during stage 2 of non-REM sleep have been significantly involved in both declarative (Clemens et al., 2005; Gais et al., 2002) and procedural (Clemens et al., 2006; Fogel & Smith, 2006; Fogel et al., 2007b; Nishida & Walker, 2007; Shabus et al., 2004; Tucker & Fishbein, 2009) memory consolidation. Moreover, Nishida & Walker attempted to distinguish between use-dependent and experience depended sleep processes. They subtracted sleep spindle EEG activity measured at a "non-learning hemisphere (left)" from that measured at a "learning hemisphere (right)" and were able to demonstrate strong positive correlations with offline memory improvement that were not evident for either hemisphere alone (Nishida & Walker, 2007). Thus, classical sleep spindles appear to represent an EEG pattern reliably associated with memory processes.

3.2 Overview of human neuroimaging data

Notably, the first human neuroimaging study almost entirely confirm previous rodent findings, which have shown that sleep-dependent memory consolidation relies on reactivation of the so-called hippocampus place cells during SWS in response to spatial or maze navigating tasks (Wilson & McNaughton, 1994). Thus, Peigneux et al. (2004) using a combination of PET and sleep EEG (PSG) methods, showed for the first time such a reactivation of hippocampal and neocortical regions in humans. At encoding during wakefulness, subjects were trained (or not) to learn and find their way inside a complex three-dimensional virtual town. Compared with the non-trained group, subjects who learned the task at encoding during wake displayed an increase in their regional cerebral blood flow (rCBF) in a bilateral pattern of neural activation, including the right and left hippocampus, the right and left parahippocampal gyri, superior parietal lobules, right and left precuneus, lingual and posterior cingulate gyri, middle and superior occipital cingulate gyri, and the anterior lobes of cerebellum. In the trained group, rCBF was consequently measured during stage 2 of non-REM sleep, SWS and REM sleep. The neural pattern of activity found at training sessions during wakefulness was reactivated only during SWS. This pattern of reactivation during SWS strongly correlated with the level of improvement on the task at recall after sleep (Peigneux et al., 2004). Three years later, Rasch et al. (2007) also used a combination of fMRI and PSG methods to investigate specifically the role for SWS in declarative memory consolidation. The authors first established a robust association between declarative learning (card place location) stimuli and a smell, olfactory stimulus (the smell of a rose). Subjects learned object locations in a two-dimensional (2D) object location memory task in the evening before sleep. During the first two periods of subsequent SWS, the odor cue was presented again (in an alternating 30 s on/30 s off mode). In a control condition, odorless vehicle was delivered. At retrieval testing after sleep, memory of card locations was distinctly enhanced when the odor was presented during SWS as compared to presentation of vehicle alone. Re-exposure to odor during SWS improved retention of memory in a hippocampus-dependent manner: bilateral reactivation of the hippocampus and medial prefrontal lobe, as measured by BOLD signal (Rasch et al., 2007). Further, an fMRI study demonstrated that compared with total sleep deprivation, post-learning sleep enhances hippocampal responses during recall of word pairs (declarative memory) 48 h after learning, thus indicating intra-hippocampal memory processing during sleep (Gais et al., 2007).. At the same time, it was shown that sleep induced a memory-related functional connectivity between the hippocampus and the medial prefrontal cortex. Six months after learning, recalling the same declarative memories reactivated the medial prefrontal cortex even more strongly than they did during encoding before sleep, thus showing that sleep leads to long lasting changes in representation of memories at a system (hippocampal-cortical) level. Although this study does not show reactivation of the hippocampus and medial prefrontal cortex during sleep, basing on previous findings, the authors assume an important role of hippocampal-cortical connectivity for sleep-dependent declarative memory consolidation (Gais et al., 2007). The last convincing evidence concerning the role for SWS in memory formation comes from a recent fMRI study where the effect of declarative memory reconsolidation on declarative memory consolidation during SWS and wake was investigated (Diekelmenn et al., 2011). By using an experimental protocol similar to that previously applied by Rasch et al. (2007), the authors aimed at reactivating memories in humans by presenting associated odor cues either during SWS or during wake. During wake, reactivation of memories was followed by an interference task to probe memory stability, and as expected (Brown & Robertson, 2007; Robertson, 2009), this reactivation resulted in destabilized memories. In contrast, reactivation during SWS immediately stabilized memories, thereby directly increasing their resistance to interference. Importantly, BOLD signal revealed quite different patterns of reactivation during SWS and wake. The reactivation during SWS was mainly seen in the hippocampus and posterior cortical regions, whereas reactivation during wake was primarily found in the prefrontal cortical areas, thus showing that reactivation of memory serves distinct functions depending on brain state: wake versus SWS (Diekelmann et al., 2011). It is to be noted that similar differences between effects of oscillating trans-cranial direct current stimulation on both EEG activity and memory processes was also shown during wake when compared to SWS, although these differences distinguished specifically verbal memory encoding from declarative memory consolidation (Kirov et al., 2009; Marshall et al., 2006; 2011).

To our knowledge, only one neuroimaging study was able to provide convincing evidence for reactivation of brain regions during REM sleep in association with sleep-dependent consolidation of procedural memory (Maquet et al., 2000). In this study, three groups of subjects learned a serial reaction time task (SRTT) during wakefulness. To verify which brain regions are activated by SRTT, one group was scanned by using of PET either during training or during the subsequent rest wake period, and was not further examined. Subjects from a second group were trained on the task during two sessions in the afternoon, and then scanned during the night after training, both during wake and during various sleep stages. This group was retested at recall after sleep to verify that sleep-dependent learning had occurred. A third group was scanned at the same time points as the second group was, however, under absence of learning (no learning condition). Sleep architecture in the latter two groups was assessed by a routine PSG, and rCBF was measured across both three groups and all time points. Interestingly, although the third group improved implicit learning component of SRTT at recall after sleep, no any changes in sleep architecture between the learning and the non-learning conditions were found. However, as measured by the rCBF, a specific pattern of brain activation found in the first group during and after learning was reactivated only in the second group, and only during REM sleep. This pattern engaged a set of brain regions located in occipital and premotor cortices (Maquet et al., 2000). A later PET study by the same group (Laureys et al., 2001) confirmed that specific brain reactivation occurs during REM sleep in relation to procedural memory consolidation (Maquet et al., 2000). The authors showed that the left premotor cortex is functionally more correlated with the left posterior parietal cortex and bilateral pre-supplementary motor area during REM sleep in subjects previously trained to a reaction time task relative to untrained subjects. The increase in functional connectivity during post-training REM sleep additionally suggests that the reactivated brain areas participate in an optimization of a network that subtends subject's visuo-motor response (Laureys et al., 2001).

Altogether, the above neuroimaging findings show that the mechanisms of memory processing during early night non-REM sleep/SWS are distinctly different from those that take place in REM sleep. The former include complex interactions between hippocampus and cortex, thus reflecting brain plasticity mechanisms at system and neural levels. The latter include local patterns of brain reactivation, which are proposed to reflect brain plasticity mechanisms at synaptic and genetic levels.

4. Sleep and cognitive functions

The strongest evidence for the important role that sleep plays in a variety of cognitive functions comes from many observations of effects of sleep loss and sleep deprivation on cognition (Killgore, 2010; Walker, 2008). The exclusively important role of sleep for cognitive functions has been best demonstrated in a study showing that even one night of total sleep deprivation results in inability to learn facts, i.e. deficient encoding of episodic memories (Yoo et al., 2007b). The neuroimaging correlates of this impaired learning ability will be presented below in the respective section.

4.1 Overview of human EEG data

Sleep spindles, the major hallmark of stage 2 of non-REM sleep, have been for long proposed to be associated with human individual cognitive abilities or intelligence. For example, Bódizs et al. (2005) found that both grouping of fast sleep spindles by cortical slow oscillation over the left frontopolar derivation (Fp1) and fast sleep spindle density over the right frontal area (Fp2, F4) during stage 2 of non-REM sleep, correlated positively with general mental ability. Further, a robust positive correlations were found between slow (< 13 Hz) and fast (> 13 Hz) spindle activity in stage 2 of non-REM sleep and both individual cognitive abilities and implicit/explicit memory-related abilities (Schabus et al., 2006). Later, Fogel et al. (2007a) showed first that number of spindles in stage 2 of non-REM sleep remains relatively stable within individuals from night to night. Second, the authors demonstrated that the number of spindles and EEG power of sigma (slow spindle) activity were positively correlated with performance intelligence quotient (PIQ), but not with verbal IQ. Also, perceptual/analytical skills measured by the PIQ accounted for most of the interindividual differences in spindles. Interestingly, in the same study, a relationship between rapid eye movements in REM sleep and VIQ in individuals with higher IQ scores was also demonstrated (Fogel et al., 2007a). However, Tucker & Fishbein (2009) demonstrated that while subject's intelligence correlated positively with pre-sleep acquisition and post-sleep retest performance on both procedural and declarative tasks, it did not correlate with over-stage 2 of non-REM sleep spindle events. These findings suggest that intelligence may not be a powerful modulator of sleep's effect on memory performance (Tucker & Fishbein, 2009).

One major question arising from the above described findings is whether sleep contributes to human intelligence in a state dependent manner (i.e., by providing neurobiological conditions for memory consolidation and reconsolidation), whether sleep is associated with intelligence in a trait dependent manner (i.e., strictly individual sleep characteristics are related to individual intelligence), or whether sleep and human intelligence are related in both ways (Geiger et al., 2011; Fogel & Smith, 2011). It has been previously proposed that sleep serves human intelligence by complex interactions between its unique physiological and mental states, and individual sleep patterns and cognitive traits (Kirov, 2007). One study has addressed this question providing some evidence that stage 2 of non-REM sleep spindle increase after learning is related to elaborate encoding before sleep, whereas individual's general learning ability is well reflected by inter-individual (trait-like) differences in absolute sleep spindle activity (Schabus et al., 2008). However,, the precise mechanisms involved in the complex association between sleep and intelligence remain so far poorly understood (Kirov, 2007). As will be seen in the paragraph below, the role for sleep in human heuristic creativity and insightful behavior can further illuminate this issue. Importantly, it has been consistently shown that sleep provides unique conditions for development of human heuristic creativity (Cai et al., 2009; Stickgold et al., 1999; Walker et al., 2002), among which the insightful behavior, as a higher form of human intelligence, is of major importance (Wagner et al., 2004; Yordanova et al., 2008; 2009; 2010; in press). Human insight refers to discovering of regularities that are out of awareness. Notably, it has been demonstrated that as twice as many subjects who had slept after initial learning of a number reduction task (NRT) gained insight into a hidden regularity relative to subjects who had been sleep deprived (Wagner et al., 2004). However, Wagner and co-authors (2004) have not objectively assessed sleep architecture by PSG. Thus, it has remained unclear how and through which mechanisms sleep promotes insight. This question was addressed in a series of later studies using the so-called split night design (Plihal & Born, 1997; 1999). The first study investigating sleep's role for insight by the split night design demonstrated that implicit knowledge acquired at encoding of NRT before sleep was transformed into insight throughout the early night sleep rich in SWS, thus pointing a role for SWS in insight (Yordanova et al., 2008). Further, the same study demonstrated that implicit learning of NRT acquired at encoding (during awakening before the second half of night) was not further transformed but was preserved by the late night sleep rich in REM sleep, thus indicating that REM sleep stabilizes implicit learning (Yordanova et al., 2008). In two later studies, Yordanova and co-authors demonstrated that SWS contributes to gaining insight in a state dependent instead of a trait-dependent manner. First, they revealed a topographic re-distribution of slow cortical potentials (SPs) indicating that a spatial reorganization occurred only after early sleep rich in SWS, but not after late sleep, and only for predictable responses on NRT. This SPs reorganization correlated with the amount of SWS (Yordanova et al., 2009). Second, they showed that only after SWS a pattern of brain activation shown as a precondition for insight (increased alpha and beta EEG desynchronization at the right hemisphere and a lack of such at the left) occurred (Yordanova et al., 2010). Finally, these authors were able to extract a specific for SWS EEG rhythm, slow (8-12 Hz) alpha activity at the right hemisphere, which was associated with transformation of implicit knowledge into insight on the NRT, and which was distinctly different form use-dependent (SWA and 12-15 Hz spindle activity) found at the left hemisphere in response to task performance (Yordanova et al., in press). Collectively, these findings strongly indicate that sleep promotes insight, as a higher form of human intelligence, in a state dependent rather than in a trait dependent way.

Finally, a recent study questioned which sleep mechanisms may play a role for abstraction of an implicit probabilistic structure in sequential stimuli using a statistical learning paradigm, and searched for a predictive relationship between the type of sleep obtained and subsequent performance improvements (abstraction). Participants who consolidated over either a night of sleep or a nap improved significantly more than those who consolidated over an equivalent period of daytime wakefulness. Importantly, PSG revealed a significant correlation between the level of improvement or abstraction and the amount of SWS obtained (Durrant et al., 2011).

4.2 Overview of human neuroimaging data

The existing so far neuroimaging data concerning sleep and cognition do not reveal patterns of brain reactivation during sleep. Instead, they reveal altered brain activities associated with impaired cognitive processes in response to sleep deprivation. One of the most important findings is presented in the study of Yoo et al. (2007b). In this study, two groups of subjects were randomly assigned to either a sleep deprivation (SD) or a sleep control (SC) group. All subjects underwent an episodic memory encoding session during fMRI scanning, in which they viewed a series of picture slides and were retested two days later (after two recovery nights of sleep) for a recognition test session (without fMRI). Compared with SC group, SD subjects displayed much worse recognition at retest after two days, though they had two nights recovery sleep. This finding clearly shows that sleep deprivation impairs learning. The fMRI scans at learning/encoding demonstrated a significant impairment of activation in the hippocampal complex in the SD relative to SC group, a region known to be of critical importance for learning of new information (Yoo et al., 2007b). Another study showed that compared with normal sleep, SD produced impairment of spatial attention that correlated with a reduced activation in the posterior cingulate cortex, as measured by fMRI (Mander et al., 2008). Similarly, it is shown that SD produces lapses of attention manifested as delayed behavioral responses to salient stimuli. To identify changes in task-related brain activation associated with lapses after SD, fMRI scans during a visual selective attention task were conducted. It was demonstrated that SD-related lapses in attention corresponded to (1) reduced ability of frontal and parietal control regions to raise activation in response to lapses, (2) dramatically reduced visual sensory cortex activation and (3) reduced thalamic activation during lapses (Chee et al., 2008). Another fMRI study by the same group tested the hypothesis of whether SD impairs short-term memory due to reduced storage capacity or whether it affects processes contributing to appropriate information encoding. Scans were conducted during performing a short-term memory visual task and during presenting varying visual array sizes without engaging memory. Whereas the magnitude of intraparietal sulcus activation and memory capacity after normal sleep were highly correlated, SD elicited a diminished pattern of activation on both tasks, indicating that deficits in both visual processing and visual attention account for loss of short-term memory capacity (Chee & Chuah, 2007). Further, an fMRI study showed that SD abolishes selective attention in association with a decreased BOLD signal found within fronto-parietal cognitive control areas (the left intraparietal sulcus and the left inferior frontal lobe) and parahippocampal place area (PPA) during a selective attention task performance. Additionally, SD resulted in a significant decrement in functional connectivity between the PPA and the two cognitive control fronto-parietal areas (Lim et al., 2010). Interestingly, a single night of SD was shown to produce a strategy shift during risky decision making such that healthy human volunteers moved from defending against losses to seeking increased gains. An fMRI assessment revealed that this change in economic preferences was correlated with the magnitude of an SD-driven increase in ventromedial prefrontal activation as well as by an SD-driven decrease in anterior insula activation during decision making (Venkatraman et al., 2011).

Regarding the above described neuroimaging findings together, it can be concluded that sleep is of critical importance for almost all, if not for all types of cognitive processes, including decision making. However, which mechanisms are responsible for substantial deficits of the many cognitive functions seen after sleep deprivation is still elusive.

5. Sleep and psychological functions

Herein, we will review existing data about sleep's role in functions different from the above described memory and cognitive ones. These include consolidation of affect, emotional regulation and dreaming mental states. As will be shown, the mechanisms, trough which sleep serves these psychological processes are distinctly different from those involved in its memory and cognitive functions. It is to be emphasized, however, that mostly REM sleep has been so far consistently and reliably associated with these human psychological processes. REM sleep characteristics are implicated for both normal psychological processes and psychopathology. Thus, REM sleep and its mental content incorporated in the co-occurring dreaming production have been proposed to aid resolution of personal emotional, affective and social conflicts (Cartwright et al., 2006; McNamara et al., 2001; 2005; 2010). Notably, REM sleep mechanisms and mental signatures have also been proposed to be involved in the pathogenesis of a number of psychopathological conditions, including posttraumatic stress disorder, anxiety, depression, schizophrenia, etc. (Benca et al., 1992; Gottesmann, 2010; Kirov & Brand, in press; Wagner et al., 2006; Walker, 2009; Walker & van der Helm, 2009). These observations are conceptualized in the so-called continuity hypothesis, according to which cognitive and emotional experiences generated, developed and used during wakefulness do continue to evolve during dreaming in REM sleep (Dumhoff & Hall, 1996; Pesant & Zadra, 2006). A recent study tested this hypothesis in both congenitally paraplegic and deaf-mute persons and matched controls. Surprisingly, perceptual representations, even of modalities not experienced during wakefulness, were quite common in dream reports not only in the control persons but also in the handicapped subjects (Voss et al., 2011). These interesting results give support to a protoconsciousness theory of REM sleep dreaming state that was recently forwarded by Hobson (2009). The REM sleep-dream protoconsciousness hypothesis proposes that development and maintenance of waking consciousness and other high-order brain functions (secondary consciousness) depends on brain activation during REM sleep (primary consciousness, i.e., simple awareness that includes perception and emotion in sleep), thus implicating for phylogenic aspects of dreaming. Accordingly, the neurobiology of REM sleep and co-occurring dreaming mentality reflect more basic (i.e., threaten, feeding, sexual, etc.) features not only in humans but also in lower species (Hobson, 2009). Interestingly, this view seems to have much in common with a previously proposed hypothesis about the psychological functions of REM sleep as an interactive genetic programming brain state (Jouvet, 1998). These two views (Hobson, 2009; Jouvet, 1998) predict that human experience during wakefulness is given more basic biological characteristics during REM sleep, which may have important adaptation roles. Also, they well fit with a more recent opinion about the memory functions of REM sleep, according to which memories consolidated during SWS undergo further transformation during REM sleep in terms of placing them in a more general and individually specific context (Walker & Stickgold, 2010).

5.1 Overview of human EEG data

Notably, human REM sleep has been so far shown to consolidate declarative (episodic or semantic) memory only when items have emotional salient components, and only when these emotional components have negative valence (Wagner et al., 2001; 2006; Nishida et al., 2009). Recently, REM sleep was shown to be very important for recalibration of the sensitivity of human brain to specific emotions (Gujar et al., 2011a).

Data concerning human sleep EEG findings about the role of REM sleep in psychological functioning are still scarce. One study investigated the effect REM sleep portion of a daily nap on episodic memory consolidation. No memorizing effects on emotionally neutral fact-based information were found. However, when episodic items were associated with negative emotional components, REM sleep strongly consolidated them. Moreover, the improvement strongly and positively correlated with all, REM sleep latency, amount of REM sleep, and importantly, with the theta (4-8 Hz) REM sleep EEG signature (Nishida et al., 2009). A more recent study tested whether boosting REM sleep EEG signatures could produce overnight improvement of memory consolidation. In this study, REM sleep EEG was potentiated by delivering theta (5 Hz) anodal trans-cranial direct current stimulation during REM sleep periods in the second half of night. The stimulation did enhanced gamma (25-45 Hz) EEG activity during REM sleep, but it did not improve either declarative or procedural memory consolidation at morning recalls. Instead, this increase in gamma EEG during REM sleep resulted in a worsened mood, as assessed by positive and negative affect scale, in the morning after sleep, accompanied by worsening on working memory, as assessed by a word fluency test (Marshall et al., 2011). Collectively, these studies demonstrate that specific REM sleep EEG rhythms are involved in affective behavior.

Interestingly, a recent study demonstrated the EEG signatures of dream recall from both REM sleep (theta, 5-7 Hz EEG activity) and stage 2 of non-REM sleep (alpha, 8-12 Hz EEG activity) (Marzano et al., 2011). These findings document different modes of mentality in REM sleep versus non-REM sleep. Furthermore, they suggest that the neurophysiological mechanisms underlying encoding and recall of episodic memories may remain the same across different states of consciousness.

5.2 Overview of human neuroimaging data

The existing so far human neuroimaging studies about the role for sleep in emotional regulation demonstrate deteriorated patterns of brain activation after total sleep deprivation (SD). By using fMRI, it has been shown that a disconnection between medial prefrontal cortex and amygdala following SD has been associated with improper response to negative emotional stimuli (Yoo et al., 2007a). Further, Sterpenich et al. (2007) showed that a successful recollection of emotional stimuli elicited larger BOLD responses in the hippocampus and various cortical areas, including the medial prefrontal cortex, in a sleep control (SC) group than in a sleep deprived (SD) group. In contrast, the recollection of negative items elicited larger responses in the amygdala and in occipital areas in the SD relative to the SC group (Sterpenich et al., 2007). A later fMRI study examined the effect of a single night SD on consolidation of aversive emotional stimuli and corresponding patterns of brain activation at retest that took place six months after encoding. At retest 6 months later, the recollection of subjects allowed to sleep, compared with SD subjects, was associated with significantly larger fMRI responses in the ventral medial prefrontal cortex (vMPFC) and precuneus, areas involved in memory retrieval, and in the extended amygdala and occipital cortex, areas involved in emotion modulation at encoding. These results suggest that sleep during the first postencoding night profoundly influences long-term systems-level consolidation of emotional memory and modifies the functional segregation and integration associated with recollection of affective memories in the long term (Sterpenich et al., 2009). Finally, using fMRI, it was recently demonstrated that SD amplifies reactivity throughout human mesolimbic reward brain networks in response to pleasure-evoking stimuli. In addition, this amplified reactivity was associated with enhanced connectivity in the early primary visual processing pathways and extended limbic regions, yet with a reduction in coupling with medial frontal and orbitofrontal regions. These neural changes were accompanied by a biased increase in the number of emotional stimuli judged as pleasant in the sleep-deprived group, the extent of which exclusively correlated with activity in mesolimbic regions (Gujar et al., 2011b). These results may offer a neural foundation on which to consider interactions between sleep loss and emotional reactivity in a variety of mood disorders (Gujar et al., 2011b).

Collectively, the above findings demonstrate sleep-related mechanisms of emotional regulation and consolidation of affective memories that partially differ from those shown to be involved in emotionally neutral memory consolidation and in the cognitive functions of sleep. The emotional "fingerprint" seems to involve mostly connections between prefrontal cortices and amygdala. However, it still remains to be revealed which sleep portions or sleep stages might have contributed to the impaired brain activation patterns after SD responsible for the behavioral results.

6. Conclusions

It is undeniable that highly specific sleep EEG rhythms and patterns of brain activation *actively* serve the memory, cognitive and psychological functions of sleep. The corresponding mechanisms involve brain plasticity at system, neural, synaptic, and genetic levels, and are closely related to the neurobiology of sleep. However, these mechanisms are *distinctly different* for certain memory, cognitive and psychological categories that sleep promotes, being *dissimilarly associated* with distinct sleep portions and sleep stages. Thus, both declarative and procedural memory consolidation and reconsolidation occur in earliest part of non-REM sleep/SWS by mechanisms of brain plasticity at system and neural levels, engaged in hippocampus-cortical relationships. Those, occurring during REM sleep appear more complex. Their pattern of brain activation engages a large set of areas, and possibly involves brain plasticity mechanisms at synaptic and genetic levels. The emotional 'fingerprint" of memory consolidation seems to be presented by connections between amygdala and cortical areas.

Further, the mechanisms involved in other cognitive functions of sleep appear different from those involved specifically in its memorizing effects. Also, it seems that sleep contributes to cognitive processes in a state dependent rather than in a trait dependent manner, but a complex interaction between both also can be suggested. Thus, since some of the EEG data imply a trait dependent role for sleep in cognitive abilities, most of the neuroimaging data indicate a state dependent role. However, these conclusions need further experimental evidence.

Importantly, different types of sleep mentality incorporated in different forms of dreaming production suggest a role for dreams in memory and cognitive processes. Data from such studies may open new perspectives of research and may provide new views about cognitive functions of sleep.

Finally, it can be concluded that the mechanisms underpinning memory, cognitive and psychological functions of sleep substantially contribute to human intelligence. Further investigation of the relationship between sleep and intelligence is clearly warranted.

7. Acknowledgment

We apologize to those whose work was not cited because of space limitations. We thank Drs. J. Yordanova and V. Kolev for their support.

8. References

Achermann, P. & Borbély, A.A. (1997). Low-Frequency (< 1 Hz) Oscillations in the Human Sleep Electroencephalogram, *Neuroscience*, 81 (1):213-222.

Amzica, F. & Steriade, M. (1997). The K-complex: its slow (<1-Hz) rhythmicity and relation to delta waves, *Neurology*, 49(4):952-959.

Anderer, P., Klösch, G., Gruber, G., Trenker, E., Pascual-Marqui, R.D., Zeitlhofer, J., Barbanoj, M.J., Rappelsberger, P. & Saletu, B. (2001). Low-resolution brain electromagnetic tomography revealed simultaneously active frontal and parietal sleep spindle sources in the human cortex, *Neuroscience*, 103(3):581-592.

Aserinsky, E. & Kleitman, N. (1953). Regularly occurring periods of eye motility, and concomitant phenomena, during sleep, *Science*, 118(3062):273-274.

Battaglia, F.P., Sutherland, G.R. & McNaughton, B.L. (2004). Hippocampal sharp wave bursts coincide with neocortical "up-state" transitions, *Learning and Memory*, 11(6): 697-704.

Benca, R.M., Obermeyer, W.H., Thisted, R.A. & Gillin, J.C. (1992). Sleep and psychiatric disorders. A meta-analysis, *Archives of General Psychiatry*, 49(8):651-668; discussion 669-670.

Bódizs, R., Kis, T., Lázár, A.S., Havrán, L., Rigó, P., Clemens, Z., Halász, P. (2005). Prediction of general mental ability based on neural oscillation measures of sleep, *Journal of Sleep Research*, 14(3):285-292.

Borbély, A.A. (1982). A two process model of sleep regulation, *Human Neurobiology*, 1(3):195-204.

Borbély, A.A. & Achermann, P. (1999). Sleep homeostasis and models of sleep regulation, *Journal of Biological Rhythms*, 14(6):557-568.

Braun, A.R., Balkin, T.J., Wesensten, N.J., Gwadry, F., Carson, R.E., Varga, M., Baldwin, P., Belenky, G. & Herscovitch, P. (1998). Dissociated pattern of activity in visual cortices and their projections during human rapid eye movement sleep, *Science*, 279(5347):91-95.

Braun, A.R., Balkin, T.J., Wesenten, N.J., Carson, R.E., Varga, M., Baldwin, P., Selbie, S., Belenky, G. & Herscovitch, P. (1997). Regional cerebral blood flow throughout the sleep-wake cycle. An H2(15)O PET study, *Brain*, 120 (Pt 7):1173-1197.

Broughton, R.J. (1987). Polysomnography: Principles and Applications in Sleep and Arousal Disorders. In: Niedermeyer, E. & Lopes da Silva, F. (Eds.), *Electroencephalography: Basic Principles, Clinical Applications and Related Fields*, pp. 765-802. Baltimore: Urban and Schwarzenberg, Baltimore.

Brown, R.M. & Robertson, E.M. (2007). Off-line processing: reciprocal interactions between declarative and procedural memories, *The Journal of Neuroscience*, 27(39):10468-10475.

Buzsáki, G. (1989) Two-stage model of memory trace formation: a role for "noisy" brain states, *Neuroscience*, 31(3):551-570

Buzsáki, G. (2006). Rhythms of the Brain, pp. 1-464, Oxford University Press, USA, ISBN 978-0-19-530106-9.

Cai, D.J., Mednick, S.A., Harrison, E.M., Kanady, J.C. & Mednick, S.C. (2009). REM, not incubation, improves creativity by priming associative networks, *Proceedings of the National Academy of Science of the USA*, 106(25):10130-10134.

Callaway, C.W., Lydic, R., Baghdoyan, H.A. & Hobson, J.A. (1987). Pontogeniculooccipital waves: spontaneous visual system activity during rapid eye movement sleep, *Cellular and Molecular Neurobiology*, 7(2):105-149.

Cantero, J.L., Atienza, M., Salas, R.M. & Dominguez-Marin, E. (2002). Effects of prolonged waking-auditory stimulation on electroencephalogram synchronization and cortical coherence during subsequent slow-wave sleep, *The Journal of Neuroscience*, 22(11):4702-4708.

Cantero, J.L., Atienza, M., Stickgold, R., Kahana, M.J., Madsen, J.R. & Kocsis, B. (2003). Sleep-dependent theta oscillations in the human hippocampus and neocortex, *The Journal of Neuroscience*, 23(34):10897-10903.

Cartwright, R., Agargun, M.Y., Kirkby, J. & Friedman, J.K. (2006). Relation of dreams to waking concerns, *Psychiatry Research*, 141(3):261-270.

Chee, M.W. & Chuah, Y.M. (2007). Functional neuroimaging and behavioral correlates of capacity decline in visual short-term memory after sleep deprivation, *Proceedings of the National Academy of Science of the USA*, 104(22):9487-9492.

Chee, M.W., Tan, J.C., Zheng, H., Parimal, S., Weissman, D.H., Zagorodnov, V. & Dinges, D.F. (2008). Lapsing during sleep deprivation is associated with distributed changes in brain activation, *The Journal of Neuroscience*, 28(21):5519-5528.

Chrobak, J.J. & Buzsáki, G. (1996). High-frequency oscillations in the output networks of the hippocampal-entorhinal axis of the freely behaving rat, *The Journal of Neuroscience*, 16(9):3056-66.

Cirelli, C. & Tononi, G. (2008). Is sleep essential? *PLoS Biology*, 6(8), e216, http://dx.doi.org./10.1371/journal.pbio.0060216

Clemens, Z., Fabó, D. & Halász, P. (2005). Overnight verbal memory retention correlates with the number of sleep spindles. *Neuroscience*, 132(2):529-535.

Clemens, Z., Fabó, D. & Halász, P. (2006). Twenty-four hours retention of visuospatial memory correlates with the number of parietal sleep spindles, *Neuroscience Letters*, 403(1-2):52-56.

Clemens, Z., Mölle, M., Eross, L., Barsi, P., Halász, P. & Born. J. (2007). Temporal coupling of parahippocampal ripples, sleep spindles and slow oscillations in humans, *Brain*, 130(Pt 11):2868-2878.

Clemens, Z., Mölle, M., Eross, L., Jakus, R., Rásonyi, G., Halász, P. & Born. J. (2011). Fine-tuned coupling between human parahippocampal ripples and sleep spindle, *European Journal of neuroscience*, 33(3):511-520.

Clemens, Z., Weiss, B., Szucs, A., Eross, L., Rásonyi, G. & Halász P. (2009). Phase coupling between rhythmic slow activity and gamma characterizes mesiotemporal rapid-eye-movement sleep in humans, *Neuroscience*, 163(1):388-396.

Crunelli, V. & Hughes, S.W. (2010). The slow (<1 Hz) rhythm of non-REM sleep: a dialogue between three cardinal oscillators, *Nature Neuroscience*, 13(1):9-17.

Csicsvari, J., Hirase, H., Czurkó, A., Mamiya, A. & Buzsáki, G. (1999). Oscillatory coupling of hippocampal pyramidal cells and interneurons in the behaving rat, *The Journal of Neuroscience*, 19(1):274-287.

Dang-Vu, T.T., Desseilles, M., Laureys, S., Degueldre, C., Perrin, F., Phillips, C., Maquet, P. & Peigneux, P. (2005). Cerebral correlates of delta waves during non-REM sleep revisited, *Neuroimage*, 28(1):14-21.

Dang-Vu, T.T., Schabus, M., Desseilles, M., Albouy, G., Boly, M., Darsaud, A., Gais, S., Rauchs, G., Sterpenich, V., Vandewalle, G., Carrier, J., Moonen, G., Balteau, E., Degueldre, C., Luxen, A., Phillips, C. & Maquet, P. (2008). Spontaneous neural activity during human slow wave sleep, *Procedings of the Nationall Academy of Science of the USA*, 105(39):15160-15165.

De Gennaro, L. & Ferrara, M. (2003). Sleep spindles: an overview, *Sleep Medicine Reviews*, 7(5):423-440.

Diekelmann, S. & Born, J. (2010). The memory function of sleep, *Nature Reviews Neuroscience*, 11(2):114-126.

Diekelmann, S., Büchel, C., Born, J. & Rasch, B. (2011). Labile or stable: opposing consequences for memory when reactivated during waking and sleep, *Nature Neuroscience*, 14(3):381-386.

Dienes, Z. & Perner, J. (1999). A theory of implicit and explicit knowledge, *Behavioral and Brain Sciences*, 22(5):735-755; discussion 755-808.

Dinges, D. F., Rogers, N. L. & Baynard, M. D. (2005). Chronic Sleep Deprivation. In: Kryger, M. H., Roth, T. & Dement, W. C. (Eds), pp. 67-76, *Principles and Practice of Sleep Medicine*, Elsevier Saunders, Philadelphia.

Domhoff, G.W. & Hall, C.S. (1996). Finding meaning in dreams: A quantitative approach, New York NY, Plenum, pp. 1-372, ISBN 13-978-0306451720.

Durrant, S.J., Taylor, C., Cairney, S. & Lewis, P.A. (2011). Sleep-dependent consolidation of statistical learning, *Neuropsychologia*, 49(5):1322-1331.

Eichenbaum, H. A. (2000). Cortical-hippocampal system for declarative memory, *Nature Reviews Neuroscience*, 1(1):41-50.

Fogel, S.M., Nader, R., Cote, K.A. & Smith, C.T. (2007a). Sleep spindles and learning potential, *Behavioral Neuroscience*, 121(1):1-10.

Fogel, S.M., Smith, C.T. & Cote, K.A. (2007b). Dissociable learning-dependent changes in REM and non-REM sleep in declarative and procedural memory systems, *Behavioral Brain Research*, 180(1):48-61.

Fogel, S.M. & Smith, C.T. (2006). Learning-dependent changes in sleep spindles and Stage 2 sleep, *Journal of Sleep Research*, 15(3):250-255.

Fogel, S.M. & Smith, C.T. The function of the sleep spindle: a physiological index of intelligence and a mechanism for sleep-dependent memory consolidation, *Neuroscience and Biobehavioral Reviews*, 35(5):1154-65.

Forkstam, C. & Petersson, K.M. (2005). Towards an explicit account of implicit learning. *Currrent Opinion in Neurology*, 18(4):435-441.

Fosse, R., Stickgold, R. & Hobson, J.A. (2001). The mind in REM sleep: reports of emotional experience, *Sleep*, 24(8):947-955.

Fosse, R., Stickgold, R. & Hobson, J.A. (2004). Thinking and hallucinating: reciprocal changes in sleep, *Psychophysiology*, 41(2):298-305.

Fröhlich, F. & McCormick, D.A. (2010). Endogenous electric fields may guide neocortical network activity, *Neuron*, 67(1):129-143.

Gais, S., Albouy, G., Boly, M., Dang-Vu, T.T., Darsaud, A., Desseilles, M., Rauchs, G., Schabus, M., Sterpenich, V., Vandewalle, G., Maquet, P. & Peigneux, P. (2007). Sleep transforms the cerebral trace of declarative memories, *Proceedings of the National Academy of Sciences of the USA*, 104(47):18778-18783.

Gais, S., Mölle, M., Helms, K. & Born, J. (2002). Learning-dependent increases in sleep spindle density, *The Journal of Neuroscience*, 22(15):6830-6834.

Geiger, A., Achermann, P. & Jenni, O.G. (2010). Sleep, Intelligence and Cognition in a Developmental Context: Differentiation Between Traits and State-dependent Aspects, In: Kerkhof, G.A. & van Dongen, H.P.A. (Eds.), *Human Sleep and Cognition. Part I, Basic Research, Progress in Brain Research*, 185:167-179.

Gottesmann, C. (1999). Neurophysiological support of consciousness during waking and sleep, *Progress in Neurobiology*, 59(5):469-508.

Gottesmann, C. (2010). The Development of the Science of Dreaming. In: Clow A. & McNamara P. (Eds.), *Dreams and Dreaming, International Review of Neurobiology*, 92:1-29.

Gujar, N., McDonald, S.A., Nishida, M. & Walker, M.P. (2011a). A role for rem sleep in recalibrating the sensitivity of the human brain to specific emotions, *Cerebral Cortex*, 21(1):115-123.

Gujar, N., Yoo, S.S., Hu, P. & Walker, M.P. (2011b). Sleep deprivation amplifies reactivity of brain reward networks, biasing the appraisal of positive emotional experiences, *The Journal of Neuroscience*, 23;31(12):4466-4474.

Hobson, J.A. (1999). Dreaming as a Delirium: How the Brain Does out of Its Mind, The MIT Press, pp. 3-287, ISBN 0-262-58179-5.

Hobson, J.A. (2005). Sleep is of the brain, by the brain and for the brain, *Nature*, 437(7063):1254-1256.

Hobson, J.A. (2009). REM sleep and dreaming: towards a theory of protoconsciousness, *Nature Reviews Neuroscience*, 10(11):803-813.

Hobson, J.A., McCarley, R.W. & Wyzinski, P.W. (1975). Sleep cycle oscillation: reciprocal discharge by two brainstem neuronal groups, *Science*, 189(4196):55-58.

Hobson, J.A., Pace-Schott, E.F. & Stickgold, R. (2000). Dreaming and the brain: toward a cognitive neuroscience of conscious states, *Behavioral and Brain Sciences*, 23(6):793-842; discussion 904-1121.

Hobson, J.A. & Pace-Schott, E.F. (2002).The cognitive neuroscience of sleep: neuronal systems, consciousness and learning. *Nature Reviews Neuroscience*, 3(9):679-693.

Huber, R., Ghilardi, M.F., Massimini, M. & Tononi, G. (2004). Local sleep and learning, *Nature*, 430(6995):78-81.

Jouvet, M. (1998). Paradoxical sleep as a programming system, *Journal of Sleep Research*, 7 (Suppl 1):1-5.

Killgore, W.D. (2010). Effects of Sleep Deprivation on Cognition. In: Kerkhof, G.A. & van Dongen, H.P.A. (Eds.), *Human Sleep and Cognition, Part I Basic Research, Progress in Brain Research*, 185:105-129.

Kirov, R. (2007). The sleeping brain, the states of consciousness, and the human intelligence, *Behavioral and Brain Sciences*, 30(2):159.

Kirov, R. & Brand, S. (in press). Nightmares as predictors of psychiatric disorders in adolescence, *Current Trends in Neurology*, Vol.5, 2011, pp. 1-12.

Kirov, R. & Moyanova, S. (2002). Distinct sleep-wake stages in rats depend differentially on age, *Neuroscience Letters*, 322(2):134-136.

Kirov, R., Weiss, C., Siebner, H.R., Born, J. & Marshall, L. (2009). Slow oscillation electrical brain stimulation during waking promotes EEG theta activity and memory encoding, *Proceedings of the National Academy of Sciences of the USA*, 106(36):15460-15465.

Laureys, S., Peigneux, P., Phillips, C., Fuchs, S., Degueldre, C., Aerts, J., Del Fiore, G., Petiau, C., Luxen, A., van der Linden, M., Cleeremans, A., Smith, C. & Maquet, P. (2001). Experience-dependent changes in cerebral functional connectivity during human rapid eye movement sleep, *Neuroscience*, 105(3):521-525.

Lim, A.S., Lozano, A.M., Moro, E., Hamani, C., Hutchison, W.D., Dostrovsky, J.O., Lang, A.E., Wennberg, R.A. & Murray, B.J. (2007). Characterization of REM-sleep associated ponto-geniculo-occipital waves in the human pons, *Sleep*, 30(7):823-827.

Lim, J., Tan, J.C., Parimal, S., Dinges, D.F. & Chee, M.W. (2010). Sleep deprivation impairs object-selective attention: a view from the ventral visual cortex, *PLoS One*, 5(2):e9087, http://dx.doi.org/10.1371/journal.pone.0009087

Mander, B.A., Reid, K.J., Davuluri, V.K., Small, D.M., Parrish, T.B., Mesulam, M.M., Zee, P.C., Gitelman, D.R. (2008). Sleep deprivation alters functioning within the neural network underlying the covert orienting of attention, *Brain Research*, 1217:148-156. Epub 2008 Apr 23.

Maquet, P., Degueldre, C., Delfiore, G., Aerts, J., Péters, J.M., Luxen, A. & Franck, G. (1997). Functional neuroanatomy of human slow wave sleep, *The Juornal of Neuroscience*, 17(8):2807-2812.

Maquet, P., Laureys, S., Peigneux, P., Fuchs, S., Petiau, C., Phillips, C., Aerts, J., Del Fiore, G., Degueldre, C., Meulemans, T., Luxen, A., Franck, G., Van Der Linden, M., Smith, C. & Cleeremans, A. (2000). Experience-dependent changes in cerebral activation during human REM sleep, *Nature Neuroscience*, 3(8):831-836.

Maquet, P., Péters, J., Aerts, J., Delfiore, G., Degueldre, C., Luxen, A. & Franck, G. (2000). Functional neuroanatomy of human rapid-eye-movement sleep and dreaming, *Nature*, 383(6596):163-166.

Marshall, L. & Born, J. (2007). The contribution of sleep to hippocampus-dependent memory consolidation, *Trends in Cognitive Sciences*, 11(10):442-450.

Marshall, L., Helgadóttir, H., Mölle, M. & Born, J. (2006). Boosting slow oscillations during sleep potentiates memory, *Nature*, 444(7119):610-613.

Marshall, L., Kirov, R., Brade, J., Mölle, M. & Born, J. (2011). Transcranial electrical currents to probe EEG brain rhythms and memory consolidation during sleep in humans, *PLoS One*, 6(2):e16905, http://dx.doi.org/10.1371/journal.pone.0016905

Marzano, C., Ferrara, M., Mauro, F., Moroni, F., Gorgoni, M., Tempesta, D., Cipolli, C. & De Gennaro, L. (2011). Recalling and forgetting dreams: theta and alpha oscillations during sleep predict subsequent dream recall, *The Journal of Neuroscience*, 31(18):6674-6683.

McCormick, D.A. & Bal, T. (1997). Sleep and arousal: thalamocortical mechanisms, *Annual Review in the Neurosciences*, 20:185-215

McNamara, P., Andresen, J., Clark, J., Zborowski, M. & Duffy, C.A. (2001).Impact of attachment styles on dream recall and dream content: a test of the attachment hypothesis of REM sleep, *Journal of Sleep Research*, 10(2):117-127.

McNamara, P., Johnson, P., McLaren, D., Harris, E., Beauharnais, C. & Auerbach, S. (2010). REM and NREM Sleep Mentation. In: Clow, A. & McNamara, P. (Eds.), *Dreams and Dreaming, International Review of Heurobiology*, 92:69-86.

McNamara, P., McLaren, D., Smith, D., Brown, A. & Stickgold, R. (2005). A "Jekyll and Hyde" within: aggressive versus friendly interactions in REM and non-REM dreams, *Psychological Science*, 16(2):130-136.

Miyauchi, S., Misaki, M., Kan, S., Fukunaga, T. & Koike, T. (2009). Human brain activity time-locked to rapid eye movements during REM sleep, *Experimental Brain Research*, 192(4):657-667.

Mölle, M., Marshall, L., Gais, S. & Born, J. (2002). Grouping of spindle activity during slow oscillations in human non-rapid eye movement sleep, *The Journal of Neuroscience*, 22(24):10941-10947.

Mölle, M., Marshall, L., Gais, S. & Born, J. (2004). Learning increases human electroencephalographic coherence during subsequent slow sleep oscillations. *Proceedings of the National Academy of Sciences of the USA*, 101(38):13963-13968.

Niedermeyer, E. (1993). The Normal EEG of the Waking Adult. In: Niedermeyer, E. & Lopes da Silva, F. (Eds.), pp. 131–152, *Electroencephalography: BasicPprinciples, Clinical Applications and Related Fields*, (3rd ed.), Baltimore, Williams & Wilkins.

Nir ,Y., Staba, R.J., Andrillon, T., Vyazovskiy, V.V., Cirelli, C., Fried, I. & Tononi, G. (2011). Regional slow waves and spindles in human sleep, *Neuron*, 70(1):153-169.

Nishida, M., Pearsall, J., Buckner, R.L. & Walker, M.P. REM sleep, prefrontal theta, and the consolidation of human emotional memory, *Cerebral Cortex*, 19(5):1158-1166.

Nishida, M. & Walker, M.P. (2007). Daytime naps, motor memory consolidation and regionally specific sleep spindles, *PLoS One*, 4;2(4):e341, http://dx.doi.org/10.1371/journal.pone.0000341

Nofzinger, E.A., Mintun, M.A., Wiseman, M., Kupfer, D.J. & Moore, R.Y. Forebrain activation in REM sleep: an FDG PET study. *Brain Research*, 770(1-2):192-201.

Pace-Schott, E.F. & Hobson, J.A. (2002). The neurobiology of sleep: genetics, cellular physiology and subcortical networks. *Nature Reviews Neuroscience*, 3(8):591-605.

Peigneux, P., Laureys, S., Fuchs, S., Collette, F., Perrin, F., Reggers, J., Phillips, C., Degueldre, C., Del Fiore, G., Aerts, J., Luxen, A. & Maquet, P. Are spatial memories strengthened in the human hippocampus during slow wave sleep? *Neuron*, 44(3):535-545.

Pesant, N. & Zadra, A. (2004). Dream content and psychological well-being: a longitudinal study of the continuity hypothesis, *Journal of Clinical Psychology*, 62(1):111-121.

Plihal, W. & Born, J. (1997). Effects of early and late nocturnal sleep on declarative and procedural memory, *Journal of Cognitive Neuroscience*, 9(4):534-547.

Plihal, W. & Born, J. (1999). Effects of early and late nocturnal sleep on priming and spatial memory, *Psychophysiology*, 36(5):571-582.

Rasch, B. & Born, J. Maintaining memories by reactivation, *Current Opinion in Neurobiology*, 17(6):698-703.

Rasch, B., Büchel, C., Gais, S. & Born, J. (2007). Odor cues during slow-wave sleep prompt declarative memory consolidation, *Science*, 315(5817):1426-1429.

Rechtschaffen, A. (1998). Current perspectives on the function of sleep, *Perspectives in Biology and Medicine*, 41(3):359-390.

Rechtschaffen, A. & Kales, A. (1968). A Manual of Standardized Terminology Techniques and Scoring System for Sleep Stages in Human Subjects. US Department of Health, Education and Welfare, Public Health Service. US Government Printing Office, Washington DC, NIH Publ. No. 204, Maryland, USA.

Reis, J., Robertson, E., Krakauer, J.W., Rothwell, J., Marshall, L., Gerloff, C., Wassermann, E., Pascual-Leone, A., Hummel, F., Celnik, P.A., Classen, J., Floel, A., Ziemann, U., Paulus, W., Siebner, H.R., Born, J. & Cohen, L.G. (2008). Consensus: Can transcranial direct current stimulation and transcranial magnetic stimulation enhance motor learning and memory formation? *Brain Stimulation*, 1(4):363-369.

Ribeiro, S., Goyal, V., Mello, C.V. & Pavlides, C. (1999). Brain gene expression during REM sleep depends on prior waking experience, *Learning & Memory*, 6(5):500-508.

Ribeiro, S., Mello, C.V., Velho, T., Gardner, T.J., Jarvis, E.D. & Pavlides, C. (2002). Induction of hippocampal long-term potentiation during waking leads to increased extrahippocampal zif-268 expression during ensuing rapid-eye-movement sleep, *The Journal of Neuroscience*, 22(24):10914-10923.

Robertson, E.M. (2009). From creation to consolidation: a novel framework for memory processing, *PLoS Biology*. 7(1):e19, http://dx.doi.org/10.1371/journal.pbio.1000019

Salih, F., Sharott, A., Khatami, R., Trottenberg, T., Schneider, G., Kupsch, A., Brown, P. & Grosse, P. (2009). Functional connectivity between motor cortex and globus pallidus in human non-REM sleep, *Journal of Physiology*, 587(Pt 5):1071-1086.

Schabus, M., Dang-Vu, T.T., Albouy, G., Balteau, E., Boly, M., Carrier, J., Darsaud, A., Degueldre, C., Desseilles, M., Gais, S., Phillips, C., Rauchs, G., Schnakers, C., Sterpenich, V., Vandewalle, G., Luxen, A. & Maquet, P. (2007). Hemodynamic cerebral correlates of sleep spindles during human non-rapid eye movement sleep, *Proceedings of the National Academy of Sciences of the USA*, 104(32):13164-13169.

Schabus, M., Gruber, G., Parapatics, S., Sauter, C., Klösch, G., Anderer, P., Klimesch, W., Saletu, B. & Zeitlhofer, J. (2004). Sleep spindles and their significance for declarative memory consolidation, *Sleep*, 27(8):1479-1485.

Schabus, M., Hödlmoser, K., Gruber, G., Sauter, C., Anderer, P., Klösch, G., Parapatics, S., Saletu, B., Klimesch, W. & Zeitlhofer, J. (2006). Sleep spindle-related activity in the human EEG and its relation to general cognitive and learning abilities, *European Journal of Neuroscience*, 23(7):1738-1746.

Schabus, M., Hoedlmoser, K., Pecherstorfer, T., Anderer, P., Gruber, G., Parapatics, S., Sauter, C., Kloesch, G., Klimesch, W., Saletu, B. & Zeitlhofer, J. (2008).

Interindividual sleep spindle differences and their relation to learning-related enhancements, *Brain Research*, 29 (1191):127-135.

Sederberg, P.B., Kahana, M.J., Howard, M.W., Donner, E.J. & Madsen, J.R. (2003). Theta and gamma oscillations during encoding predict subsequent recall, *The Journal of Neuroscience*, 23(34):10809-10814.

Sejnowski, T.J. & Destexhe, A. (1998). Why do we sleep? *Brain Research*, 886(1-2):208-223.

Siapas, A.G. & Wilson, M.A. (1998). Coordinated interactions between hippocampal ripples and cortical spindles during slow-wave sleep, *Neuron*, 21(5):1123-1128.

Siegel, J.M. (2009). Sleep viewed as a state of adaptive inactivity, *Nature Reviews Neuroscience*, 10(10):747-753

Sinton, C.M. & McCarley, R.W. (2000). Neuroanatomical and neurophysiological aspects of sleep: basic science and clinical relevance, *Seminars of Clinical Neuropsychiatry*, 5(1):6-19.

Sirota, A., Csicsvari, J., Buhl, D. & Buzsáki, G. (2003). Communication between neocortex and hippocampus during sleep in rodents, *Proceedings of the National Academy of Sciences of the USA*, 100(4):2065-2069.

Steriade, M. (2001). Impact of network activities on neuronal properties in corticothalamic systems, *The Journal of Neuroscience*, 86(1):1-39.

Steriade, M. (2006). Grouping of brain rhythms in corticothalamic systems, *Neuroscience*, 137(4):1087-1106.

Steriade, M., Nuñez, A. & Amzica, F. (1993). A novel slow (< 1 Hz) oscillation of neocortical neurons in vivo: depolarizing and hyperpolarizing components, *The Journal of Neuroscience*, 13(8):3252-3265.

Steriade, M. & Timofeev, I. (2003). Neuronal plasticity in thalamocortical networks during sleep and waking oscillations, *Neuron*, 37(4):563-576.

Sterpenich, V., Albouy, G., Boly, M., Vandewalle, G., Darsaud, A., Balteau, E., Dang-Vu, T.T., Desseilles, M., D'Argembeau, A., Gais, S., Rauchs, G., Schabus, M., Degueldre, C., Luxen, A., Collette, F. & Maquet, P. (2007). Sleep-related hippocampo-cortical interplay during emotional memory recollection, *PLoS Biology*, 5(11):e282. http://dx.plos.org/10.1371/journal.pbio.0050282

Sterpenich, V., Albouy, G., Darsaud, A., Schmidt, C., Vandewalle, G., Dang Vu, T.T., Desseilles, M., Phillips, C., Degueldre, C., Balteau, E., Collette, F., Luxen, A. & Maquet, P. (2009). Sleep promotes the neural reorganization of remote emotional memory, *The Journal of Neuroscience*, 29(16):5143-5152.

Stickgold, R. (2005). Sleep-dependent memory consolidation, *Nature*, 437(7063):1272-1278.

Stickgold, R., Hobson, J.A., Fosse, R. & Fosse, M. (2001). Sleep, learning, and dreams: off-line memory reprocessing, *Science*, 294(5544):1052-1057.

Stickgold, R., Scott, L., Rittenhouse, C. & Hobson, J.A. (1999). Sleep-induced changes in associative memory, *Journal of Cognitive Neuroscience*, 11(2):182-193.

Tononi, G. & Cirelli, C. (2006). Sleep function and synaptic homeostasis. *Sleep Medicine Reviews*, 10(1):49-62.

Tucker, M.A. & Fishbein, W. (2009). The impact of sleep duration and subject intelligence on declarative and motor memory performance: how much is enough? *Journal of Sleep Research*, 18(3):304-312.

Tulving, E. (1985). How Many Memory Systems are there? Reprinted from *American Psychologist*, 40(4), pp.385-398, Printed in U.S.A.

Venkatraman, V., Huettel, S.A., Chuah, L.Y., Payne, J.W. & Chee, M.W. (2011). Sleep deprivation biases the neural mechanisms underlying economic preferences, *The Journal of Neuroscience*, 31(10):3712-3718.

Voss, U., Tuin, I., Schermelleh-Engel, K. & Hobson, A. (2011). Waking and dreaming: Related but structurally independent. Dream reports of congenitally paraplegic and deaf-mute persons, *Consciousness and Cognition*, 20(3):673-687.

Wagner, U., Gais, S. & Born, J. (2001). Emotional memory formation is enhanced across sleep intervals with high amounts of rapid eye movement sleep, *Learning and Memory*, 8(2):112-119.

Wagner, U., Gais, S., Haider, H., Verleger, R. & Born, J. (2004). Sleep inspires insight, *Nature*, 427(6972):352-355.

Wagner, U., Hallschmid, M., Rasch, B. & Born, J. (2006). Brief sleep after learning keeps emotional memories alive for years, *Biological Psychiatry*, 60(7):788-790.

Walker MP. (2008). Cognitive consequences of sleep and sleep loss, *Sleep Medicine*, 9(Suppl 1):S29-S34.

Walker MP. (2009). The role of sleep in cognition and emotion, *Annals of the New York Academy of Sciences*, 1156:168-197.

Walker, M.P., Liston, C., Hobson, J.A. & Stickgold, R. (2002). Cognitive flexibility across the sleep-wake cycle: REM-sleep enhancement of anagram problem solving, *Brain Research Cognitive Brain Research*, 14(3):317-324.

Walker, M.P. & Stickgold, R. (2006). Sleep, memory, and plasticity. *Annual Review of Psychology*, 57:139-166.

Walker, M.P. & Stickgold, R. (2010). Overnight alchemy: sleep-dependent memory evolution, *Nature Reviews Neuroscience*, 11(3):218; author reply 218.

Walker, M.P. & van der Helm, E. (2009). Overnight therapy? The role of sleep in emotional brain processing, *Psychological Bulletin*, 135(5):731-748.

Wilhelm, I., Diekelmann, S., Molzow, I., Ayoub, A., Mölle, M. & Born, J. (2011). Sleep selectively enhances memory expected to be of future relevance, *The Journal of Neuroscience*, 31(5):1563-1569.

Wilson, M.A. & McNaughton, B.L. (1994). Reactivation of hippocampal ensemble memories during sleep, *Science*, 265(5172):676-679.

Yoo, S.S., Gujar, N., Hu, P., Jolesz, F.A. & Walker, M.P. (2007a). The human emotional brain without sleep--a prefrontal amygdala disconnect, *Current Biology*, 17(20):R877-878.

Yoo, S.S., Hu, P.T., Gujar, N., Jolesz, F.A. & Walker, M.P. (2007b). A deficit in the ability to form new human memories without sleep, *Nature Neuroscience*, 10(3):385-392.

Yordanova, J., Kolev, V., Verleger, R., Bataghva, Z., Born, J. & Wagner, U. (2008). Shifting from implicit to explicit knowledge: different roles of early- and late-night sleep, *Learning and Memory*, 15(7):508-515.

Yordanova, J., Kolev, V., Wagner, U., Born, J. & Verleger, R. (in press). Increased alpha (8-12 Hz) activity during slow-wave sleep as a marker for the transition from implicit knowledge to explicit insight, *Journal of Cognitive Neuroscience*.

Yordanova, J., Kolev, V., Wagner, U. & Verleger, R. (2009). Covert reorganization of implicit task representations by slow wave sleep, *PLoS One*, 4(5):e5675.

http://dx.plos.org/10.1371/journal.pone.0005675

Yordanova, J., Kolev, V., Wagner, U. & Verleger, R. (2010). Differential associations of early-
and late-night sleep with functional brain states promoting insight to abstract task
regularity, *PLoS One*, 5(2):e9442. http://dx.plos.org/10.1371/journal.pone.0009442

9

Neuroimaging and Outcome Assessment in Vegetative and Minimally Conscious State

Silvia Marino, Rosella Ciurleo, Annalisa Baglieri, Francesco Corallo,
Rosaria De Luca, Simona De Salvo, Silvia Guerrera, Francesca Timpano,
Placido Bramanti and Nicola De Stefano

IRCCS Centro Neurolesi "Bonino-Pulejo", Messina,
Dept. of Neurology, Neurosurgery & Behavioral Sciences, University of Siena, Siena,
Italy

1. Introduction

Consciousness is a multifaceted concept that has two dimensions: arousal, or wakefulness (i.e., level of consciousness), and awareness (i.e., content of consciousness) (Laureys et al., 2004). An accurate and reliable assessment of the arousal and awareness of consciousness in patients with severe brain damage is of greatest importance for the differential diagnosis of low levels consciousness patients and for outcome evaluation. Following coma, some patients permanently lose all brainstem function (brain death), some progress to "wakeful unawareness" (vegetative state - VS), whereas others recover typically and progress through different stages before fully or partly recovering consciousness (minimally conscious state - MCS). Patients in VS can open their eyes and exhibit basic orienting responses, but show no conscious, purposeful activity. Reflex and other movements are seen, mediated by brainstem, spinal cord, and brainstem-diencephalic arousal systems (Laureys et al., 2004). VS can occur after patients emerge from an acute catastrophic brain insult causing coma, or can also be seen in degenerative or congenital nervous system disorders. The two common findings are necrosis of the cerebral cortex, thalamus and brainstem (usually after anoxic injury) and diffuse axonal injury (usually after trauma), although other pathological findings can be seen in degenerative and other disorders (Laureys, 2008). The MCS patients do not meet diagnostic criteria for coma or VS because they demonstrate some inconsistent but clear evidence of consciousness (Laureys et al., 2008; Giacino et al., 2002). In the MCS, there is variable impaired function of the cerebral cortex, diencephalons and upper brainstem. This allows occasional conscious behaviours to occur, unlike in VS or coma. Patients may enter the MCS as they emerge from coma or VS, or they can become minimally conscious as a result of acute injury or chronic degenerative diseases. Recent studies suggest a number of potential clinical and rehabilitative applications of magnetic resonance (MR) techniques. Although bedside clinical examination remains the criterion standard for establishing diagnosis, MR may provide an adjunctive diagnostic role when behavioural findings are very limited or ambiguous. The future of diagnostic and prognostic assessment of patients with disorders of consciousness (DOC) envisions a battery of neurobehavioral and neuroimaging techniques (such as structural and functional MR imaging (MRI and fMRI), MR spectroscopy (MRS), diffusion tensor imaging (DTI), fiber tracking, positron emission tomography (PET)) that serve as complementary clinical tools that may help differentiate the effects of underarousal, sensory impairment, motor dysfunction, and cognitive disturbance in the search for potential causes of behavioural unresponsiveness.

2. Magnetic Resonance and Magnetization Transfer Imaging

The morphological MRI acquisitions usually include non-contrast-enhanced sagittal T1, axial diffusion, axial fluid attenuated inversion recovery (FLAIR), axial T2-SE, coronal T2 sequences and a 3D T1-weighted volume acquisition. FLAIR and T2-SE sequences permit to detect brain edema, contusion, hematoma, herniation, subarachnoid hemorrhage, or hydrocephalus. T2 sequences are useful in detecting hemorrhagic diffuse axonal injuries (DAI). The total number of lesions detected by FLAIR and T2 are shown to be inversely correlated with Glasgow Outcome Scale (GOS) of traumatic coma patients; while the 3D T1 sequence provides an opportunity to evaluate the brain atrophy during the follow up of these patients. A lot of studies performed on traumatic coma patients with conventional MRI showed that lesions of the pons, midbrain, and basal ganglia were predictive of poor outcome especially when they are bilateral. Despite their encouraging results, these studies fail to explain why some patients in VS or with long-term marked cognitive impairments have no or minimal lesions on conventional MRI examination. This raises the question of the lack of specificity and insufficient sensitivity of conventional MR sequences which fail to reveal lesions such as ischemic axonal injuries. Therefore, it is clear that morphological and conventional MRI alone cannot be considered as a reliable tool to assess consciousness disorders severity or to predict their evolution and outcome (Tshibanda et al., 2009). Several studies investigated patients in VS and in MCS using non-conventional, quantitative and volumetric MR techniques, useful to provide information about the anatomical patterns, the prognosis and the outcome of these patients. Ammermann et al. (2007) have used volumetric analysis of MRI to determine the pattern of lesions in 12 patients with a severe neurological impairment after acute ischemic injury. At the time of scanning, the patients were either in VS or in an early remising state, that is MCS. Lesions were classified as having been present in the gray and/or white matter in four different brain regions (frontal, parietal, temporal, occipital). An additional separate evaluation was performed for the basal ganglia, thalamus, hippocampus, cerebellum, and brainstem. The total clinical follow-up period of all patients from the time of the causative event lasted for at least 5 months. The clinical outcomes were reported according to the Rancho Los Amigos Cognitive Scale (RLACS) as a universal guide to assess a patient's level of functioning. The final RLACS levels were correlated to the MRI lesion size with a Spearman correlation. All patients demonstrated extensive white matter lesions, with the largest lesions observed in the frontal and occipital lobe. A preferential involvement of the white matter located in the periventricular area and in the subcortical regions below the motor and internal temporal cortices was found, in addition to the classifically described lesions of the striatum, motor and occipital cortices. Lesion magnitude showed an association with the severity of the outcome as quantitatively assessed by RLACS. With respect to gray matter lesions, the vulnerability pattern observed included frontal and occipital and in some cases parietal cortical areas, moreover in most cases the thalamus. Additionally, almost all of patients showed lesions of the hippocampus or lesions to the basal ganglia. An association between the extent of the MRI defined lesions located within the white matter and the clinical outcomes of the patients was found. All patients in the most unfavorable class III clinical outcome group (i.e. persistent VS) exhibited white matter lesions exceeding 2/3 of the volume of at least one lobe, most frequently the occipital lobe.

Moreover, Juengling et al. (2005) investigated 5 patients in persistent VS due to prolonged cerebral hypoxia of non-traumatic origin, using combined Voxel-Based Morphometry (VBM) of 3D MRI and FDG-PET analysis. In the analysis of the regional distribution of gray matter atrophy, VBM revealed multiple areas of significantly decreased gray matter density at p<.001, corrected for multiple comparisons. Those were localized in multiple cortical areas, in particular including inferior parietal lobe, superior and medial frontal lobe, paracentral lobule, superior and medial temporal lobe, the cingulum, and the fusiform gyrus. Thalamic changes were limited to small voxel clusters in dorso-medial areas. These structural atrophic changes were compared with the local distribution of functional loss as assessed by regional hypometabolism in the FDG-PET group analysis. At the threshold pb0.001 (corrected for multiple comparisons), PET showed a widespread pattern of hypometabolic areas. In particular, the parietal and frontotemporal cortices, the cuneus/precuneus, the cingulum, the frontal medial and precentral gyrus, and the transverse temporal gyrus were involved, additionally the bilateral thalamus (mainly dorso-medial subnucleus). All changes were, similar to the VBM results, nearly symmetrical. Improved understanding of this complex lesion pattern gained by in vivo group analyses like here might help to provide deeper insights into the general pathoanatomy of patients in the persistent VS.

Using high-resolution T1-weighted magnetic resonance images and a novel approach to shape analysis applied SIENAX software, Fernandez-Espejo et al. (2010) investigated thalamic global and regional changes in a sample of patients in a VS or an MCS. They found that total thalamic volume was significantly lower in patients than in healthy volunteers. Shape analysis revealed significant bilateral regional atrophy in the dorso-medial body in patients compared to controls; this atrophy was more widespread in VS than in MCS patients. Lower thalamic volume was significantly correlated with worsening of Disability Rating Scale (DRS) scores. Shape analysis suggested that the dorso-medial nucleus and the internal medullar lamina were the main regions responsible for this correlation. These findings suggest that MCS and VS patients present different patterns of regional thalamic abnormalities. In particular, VS patients showed a more widespread pattern of atrophy than controls, producing differences in global thalamic volume. MCS patients did not show volumetric differences compared to controls, and regionally they showed a less pronounced inward collapse in both the dorsal and ventral areas, with the anterior-ventral body significantly spared. Neuropathological studies have demonstrated that thalamic damage is less common in MCS than in VS patients (Jennett et al., 2001).

Another quantitative RM technique is the Magnetization Transfer Imaging (MTI). The MTI relies on the principle that protons bound in structures exhibit T1 relaxation coupling with protons in the aqueous phase. When an off-resonance saturation pulse is applied, it selectively saturates those protons that are bound in macromolecules. These protons subsequently exchange longitudinal magnetization with free water protons, leading to a reduction in the detected signal intensity (Sinson et al., 2001). The MTI may provide a quantitative index of the structural integrity of tissue and might be useful to study the outcome of patients with low levels of consciousness.

However, further studies, on larger groups of patients, need to be performed to confirm the usefulness of quantitative MRI in the assessment of the eventual neurological prognosis and outcome of these challenging patients.

3. Functional Magnetic Resonance Imaging and Positron Emission Tomography

At present a diagnosis of VS or MCS is made using prognostic markers from the patient's clinical history supported by detailed neurological and behavioral assessment by a multidisciplinary team over several weeks. However, the behavioral assessment of these patients predominately relies upon the subjective interpretation of observed spontaneous and volitional behavior. A diagnosis of VS is supported if the patient demonstrates no evidence of awareness of self or environment, no evidence of sustained, reproducible, purposeful or voluntary behavioral response to visual, auditory, tactile or noxious stimuli and critically no evidence of language comprehension or expression (MSTF, 1994). In contrast the patient in MCS demonstrates partial preservation of awareness of self and environment, responding intermittently, but reproducibly, to verbal command and therefore demonstrating some degree of basic language comprehension (Giacino et al., 2002).

PET and recently fMRI, by measurement of cerebral metabolism and brain activations in response to sensory stimuli, can provide important MR indices on the presence and location of any residual brain function.

PET is the most sensitive method to image trace amounts of molecules in vivo. Therefore this technique is used to measure in man or in the living animal biochemical and physiological processes in any organ with three dimensional resolution. The last 25 years have seen a rapid and still ongoing development in the production of positron emitters, radiochemical labeling techniques, tomograph technology and image reconstruction algorithms. Because of the possibility to see and measure quantitatively physiological disorders in an early stage, before permanent morphological damage has occurred, which will only then be visible in x-ray or magnetic resonance computer tomography, PET is finally finding its way from a sophisticated research tool into routine clinical diagnosis.

Resting cerebral metabolism derived from quantitative glucose uptake provides an indirect assessment of neuronal activity against which brain states may be compared quantitatively (Levy et al., 1987). All previous quantitative [18F] fluorodeoxyglucose–positron emission tomograph (FDG-PET) investigations of VS have correlated the condition with a global reduction of brain metabolic activity: Laureys et al. (1999) have assessed regional cerebral glucose metabolism (rCMRGlu) and effective cortical connectivity in four patients in VS by means of statistical parametric mapping and FDG-PET. Results showed a common pattern of impaired rCMRGlu in the prefrontal, premotor, and parietotemporal association areas and posterior cingulate cortex/precuneus in VS. In a next step, they demonstrated that in VS patients various prefrontal and premotor areas have in common that they were less tightly connected with the posterior cingulate cortex than in normal controls. Schiff et al. (2005) have described the first evidence of reciprocal clinical–pathological correlation with regional differences of quantitative cerebral metabolism. They studied five patients in VS with different behavioral features employing FDG-PET, MRI and magnetoencephalographic (MEG) responses to sensory stimulation. Each patient's brain expressed a unique metabolic pattern. The specific patterns of preserved metabolic activity identified in these patients reflect novel evidence of the modular nature of individual functional networks that underlie conscious brain function. In three of the five patients, co-registered PET/MRI correlate islands of relatively preserved brain metabolism with isolated fragments of behavior. Two patients had suffered anoxic injuries and demonstrated marked decreases in overall cerebral metabolism. Two other patients with non-anoxic, multifocal brain injuries demonstrated several isolated brain regions with relatively higher metabolic rates. A single patient who suffered severe injury to the tegmental mesencephalon and paramedian thalamus showed widely preserved cortical metabolism. The variations in cerebral metabolism in chronic VS patients indicate that some cerebral regions can retain partial function in catastrophically injured brains.

fMRI is based on the increase in blood flow to the local vasculature that accompanies neural activity in the brain. This result in a corresponding local reduction in deoxyhemoglobin because the increase in blood flow occurs without an increase of similar magnitude in oxygen extraction (Roy & Sherrington, 1890; Fox & Raichle, 1985). Since deoxyhemoglobin is paramagnetic, it alters the T2 weighted magnetic resonance image signal (Ogawa et al, 1990). Thus, deoxyhemoglobin is sometimes referred to as an endogenous contrast enhancing agent, and serves as the source of the signal for fMRI. Using an appropriate imaging sequence, human cortical functions can be observed without the use of exogenous contrast enhancing agents on a clinical strength (1.5 T) scanner (Bandettini et al., 1992, 1993; Schneider et al, 1993).

Functional activity of the brain determined from the magnetic resonance signal has confirmed known anatomically distinct processing areas in the visual cortex (Schneider, et al, 1993), the motor cortex, and Broca's area of speech and language-related activities (Hinke et al., 1993; Kim et al., 1995). Further, a rapidly emerging body of literature documents corresponding findings between fMRI and conventional electrophysiological techniques to localize specific functions of the human brain (Atlas et al., 1996; Detre, et al, 1995; George, et al, 1995). Consequently, the number of medical and research centers with fMRI capabilities and investigational programs continues to escalate.

Several fMRI studies in the VS have confirmed the findings of previous PET studies. Di et al. (2007) used fMRI to evaluate differences between seven VS and four MCS patients in brain activation occurring in response to the presentation of the patient's own name, spoken by familiar voice (SON-FV). They prospectively studied residual cerebral activation to SON-FV in seven patients with VS and four with MCS. Two patients with VS failed to show any significant cerebral activation. Three patients with VS showed SON-FV induced activation within the primary auditory cortex. Only two of the VS patients, and all four MCS patients, showed activation not only in the primary auditory cortex but also in hierarchically higher-order associative temporal areas.

Three months after fMRI examination, these two VS patients had progressed to the MCS. This study showed that fMRI measurement might be a useful tool for pre-clinically distinguishing MCS-like cognitive processing in some patients behavioural classified as vegetative. Schiff et al. (2005) have tested the hypothesis that MCS patients retain active cerebral networks that underlie cognitive function. fMRI was employed to investigate cortical responses in two male adults with severe brain injuries resulting to MCS and in seven healthy volunteers. Three passive stimulation tasks were performed: tactile stimulation, auditory narratives of familiar events presented by a familiar person, and the same auditory passages without language-related content. Results have showed a residual brain activity of cortical systems involved in a potential cognitive and sensory function despite their inability to follow simple instructions or communicate reliably.

In conclusion, results of these studies we analyzed confirm the idea that PET and fMRI activation profiles may constitute useful adjunctive diagnostic methods when behavioral findings are very limited or ambiguous, helping in differential diagnosis, prognostic assessment and identification of pathophysiological mechanism.

4. Diffusion Tensor Imaging

Diffusion tensor imaging (DTI) is an emerging technique that complements traditional MRI and may be able to provide erstwhile unavailable information about the pathological substrates of DOC. DTI is a modified MRI technique that is sensitive to microscopic, three-dimensional water motion within tissue. In cerebrospinal fluid, water motion is isotropic, i.e., roughly equivalent in all directions. In white matter, however, water diffuses in a highly directional or anisotropic manner. Due to the structure and insulation characteristics of myelinated fibers, water in these white matter bundles is largely restricted to diffusion along the axis of the bundle. DTI can thus be used to calculate two basic properties: the overall amount of diffusion and the anisotropy (Douaud et al., 2007; Benson et al., 2007; Kraus et al., 2007; Ringman et al., 2007; O'Sullivan et al., 2004). It is only very recently that DTI has been used to evaluate white matter integrity in patients with DOC. For example, Voss et al. (2006) described two patients with traumatic brain injury: one who had remained MCS for 6 years and one who had recovered expressive language after 19 years diagnosed as MCS. In both cases, widespread changes in white matter integrity were observed. Interestingly, however, the increased anisotropy and directionality in the bilateral medial parieto-occipital regions that was observed in the second patient reduced to normal values in a follow-up scan performed 18 months later. This coincided with increased metabolic activity, leading the authors to interpret these observations as evidence of axonal regrowth in this region. Although this is certainly a landmark finding in two high spectrum MCS patients, it remains to be seen whether DTI has any diagnostic or prognostic utility in a broader group of patients with disorders of consciousness. To this end, Tollard et al. (2009) and Perlbarg et al. (2009) have recently demonstrated that DTI measures in sub-acute severe traumatic brain injury may be a relevant biomarker for predicting the recovery of consciousness at 1 year. However, VS and MCS patients were classified in the same outcome category and potential differences between these two groups were not investigated. Although, in this context DTI has been generally used to address specific clinical problems, the study of white matter integrity in behaviorally defined states has a more basic relevance to understanding the relationship between brain and behavior in both health and disease. For example, in healthy volunteers, DTI techniques have been used recently to examine how structural changes underpin the behavioral changes that are related to learning a complex skill (Scholz et al., 2009). In a very recent study (Espejo et al., 2011), the integrity of white and grey matter regions was assessed in a group of 25 VS and MCS patients in vivo. In accordance with previous post-mortem work (Jennett et al., 2001; Adams et al., 1999) significant changes were observed in the integrity of the tissue in subcortical, thalamic and brainstem regions in the patients when compared to healthy volunteers. The precise location of this damage was not different between the MCS and VS sub-groups, which, again, accords well with previous post-mortem studies. However, an analysis of the MD values within two of these regions of interest (subcortical white matter and thalami), revealed significant differences between the patients meeting the clinical (behavioral) criteria defining VS and those who met the criteria defining MCS. Specifically, the VS patient group exhibited a decrease in the peak height of the histograms derived from the subcortical white matter and the thalami and an increase in the peak width of the thalamic histogram.

In addition, DTI may be a valuable biomarker for the severity of tissue injury and a predictor for outcome. It reveals changes in the WM that are correlated with both acute GCS and Rankin scores at discharge (Huisman et al., 2004). Significant early reduction of anisotropy was observed in WM structures, in particular in the internal capsule and the corpus callosum, which are the sites most commonly involved by DAI (Arfanakis et al., 2002). Moreover, several regions recovered normal values of anisotropy 1 month after the injury (Arfanakis et al., 2002). Xu et al. (2007) found significant differences in the corpus callosum, internal and external capsule, superior and inferior longitudinal fascicles, and the fornix in TBI patients. They showed that FA and ADC measurements offered superior sensitivity compared to conventional MRI diagnosis of DAI. Salmond et al. (2006) reported increased diffusivity in TBI patients at least 6 months after their injury in the cerebellum, frontal, insula, cingulate, parietal, temporal, and occipital lobes. The anisotropy seems to be reduced both in the major WM tracts such as the corpus callosum and the internal and external capsule, and the associative fibers underlying the cortex. DTI has a number of advantages as an imaging biomarker of brain injury: first, it can be used to evaluate brain trauma in an unconscious or sedated patient; second, it could permit the evaluation of responses to treatment even when the clinical scores are inadequate for assessing the patient; third, quantitative DTI measurements are unlikely to be tainted by adverse central nervous system (CNS) effects of hypnotic drugs, unlike clinical scores; and fourth, DTI may be an important alternative marker, as low initial Glasgow Come Scale scores are of limited value in predicting the prognosis (Huisman et al., 2004). Finally, Perlbarg et al. (2009) showed significant FA differences between favorable and unfavorable 1-year outcome groups around four FA tracks: in inferior longitudinal fasciculus, posterior limb of the internal capsule, cerebral peduncle, and posterior corpus callosum.

5. Magnetic Resonance Spectroscopy

Proton MRS (^{1}H-MRS) is a non-invasive imaging technique that enables in vivo quantification of certain neurochemical compounds. Using the same equipment utilized for the conventional MRI, single-voxel ^{1}H-MRS and multi-voxel Imaging (^{1}H-MRSI) or Chemical Shift Imaging (CSI) provide metabolic information on brain damage that may not be visible with the conventional structural imaging methods. Then ^{1}H-MRS, added to traditional MRI, offers the possibility to study the brain activity combining information on structure and function.

Classically, the exploration of DOC is performed on 1,5 or 3 Tesla MR scanners and at intermediate or long echo time (TE) (135-288 ms). Long TE ^{1}H-MRS detects the signal arising from four metabolites: N-acetyl-aspartate containing compounds (NAA), choline-containing compounds (Cho), creatine + phosphocreatine (Cre) and lactate (Lac). Short TE ^{1}H-MRS identifies peaks from mobile lipids, Lac, alanine, NAA, Glutamate/Glutamine (Glx), γ-aminobutyric acid, Cre, Cho, myo-inositol, and scyllo-inositol (Figure 1).

NAA, which resonates at 2.02 parts per million (ppm), represents the largest proton metabolic concentration in the human brain after water. Indeed the concentration of NAA reaches on the order of 10 μmol/g. NAA is widely interpreted as a neuronal marker and implicated in several neuronal processes, mitochondrial functioning and osmoregulation.

NAA synthesis occurs in mitochondria and requires acetyl-CoA and L-aspartic acid as substrates. NAA has been proposed to serve as a mitochondrial shuttle of acetyl-CoA used for fatty acid synthesis. Its peak decreases when there is neuron suffering or loss. The Cho peak (3.2 ppm) represents a combination of several choline-containing compounds, including free Cho, phosphorylcholine and glycerophosphorylcholine, and to a small extent acetylcholine. Free Cho acts as a precursor to acetylcholine, while glycerophosphorylcholine is a product of breakdown of membrane phosphatidylcholine and acts as an osmoregulator. Its peak increases when there is greater membrane turnover, cell proliferation or inflammatory process. The peak of Cre at 3.03 ppm represents total creatine and phosphocreatine supplies phosphate for conversion of ADP to ATP in creatine kinase reaction. Indeed these metabolites buffer the energy use and energy storage of cells. The level of total Cre mainly remains constant in many neuronal diseases. Thus, total Cre is often used as an internal reference (i.e., a denominator in metabolite signal ratio). The Lac (1.3 ppm) is an end product of anaerobic glycolysis, thus increase in Lac concentrations often serves as an index of altered oxidative metabolism, i.e., in ischemia, hypoxia, and cancer. Increases of Lac in the brain are often accompanied by decreased intracellular pH and high-energy phosphates. The proposed role of Lac is a source of energy for neurons and the transport of Lac plays an essential role in the concept of metabolic coupling between neurons and glia. Glutamate (Glu) is the highest excitatory neurotransmitter in concentration in the CNS. Its peak increases when neuronal and astrocytic activation impairs mitochondrial function and energy utilization. Indeed this process impairs Glu transport and its following enhancement is associated to cellular toxicity.

^{1}H-MRS has been used for at least 15 years in the exploration of patients with altered consciousness, both to investigate the mechanisms of vigilance and to predict the possibilities of regaining consciousness.

Predicting outcome of patients with DOC is an integral part of clinical care, facilitating medical decision making and therapeutic intervention. Current neurological and neurophysiological methods do not enable prediction of outcome of these patients in early stages. Although conventional neuroimaging can provide important information for acute clinical management, its prognostic value is limited, particularly at early stage of injury resolution, owing to its poor sensitivity.

Several studies present in literature have demonstrated the value of ^{1}H-MRS as an accurate tool to predict patient's clinical outcome. Indeed many investigators have shown that correlation exists between metabolite changes and outcome of patients with DOC.

Previous studies using single-voxel technique have shown in brain-injured subjects a significant correlation between unfavorable outcome and reduction of marker NAA in occipitoparietal white and gray matter (WM and GM) (Brooks et al., 2000; Friedman et al., 1999; Ross et al., 1998; Yoon et al., 2005), frontal WM (Garnett et al., 2000), parietal WM (Shutter et al., 2004), brainstem (Carpentier et al., 2006), splenium of the corpus callosum (Sinson et al., 2001; Cecil et al., 1998), and thalamus (Uzan et al., 2003), increase in choline a marker for cell membrane disruption in frontal WM (Garnett et al., 2000) and occipitoparietal WM and GM (Brooks et al., 2000; Cecil et al., 1998; Ross et al., 1998; Yoon et al., 2005), and increase in Glx in occipital GM and parietal WM (Shutter et al., 2004).

In particular, NAA levels seem to discriminate patients who recovered from coma from those who died or remained in persistent VS (Ricci et al., 1997). Uzan et al. (2003) carried out a thalamic proton MRS in patients in VS resulting from severe TBI. They found that

NAA/Cr ratios were able to differentiate patients in VS who recovered awareness from those who remained in persistent VS. However, this alteration was not found in the thalamus of patients in VS resulting from mild TBI (Kirov et al., 2007).

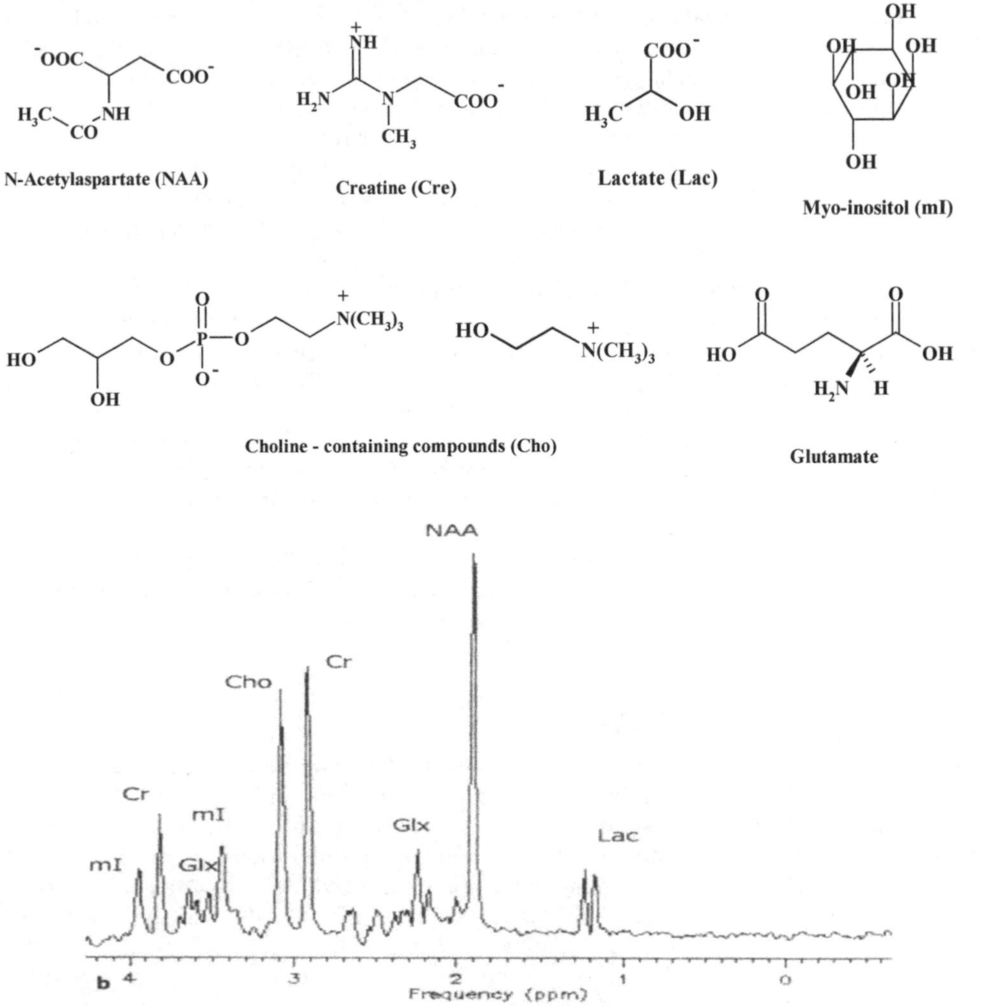

Fig. 1. Chemical structure and spectrum of main cerebral metabolites detected by ^{1}H-MRS.

In some studies has been shown that the combination of imaging techniques may be useful to predict the long-term neurological outcome. A ^{1}H-MRS study in the pons allowed separating of patients who recovered from patients with severe neurological impairment, death or in VS. In addition, ^{1}H-MRS metabolic alterations were not correlated with anatomical MRI lesions, suggesting that these two techniques are strongly complementarity (Carpentier et al., 2006). Tollard et al. (2009) reported the first study on patients with TBI based on a combined quantitative analysis of ^{1}H-MRS and DTI. This combined analysis was

97% specific for predicting an unfavorable outcome after 1 year, compared with 85% for DTI and 75% for ^{1}H-MRS. Similarly, sensitivity was better with the combined analysis (86%) than with either DTI (79%) or MRS (75%).

To study metabolite changes from a wider area of the brain, with the advantage of identifying more anatomical and functional details, a few investigators have used ^{1}H-MRSI (Holshouser et al., 2006; Marino et al. 2007; Shutter et al., 2006; Signoretti et al., 2002, 2008). This technique has an advantage over single-voxel ^{1}H-MRS because generates individual spectra from multiple voxels at the same time. Also ^{1}H-MRSI studies have highlighted close correlation between metabolite alterations and potential recovery.

Neurometabolite concentrations obtained soon after injury may be useful for predicting individual outcome. The decrease of NAA and the increase of Lac, seen by Marino et al. (2007) early after brain injury, were correlated with GOS score. Then these ^{1}H-MRS data may be, at this stage, a reliable index of injury severity and disease outcome.

However it is need to note that ^{1}H-MRS studies in patients with DOC are heterogeneous in terms of patient nature, injury types, time from cerebral damage, voxel location, methods and timing outcome assessment. In addition, in many studies the metabolite concentrations were expressed in terms of semiquantitative ratios. The assumption that the concentration of Cr as reference metabolite remains constant may be incorrect, especially in acute conditions. It is therefore advisable to obtain concentration expressed in standard units by applying absolute quantification. Some studies have expressed metabolite concentrations in term of absolute quantification (Brook et al., 2000; Friedman et al., 1999; Marino et al. 2007; Ross et al., 2000; Shutter et al., 2004).

Data reported so far demonstrate that MRS measure have the potential to provide new and important biological brain markers able to predict clinical outcome, helping in the therapeutic interventions, clinical and rehabilitative management of these patients, as well as to assist with family education.

6. Neurophysiological techniques

The neurophysiological approach to patients with DOC allows the recording of electrical activities of both CNS and Peripheral Nervous System (PNS) and provides a functional assessment, which can be integrated with data obtained mainly from morphological neuroimaging techniques (CT and MRI). The combined use of various neurophysiological examinations, such as Electroencephalogram (EEG), Evoked Related Potentials (ERPs), Transcranial Magnetic Stimulation (TMS), Deep Brain Stimulation (DBS), EEG in association with fMRI, contributes to the topographic and functional diagnosis of the various anatomical structures of the injured CNS and the PNS. The electrophysiological signals recorded from electrodes placed on the surface of the scalp reflect spatially the average post-synaptic potential originated by large neuronal populations. Experimental evidence and clinical observations suggest functional correlations among the neural mechanisms of sensory information, cognitive performance, sleep-wake cycle, alertness and electrophysiological signals generated by neuronal activity. A greater amount of patients can be assessed with electrophysiological techniques, including those who may not have access to a MRI due to geographic, financial, or physical (i.e., metal plates or pins) impairment.

The electroencephalogram in patients in VS has shown a spectrum of abnormalities with changes during the wake-sleep cycle. Patterns have included delta and theta activity and spindle and alpha-like rhythms, but they are more diffusely distributed than in the typical posterior regions and are not reactive to sound, pain, and light stimuli (Chokroverty, 1975; Huges, 1978). During sleep, fewer muscle twitches are observed, but a REM sleep remains (Oksenberg et al., 2001). In most patients, the transition from wakefulness to sleep is accompanied by some desynchronization of the background activity. Very-low-voltage EEG activity is all that can be detected in some patients. In others, persistent alpha activity is the most remarkable feature. In around 10% of patients with VS, the EEG is nearly normal late in the course of disease but without evidence of vision-induced alpha blocking (Danze et al., 1989). There have been occasional reports of isoelectric EEGs in patients in a VS, although it has not been confirmed (Higashi et al., 1977; Mizrahi et al., 1985). Typical epileptiform activity is unusual in patients in VS, as seizure activity is (The Multi-Society Task Force on PVS, 1994). Clinical recovery from the vegetative state may be paralleled by diminished delta and theta activity and reappearance of reactive alpha rhythm. Indeed, Babiloni (2009) has observed that occipital source power in the alpha band (8-13 Hz) of resting EEG, when calculated with low-resolution electromagnetic tomography (LORETA), is correlated with recovery outcome at 3-month follow-up in a group of VS patients; those who made a behavioural recovery had higher resting alpha band power than those who did not make a significant recovery.

The EEG in MCS shows diffuse slowing brain activity, mainly of the theta band, and in most cases responsive to external stimuli. However, there are insufficient data as well as the typical pattern of MCS concerns. Evoked potentials have been studied in patients in a VS and showed normal brainstem auditory responses but abnormal somatosensory responses: prolonged conduction time or absence of scalp potentials. ERPs are more useful than EEG in the differential diagnosis between VS and MCS. ERPs studies focusing on the assessment of conscious awareness have frequently examined four specific components: the N100, the mismatch negativity (MMN), the P300, and the N400 (Connoly & D'Arcy, 2000).

In a recent work, the authors focused on the prediction of consciousness recovery in patients with post-traumatic VS. They used a classical two-stimulus oddball task to elicit the P300 using the patient's own name as deviant and a pure tone as standard stimulus ("subject's own name" paradigm). There is evidence that the amplitude of the P300 wave increases when more salient stimuli are used, such as the own first name instead of visual or auditory deviants. The authors found that P300 is a strong predictor of future recovery of consciousness in VS. This finding is in line with several studies that have confirmed the utility of P300 evoked by deviant tones to predict awakening and favourable outcome from coma and VS (Cavinato et al., 2009). In another study Cavinato et al., (2011) continue to using the "subject's own name" paradigm, but add a pure tone and an "other first name" paradigm. The authors instructed their patients to count the occurrence of deviant stimuli to better differentiate between patients in VS and MCS. The study indicates that in 6 out of 11 patients fulfilling the behavioral criteria for VS a reliable P300 component could be observed in all two conditions. These findings corroborate earlier reports showing that 38% of patients in VS generate a P300 wave. The patients in MCS exhibit significantly longer P300 latencies for the "subject's own name" and the "other first name" paradigms than patients in VS. The increase of P300 latencies for more complex and salient paradigms in MCS but not in VS might help in the difficult differential diagnosis of MCS vs. VS.

The TMS, for high temporal resolution, was proposed as an additional functional imaging technique for the study of cognitive function. To date only some studies have assessed VS and MCS patients with TMS. Moosavi et al. (1999) applied TMS to the hand and leg motor area in 19 patients, few months after severe anoxic brain injury. Eleven patients were in VS, while eight patients were in MCS. The VS patient group differed from the MCS patient group in having a higher threshold, longer duration, and greater irregularity in the form of the response, while the threshold, form, and latency of motor evoked potentials (MEPs) from the MCS group were similar to healthy control subjects. In another study, TMS is used to monitor recovery. The authors examined MEPs from upper and lower limbs in 27 patients in the subacute period and then at 6 and 12 months post – ictus. During the study period, the authors observed an overall trend toward an increase and decrease of latency of MEPs. MEPs from upper and lower limbs progressively normalized in all patients, and at one year after trauma, only 12% of patients had mild abnormalities in MEP responses (Mazzini et al., 1999).

TMS elicited MEP responses in the majority of severely brain damage patients, and a trend toward an increase of amplitude and decrease of latency of MEPs could be observed during the recovery period.

DBS works on reactivating the cortex, aiming to produce a functional recovery. In study of Yamamoto et al. (2010) patients in VS were treated with DBS. Eight of the patients recovered from VS and were able to obey verbal commands at 13 and 10 months in the case of head trauma and a year and a half in the case of vascular disease after comatose brain injury, and no patients without DBS recovered from VS spontaneously within 24 months after brain injury.

In the last years the interest in using of neurophysiological investigations (EEG and EPs) in association with fMRI, has grown: the combination of these different neuroimaging techniques allows study of different components of the brain's activity (e.g., neurovascular coupling, electromagnetic activity) with both a high temporal and spatial resolution (Gosseries et al., 2008).

Clinical neurophysiology procedures are useful as easily performed, non invasive and repeatable at the bed side. These methods provide irreplaceable data about the degree of neuronal dysfunctions and their evolution, and gave also information to assess the outcome.

7. Cognitive recovery

A diagnosis of VS is made if a patient demonstrates no evidence of awareness of self or environment. No evidence of sustained, reproducible, purposeful or voluntary behavioral response to visual, auditory, tactile, or noxious stimuli and critically no evidence of language comprehension or expression. In contrast, the patient in a MCS demonstrates partial preservation of awareness of self and environment, responding intermittently, but reproducibly, to verbal command and therefore demonstrating some degree of basic language comprehension (Coleman et al., 2007).

VS and MCS patients may permanently remain in their clinical condition, or may partly or fully recover consciousness through different stages (Laureys et al., 2004). In this view, it's very important evaluate the residual cognitive across the time. In fact, it allows to make a differential diagnosis between VS and MCS, to monitoring functional changes of the patients, in order to customize the treatment, and, at least, to have a baseline evaluation of the patients in case of consciousness recovery. Nevertheless, the assessment of residual brain functions and the degree of recovery of these patients remain, still today, an opened issue in the medical field. To date, there have been no detailed studies of these patients evaluating cognitive changes and recovery over time through a specific neuropsychological battery (Neumann & Kotchoubey, 2004). This might suggest a new and possible way to further investigate the potential outcome of these challenging patients.

In this paragraph we try to identify some markers of consciousness with prognostic value, based on literature review. As it has been clearly established in clinical practice, significant spontaneous recovery frequently occurs during the subacute period (Wilson et al., 2002; Giacino & Trott 2004). Two factors can facilitate cognitive recovery of these patients: young age and immediate medical assistance after the injury.

Literature findings demonstrated that no clinical tools strongly predicted good outcome. In contrast, complementary examinations such as electrophysiological and functional neuroimaging studies objectively measure residual brain functions and are indicative of recovery of consciousness.

Several studies explore the prognostic validity of behavioural assessment scales (i.e. GOS, Coma Recovery Scale, Wessex Head Injury Matrix, Western Neuro Sensory Stimulation Profile, DRS, Functional Independence Measure), electrophysiological measures (ERPs), and functional neuroimaging (PET, fMRI), to predict outcome in patients with low levels of consciousness. Particular progress towards addressing this objective has been made using brain imaging techniques such as PET and fMRI. Schiff et al. (2002) suggested that rather than a complete loss of cortical function some patients retain "island" of preserved cognitive functions. PET and fMRI studies suggest that a higher-level associative cortical activation seems to predict recovery of consciousness with a 93% specificity and 69% sensitivity (Di et al., 2008). PET work has identified preserved responses to a variety of sensory stimuli, including photographs of familiar people, noxious, tactile (Laureys et al. 2000; Owen et al., 2002; Boly et al., 2004) in some vegetative and minimally conscious patients. Some studies underline the importance of the cognitive ERPs in the assessment of residual functions in comatose, VS, or MCS patients. As a general rule, early ERPs (such as the absence of cortical response on somatosensory evoked-potentials) predict bad outcome, while cognitive ERPs are indicative of recovery of consciousness (Vanhaudenhuyse et al., 2007). Moreover, auditory cognitive ERPs are useful to investigate residual cognitive functions, such as echoic memory (Mismatch Negativity), acoustical and semantic discrimination (P300), and incongruent language detection (N400). In VS patients, cognitive potential are more frequently obtained when using stimuli that are more ecologic or have an emotional content (such as the patients' own name) than when using classical sine tones.

Electrophysiological and functional neuroimaging studies may provide useful and objective information to the outcome and possibly cognition of patients with low levels of consciousness (Di et al., 2007). To date, there have been no detailed studies of these patients combining and correlating specific neuropsychological tools and functional imaging, in order to evaluate the cognitive changes and recovery over time (Bekinschtein et al, 2005). In spite of the important findings, functional neuroimaging cannot, and should not replace, clinical and behavioural evaluation as the criterion standard for assessment of patients with DOC. It offers an objective method of differentiating brain activity measured at rest and during external stimulation, but further studies are needed to assess the temporal evolution of individual patients' somatosensory and cognitive processing (Giacino et al., 2006). Despite converging agreement about the definition of persistent vegetative state, recent reports have raised concerns about the accuracy of diagnosis in some patients, and the extent to which, in a selection of cases, residual cognitive functions may remain undetected. Objective assessment of residual cognitive function can be extremely difficult as motor responses may be minimal, inconsistent, and difficult to document in many patients, or may be undetectable in others because no cognitive output is possible (Owen et al., 2002). There are no standards of care to guide the selection of rehabilitation assessment and treatment procedures for patients with DOC (Neumann & Kotchoubey, 2004). Cognition abilities with theory of mind tasks, decision-making tasks, social performance tests and expanded cognitive assessment, to further characterize post-traumatic or hypoxic-ischemic brain damaged vegetative patients after recovery remain under evaluation at this time. The cognitive recovery in patients with DOC is a continual process rather than a step-by-step phenomenon and confirms that a good recovery assessment should include objective measures of behavioural, cognitive and functional domains, and neurophysiological data to support diagnosis. Survivors from a coma frequently suffer from long-lasting disability, which is mainly related to cognitive deficits. Such deficits include slowed information processing, deficits of learning and memory, of attention, of working memory, and of executive functions, associated with behavioral and personality modifications (Azouvi et al., 2009). An accurate cognitive assessment during the very first phase of the convalescence, when it is possible, is the first step for the management and the implementation of an individual and effective treatment.

Appropriate management requires an experienced inter-disciplinary as opposed to multidisciplinary team working style, whose skill repertoire equips them to recognize often-subtle improvements in cognitive function and act to maximize individual patient's quality of life. The current paucity of service provision for this vulnerable group of patients is highlighted. In fact, predicting the chances of recovery of consciousness and communication in patients who survive their coma, but transit in a VS or MCS remains a major challenge for their medical caregivers. Very few studies have examined the slow neuronal changes underlying functional recovery of consciousness from severe chronic brain damage.

8. Prognosis and rehabilitation

Determining the accurate prognosis of VS and MCS is a critical step in counseling families and determining appropriate treatment. Previous studies of prognosis in VS were limited by several factors: 1) because there were no accepted diagnostic criteria for MCS prior to 2002, some patients in MCS in those studies may have been diagnosed with VS; 2) it is more accurate to determine prognosis by the etiology of brain damage than merely by categorization in a clinical syndrome; and 3) retrospective experiential analysis of outcomes, such us that by the Multi-Society Task Force, committed the fallacy of the self-fulfilling prophecy because they included patients in their survival data who died primarily because their life-sustaining therapy was discontinued (Bernat et al., 2010). Nevertheless, the prognostic guidelines published in 1994 by Multi-Society Task Force on PVS have been generally accepted, showing a very low probability of recovering awareness once VS has been present for a year following TBI or for 3 months following hypoxic-ischemic neuronal injury (Bernat et al., 2009).Two recently published studies of prognosis in VS add useful data. Luautè and colleagues (Luautè et al., 2010), confirmed the prognostic guidelines of the Multi- Society Task Force in all the patients in VS. They studied and showed that age greater than 39 years and absence of the middle-latency auditory evoked potentials were independent early predictors of poor outcome irrespective of pathogenesis. Estraneo and colleagues (Estraneo et al., 2010), found that 88% of patients in VS in their serious conformed to the Multi- Society Task Force prognostic guidelines but 12% made late recoveries of awareness but only to the point of severe disability with MCS, most of whom had TBI. Because of varying pathophysiologies, prognostic indicators for MCS as a group have been difficult to establish whereas prognostic indicators in individual pathophysiologic subsets of

MCS (e.g. patients in MCS from TBI) have been more reliable (Bernat et al.,2010). The appropriate level of treatment of patients with chronic DOC depends on their diagnosis, prognosis and prior stated treatment values and preferences. Specialized neurorehabilitation units are the optimal treatment for patients with chronic DOC , at least until they are no longer improving. Patients have better functional out comes when treated by skilled personnel who have been trained in neurorehabilitation. The difference between patients in VS and patients in MCS in their response to stimulatory treatment is noteworthy: patients in VS rarely improve as a consequence of stimulation but patients in MCS may improve to some extent. Treatment modalities that have been studied include environmental and sensory stimuli such as sounds, smells, touch, images and music. Pharmacologic stimuli include treatment with stimulants, levodopa, and dopamine agonists (by stimulating intact dopaminergic thalamic neurons), and selective serotonin reuptake inhibitor antidepressants. Electrical stimuli include deep brain stimulation of medical thalamic nuclei. Each of these modalities has been reported to improve functional responsiveness in some patients in MCS though there are few controlled studies. These therapies are also widely tried in patients in VS but a meta-analysis of their outcomes showed no consistent benefits (Bernat, 2006).

9. Sensory stimulation procedure

The use of unimodal and multimodal sensory stimulation for the treatment of comatose patient, both in the acute and prolonged states, has been advocated (Johnson et al., 1988). The rationale behind the use of these techniques is that all aspects of the patient must be treated; it is insufficient to attend to the maintenance of bodily well being alone. Sensory stimulation should at the least not have any ill-effects on the patient and could enhance the processes of recovery. S.L. Wilson et al. (1991) have observed patients diagnosed as being in prolonged coma, routinely treated according to a sensory stimulation protocol. They reported an evaluation of the efficacy of this procedure using the comparison of behavioral measures taken immediately prior and post-stimulation. Sensory stimulation treatment appears to be widely used with patients who are in VS arising from traumatic causes, but the term has to be regarded as generic rather than specific since sensory stimulation procedures appear to differ widely in content (Wilson et al., 1993). A number of studies have been published evaluating the effects of these treatment; some have methodological flaws, but the major difficulty in evaluating any treatment with this group of patients is getting sufficient subjects, so most of the published studies use relatively small numbers. Ideally, a large-scale matched control study would be looked for, which examined rate of recovery and long-term outcome. If sensory stimulation is rejected on the basis of lack of empirical evidence, then logically many other treatments used with medical settings should also be rejected. In real life, however, where definitive empirical evidence is not yet available, then clinicians can reasonably make decisions on treatment by combining clinical experience with inferences from scientific knowledge concerning related populations. For example, stimulation treatments which involve the use of some constant background stimulation within the patient's environment, such as TV or radio, have been justifiably criticized. As Wood points out, it is likely to be damaged within the brain that mediate selective attention are highly likely to be damaged within these patients; therefore it is unlikely they are going to be able to differentiate between stimuli in a situation where they are being bombarded with sensory input. In addition, habituation may exacerbate the problem.

10. Neuroimaging of self-consciousness and recovery

A recent meta-analysis by Northoff et al. (2006) of 27 PET and fMRI studies comparing hemodynamic brain responses obtained during active paradigms comparing processing of stimuli related to the self with those of non-self-referential stimuli identified activation in cortical midline structures in all studies and occurring across all functional domains (e.g. verbal, spatial, emotional, and facial). Cluster and factor analyses indicated functional specialization into ventral, dorsal, and posterior cortical midline areas. The latter encompasses the posterior cingulate cortex and adjacent precuneus and is considered to be involved in self-integration – that is linkage of self-referential stimuli to the personal context (Northoff et al., 2004). Neuroimaging studies during tasks involving self-processing (i.e. self-reflection, self-perspective and free thoughts) have also reported the activation of the medial prefrontal areas. Gusnard, Akbudak, Shulman , and Raichle (2001) for example showed medial frontal activation when subjects had to make two judgments in response to pleasant *vs* unpleasant pictures (i.e. self-referential) as compared to indoors *vs* outdoors pictures (i.e. not self-referential). The same area was also shown to be engaged when subjects had to make self-referential judgments about trait adjectives (i.e. self-referential processing) as compared to when they had to make case judgments (Kelley et al., 2002) and when subjects responded to statements requiring knowledge of, and reflection on, their own abilities, traits and attitudes , i.e. self-reflective thought (Johnson et al., 2002). Taking a self–perspective (i.e. being the agent of an history) also activated medial prefrontal/anterior cingulate cortices (Vogeley et al., 2001). Finally, activation of the mesiofrontal areas was describes in studies dealing with the conscious resting state, i.e. free thought (Mazoyer et al., 2001), a brain state which "instantiates functions that are integral to the self". The recovery of consciousness of one VS patient has previously been linked to an increase in the functional connectivity within fronto-parietal network, (Laureys et al, 1999) encompassing the areas known to be most active in resting–state conditions (Gusnard et al., 2001). A growing body of evidence from Positron emission tomography (PET) and fMRI studies of healthy volunteers in a variety of altered states of consciousness has emphasized the role of this "default-mode" network in the genesis of awareness. In keeping with this, functional impairments to this network have been observed during sleepwalking, absence of seizures, deep sleep and anesthesia (Bassetti et al., 2000). fMRI has also proved its utility in identifying a number of cognitive functions which may be preserved in DOC patients, the results of which have, in some cases, proved prognostic of positive outcomes (Owen et al., 2008). In one such fMRI study investigating language processing. Coleman et. al found evidence of speech processing in three out of seven behaviorally non-communicative VS patients (Coleman et al., 2007). Six months after the scan, each of these patients had made a marked behavioral recovery relative to those patients who did not demonstrate comparable activations. Similar findings have also been reported for the neural responses observed when patients hear their own name (Di et al., 2007). Multimodal imaging approach can provide a powerful tool for assessing the mechanisms involved in the recovery of consciousness in DOC patients. Further longitudinal studies with large cohorts will prove useful in assessing its full value in predicting outcome. Such insights may then provide guidance for decisions relating to rehabilitation programs by those orientating these towards the effective stimulation of those functions that appear preserved, in order to maintain their integrity.

11. Conclusions

Patients with severe brain damage who are unable to communicate present several ethical concerns. Foremost is the concern that diagnostic and prognostic accuracy is certain, as treatment decisions typically include the possibility of withdrawal of life-support. Although imaging techniques have the potential to improve both diagnostic and prognostic accuracy, careful and repeated neurological assessment by a trained examiner remains best practice. Accurate clinical assessments of patients in these conditions must be obtained before they undergo neuroimaging. Moreover, in reports of neuroimaging studies, all relevant clinical details must be available for comparisons between studies.

Ethical concerns are commonly raised about the participation of patients with severe brain damage in neuroimaging studies. By definition, unconscious or minimally conscious patients cannot give informed consent to participate in clinical research and written approval must typically be obtained from family or legal representatives depending on governmental and hospital guidelines. Nonetheless, researchers studying these patients have been refused grants, ethics committee approval, and research publication; these decisions tend to be made on the basis that studies of patients who cannot provide consent are unethical. We prefer an ethical framework that balances access to research with medical advances alongside protection for defenseless patients. Severe brain damage represents an immense social and economic problem that warrants further research. Unconscious, minimally conscious, and locked-in patients deserve special procedural protections. However, it is important to stress that they are also at risk of being denied therapy that may be life-saving if clinical research cannot be done on these patient groups.

Patients who are in coma, VS, MCS, or locked-in syndrome present unique problems for diagnosis, prognosis, treatment, and everyday management. At the patient's bedside, assessment of cognitive function is difficult because voluntary movements may be very small, inconsistent, and easily exhausted. Functional neuroimaging will never replace the clinical assessment of patients with altered states of consciousness. Nevertheless, using population norms it can provide an objective measure of the regional distribution of cerebral activity at rest and under various conditions of stimulation. The quantification of brain activity differentiates patients who sometimes only differ by a brief and small movement of a finger. In our opinion, PET, MRS and fMRI will increase substantially our understanding of patients with severe brain damage.

12. References

Adams, J.H.; Jennett, B.; McLellan, D.R.; Murray, L.S. & Graham D.I. The neuropathology of the vegetative state after head injury. *Journal of Clinical Pathology*, Vol. 52, No. 11, *(November 1999), pp. 804-806,* ISSN 1472-4146

Ammermann, H.; Kassube, K.J.; Lotze, M.; Gut, E.; Kaps, M. et al. MRI brain lesion patterns in patients in anoxia-induced vegetative state. *Journal of the Neurological Sciences*, vol. 260, N° 1-2, (September 2007), pp. 65-70, ISSN 0022-510X

Arfanakis K.; Haughton V.M.; Carew J.D.; Rogers, B.P.; Dempsey, R.J. et al. Diffusion tensor MR imaging in diffuse axonal injury. *American Journal of Neuroradiology*, Vol.23, No.5, (May 2002), pp. 794-802, ISSN 1936-959X

Atlas, S.W.; Howard, I.I.R.S.; Maldijian, J.; Alsop, D.; Detre, J.A. et al. Functional magnetic resonance imaging of regional brain activity in patients with intracerebral gliomas:

findings and implications for clinical management. *Neurosurgery*, Vol.38, No2, (February 1996), pp. 329-338, ISSN 0148-396X

Azouvi, P.; Vallat-Azouvi, C. & Belmont, A. Cognitive deficits after traumatic coma. *Progress in brain research*, Vol. 117, (October 2009), pp. 89-110, ISSN 0079-6123

Babiloni, C.; Sarà, M.; Vecchio, F.; Pistoia, F.; Sebastiano, F. et al. Cortical sources of resting-state alpha rhythms are abnormal in persistent vegetative state patients. *Clinical Neurophysiology*, Vol. 120, No. 4, (April 2009), pp. 719-729, ISSN 1388-2457

Bandettini, P.A.; Jesmanowicz, A.; Wong, E.C. & Hyde, J.S. Processing strategies for time-course data sets in functional MRI of the human brain. *Magnetic Resonance in Medicine*, Vol.30, No2, (August 1993), pp. 161-173, ISSN 0740-3194

Bassetti, C.; Vella, S.; Donati, F.; Wielepp, P. & Weder, B. SPECT during sleepwalking. *Lancet*, (August 2000), Vol. 356, No. 9, pp. 484-485, ISSN 0140-6736

Bekinschtein, T.; Tiberti, C.; Niklison, J.; Tamashiro, M.; Ron, M. et al. Assessing level of consciousness and cognitive changes from vegetative state to full recovery. *Neuropsychological rehabilitation*, Vol. 15, No. 3/4, (July-September 2005), pp. 307-322, ISSN 0960-2011

Benson, R.; Meda, S.; Vasudevan, S.; Kou, Z.; Govindarajan, K.A. et al. Global white matter analysis of diffusion tensor images is predictive of injury severity in traumatic brain injury. *Journal of Neurotrauma*, Vol. 24, No. 3, (March 2007), pp. 446-459, 0897-7151

Bernat, J.L. Chronic disorders of consciousness. *Lancet*, (June 2006) Vol. 367, No. 9528, pp.1181-1192, ISSN 0140-6736

Bernat, J.L. Chronic consciousness disorders. *Annual Review of Medicine*, (February 2009), Vol. 60, No. 1, pp. 381-392, ISSN 0066-4219

Bernat, J.L. The natural history of chronic disorders of consciousness. *Neurology*, (July 2010), Vol. 75, No. 3, pp. 206-207, ISSN 0028-3878

Boly, M.; Faymonville, M.; Damas, P.; Lambermont, B.; Del Fiore, G. et al. Auditory processing in severely brain injured patients: differences between the minimally conscious state and the vegetative state. *Archives of neurology*, Vol. 61, No. 2, (February 2004), pp. 233-238, ISSN 0003-9942

Brooks, W.M.; Stidley, C.A.; Petropoulos, H.; Jung, R.E.; Weers, D.C. et al. Metabolic and cognitive to human traumatic brain injury: a quantitative proton magnetic resonance study. *Journal of Neurotrauma*, Vol.17, No.8, (August 2000), pp. 629-640, ISSN 0897-7151

Carpentier, A.; Galanaud, D.; Puybasset, L.; Mullar, J.C.; Lescot, T. et al. Early morphologic and spectroscopic magnetic resonance in severe traumatic brain injuries can detect "invisible brain stem damage" and predict "vegetative states". *Journal of Neurotrauma*, Vol.23, No.5, (May 2006), pp. 674-685, ISSN 0897-7151

Cavinato, M.; Freo, U.; Ori, C.; Zorzi, M.; Tonin, P. et al. Post-acute P300 predicts recovery of consciousness from traumatic vegetative state. *Brain Injury*, Vol.23, No. 12, (November 2009), pp. 973-80, ISSN 0269-9052

Cavinato, M.; Volpato, C.; Silvoni, S.; Sacchetto, M.; Merico, A. et al. Event-related brain potential modulation in patients with severe brain damage. *Clinical Neurophysiology*, Vol. 122, No. 4, (April 2011), pp. 719-24, ISSN 1388-2457

Cecil, K.M.; Hills, E.C.; Sandel, M.E.; Smith, D.H.; McIntosh, T.K. et al. Proton magnetic resonance spectroscopy for detection of axonal injury in the splenium of the corpus callosum of brain-injured patients. *Journal of Neurosurgery*, Vol.88, No.5, (May 1998), pp. 795-801, ISSN 0022-3085

Chokroverty, S. "Alpha-like rhythms" in electroencephalograms in coma after cardiac arrest. *Neurology*, Vol. 25, No. 7, (July 1975), pp. 655-663, ISSN 0028-3878

Coleman, M.R.; Rodd, J.M.; Davis, M.H.; Johnsrude, I.S.; Menon, D.K. et al. Do vegetative patients retain aspects of language comprehension? Evidence from fMRI. *Brain*, Vol. 130, No. 10, (September 2007), pp. 2494-2507, ISSN 0006-8950

Connolly, J.F. & D'Arcy, R.C. Innovations in neuropsychological assessment using event-related brain potentials. *International Journal of Psychophysiology*, Vol. 37, No. 1, (July 2000), pp. 31-47, ISSN 0167-8760

Danze, F.; Brule, J.F. & Haddad, K. Chronic vegetative state after severe head injury: clinical study; electrophysiological investigations and CT scan in 15 cases. *Neurosurgical Review*, Vol. 12, No.1, (March 1989), pp. 477-499, ISSN 0344-5607

De Young, S. & Grass, R.B. Coma recovery program. *Rehabilitation Nursing*, (March 1987), Vol. 12, No 7, pp. 121-124, ISSN 0278-4807

Di, H.; Boly, M.; Weng, X.; Ledoux, D. & Laureys, S. Neuroimaging activation studies in the vegetative state: predictors of recovery. *Clinical Medicine*, Vol. 8, No. 5, (October 2008), pp. 502-507, ISSN 1473-4893

Di, H.; Yu, S.M.; Weng, X.C.; Laureys, S.; Yu, D. et al. Cerebral response to patient's own name in the vegetative and minimally conscious state. *Neurology*, Vol. 68, No. 12, (March 2007), pp. 895–899, ISSN 0028-3878

Douaud, G.; Smith, S.; Jenkinson, M.; Behrens, T.; Johansen-Berg, H. et al. Anatomically related grey and whitematter abnormalities in adolescent-onset schizophrenia. *Brain*, Vol.130, No.9, (September 2007), pp. 2375-2386, ISSN 0006-8950

Estraneo, A.; Moretta, P.; Loreto,V.; Lanzillo, B.; Santoro L. et al. Late recovery after traumatic, anoxic or hemorrhagic long-lasting vegetative state. *Neurology*, (July 2010), Vol. 75, No. 3 pp. 239-245, ISSN 0028-3878

Fernandez-Espejo, D.; Junque, C.; Bernabeu, M.; Roig-Rovira, T.; Vendrell P. et al. Reductions of thalamic volume and regional shape changes in the vegetative and the minimally conscious states. *Journal of Neurotrauma*, vol. 27, N° 7, (July 2010), pp. 1187–1193, ISSN 0897-7151

Fernández-Espejo, D; Bekinschtein, T.; Monti, M.M.; Pickard, J.D.; Junque, C. et al. Diffusion weighted imaging distinguishes the vegetative state from the minimally conscious state. *Neuroimage*, Vol.51, No.1, (January 2011), pp. 103-112, ISSN 1053-8119

Fox, P.T. & Raichle, M.E. Stimulus rate determines regional brain blood flow in striate cortex. *Annals of Neurology*, Vol.17, No3, (March 1985), pp.303-305, ISSN 0364-5134

Friedman, S.D.; Brooks, W.M.; Jung, R.E.; Chiulli, S.J.; Sloan, J.H. et al. Quantitative proton MRS predicts outcome after traumatic brain injury. *Neurology*, Vol.52, No.7, (April 1999), pp. 1384-1391, ISSN 0028-3878

Garnett, M.R.; Blamire, A.M.; Corkill, R.G.; Cadoux-Hudson, T.A.D.; Rajagopalan B. et al. Early proton magnetic resonance spectroscopy in normal-appearing brain correlates with outcome in patients following traumatic brain injury. *Brain*, Vol.123, No.10, (October 2000), pp. 2046-2054, ISSN 0006-8950

George, J.S.; Aine, C.J.; Mosher, J.C.; Schmidt, M.D.; Ranken, D.M. et al., Mapping function in the human brain with magneto encephalography, anatomical magnetic resonance imaging, and functional magnetic resonance imaging. *Journal of Clinical Neurophysiology,* Vol.12, No5, (September 1995), pp. 406-429 ISSN 1676-2649

Giacino, J.Y.; Ashwal, S.; Childs, N.; Cranford, R.; Jennett, B. et al. The minimally conscious state: definition and diagnostic criteria. *Neurology,* Vol. 58, No.3, (February 2002), pp. 349-353, ISSN 0028-3878

Giacino, J.T. & Trott, C.T. Rehabilitative management of patients with disorders of consciousness: Grand rounds. *Journal of head trauma rehabilitation,* Vol. 19, No. 3, (May-June 2004) pp. 254-265, ISSN 1550-509X

Giacino, J.T.; Hirsch, J.; Schiff, N. & Laureys, S. Functional neuroimaging for assessment and rehabilitation planning in patients with disorders of consciousness. *Archives of physical medicine and rehabilitation,* Vol. 87, Suppl. 2, (December 2006), pp. S67-S75, ISSN 0003-9993

Gosseries, O.; Demertzi, A.; Noirhomme, Q.; Tshibanda, J.; Boly, M. et al. Functional neuroimaging (fMRI, PET and MEG): what do we measure? *Revue Medical de Liege,* Vol. 63, No. 5-6, (May-Jun 2008), pp.231-7, ISSN 0370-629X

Gusnard, D.A. & Raichle, M.E. Searching for a baseline: functional imaging and the resting human brain. *Nature Reviews Neuroscience,* (October 2001), Vol. 2, No. 2, pp. 685-694, ISSN 1471-003X

Higashi, K.; Sakata, Y.; Hatano, M.; Abiko, S.; Ihara,K. et al. Epidemiological studies on patients with a persistent vegetative state. *Journal of Neurology, Neurosurgery & Psychiatry,* Vol. 40, No. 9, (September 1977), pp. 876-885, ISSN 0022-3050

Hinke, R.M.; Hu, X.; Stillman, A.E.; Kim, S.G.; Merkle, H. et al. Functional magnetic resonance imaging of Broca's area during internal speech. *NeuroReport,* Vol.4, No6, (June 1993) pp. 675-678 ISSN 0959-4965

Holshouser, B.A.; Tong, K.A.; Ashwal, S.; Oyoyo, U.; Ghamsary, M. et al. Prospective longitudinal proton magnetic resonance spectroscopic imaging in adult traumatic brain injury. *Journal of Magnetic Resonance Imaging,* Vol.24, No.1, (July 2006), pp. 33-40, ISSN 1522-2586

Hughes J.R. Limitations of the EEG in coma and brain death. *Annals of the New York Academy Sciences,* Vol. 315, No. 1, (November 1978), pp. 121-136, ISSN 0077-8923

Huisman, T. A.; Schwamm, L. H.; Schaefer, P. W.; Koroshetz, W.J.; Shetty-Alva, N. et al. Diffusion tensor imaging as potential biomarker of white matter injury in diffuse axonal injury. *American Journal of Neuroradiology,* Vol.25, No.3, (March 2004), pp. 370-376, ISSN 1936-959X

Jennett, B.; Adams, J.H.; Murray, L.S. & Graham, D.I. Neuropathology in vegetative and severely disabled patients after head injury. *Neurology,* vol. 56, N° 4, (February 2001), pp. 486–490, ISSN 0028-3878

Johnson, D.A. & Roethig-Johnston, K. Coma stimulation: a challenge to occupational therapy. *British Journal of Occupational Therapy.* (April 1988), Vol. 51, No 5, pp. 88-90, ISSN 1477-6006

Juengling, F.D.; Kassubek, J.; Huppertz, H.; Krause, T. & Els, T. Separating functional and structural damage in persistent vegetative state using combined voxel-based analysis of 3-D MRI and FDG-PET. *Journal of the Neurological Sciences,* vol. 228, N° 2, (February 2005), pp. 179– 184, ISSN 0022-510X

Kaisti, K.K.; Metsahonkala, L.; Teras, M.; Oikonen, V.; Aalto, S. et al. Effects of surgical levels of propofol and sevoflurane anesthesia on cerebral blood flow in healthy subjects studied with positron emission tomography. *Anesthesiology,* (June 2002), Vol. 96, No. 6, pp. 1358-1370, ISSN 1528-1175

Kim, K.; Hirsch, J.; DeLaPaz, R.L.; Relkin, N. & Lee, K.M. Comparison of cortical areas activated by primary and secondary languages in human brain using functional magnetic resonance imaging (fMRI). *Abstracts: Society of Neuroscience,* Vol.21, No3, (1993), pp.1763, ISSN 0270-6474

Kirov, I.; Fleysher, L.; Babb, J.S.; Silver, J.M.; Grossman, R.I. et al. Characterizing "mild" in traumatic brain injury with proton MR spectroscopy in the thalamus: initial findings. *Brain Injury,* Vol.21, No.11, (October 2007), pp. 1147-1154, ISSN 0269-9052

Kraus, M.F.; Susmaras, T.; Caughlin, B.P.; Walker, C.J.; Sweeney J.A. et al. White matter integrity and cognition in chronic traumatic brain injury: A diffusion tensor imaging study. *Brain,* Vol.130, No.19, (October 2007), pp. 250-2519, ISSN 0006-8950

Laureys, S.; Goldman, S.; Phillips. C.; Van Bogaert, P.; Aerts, J. et al. Impaired effective cortical connectivity in vegetative state: preliminary investigation using PET. *Neuroimage,* Vol.9, No4, (April 1999), pp.377–82, ISSN 1053-8119

Laureys, S.; Lemaire, C.; Maquet, P.; Phillips, C. & Franck, G. Cerebral metabolism during vegetative state and after recovery to consciousness. *Journal of Neurology, Neurosurgery & Psychiatry,* (April 1999), Vol. 67, No. 10, p. 121, ISSN 0022-3050

Laureys, S.; Faymonville, M.E.; Luxen, A.; Lamy, M.; Franck, G. et al. Restoration of thalamocortical connectivity after recovery from persistent vegetative state. *Lancet,* (May 2000), Vol. 355, No. 9217, pp. 1790-1791, ISSN 0140-6736

Laureys, S.; Faymonville, M.E.; Degueldre, C.; Fiore, G.D.; Damas, P. et al. Auditory processing in the vegetative state. *Brain,* Vol. 123, No. 8, (August 2000), pp. 1589-601, ISSN 0006-8950

Laureys, S.; Owen, A.M. & Schiff, N.D. Brain function in coma, vegetative state, and related disorders. *Lancet Neurology,* Vol. 3, No. 9, (Spetember 2004), pp. 537-546, ISSN 0028-3878

Laureys, S. & Boly, M. The changing spectrum of coma. *Nature Clinical Practice Neurology,* Vol.10, No.10, (October 2008), pp. 544-546, ISSN 1745-8358

Levy, D.E.; Sidtis, J.J.; Rottenberg, D.A.; Jarden, J.O.; Strother, S.C.; Dhawan, V. et al. Differences in cerebral blood flow and glucose utilization in vegetative versus locked-in patients. *Annals of Neurology,* Vol.22, No6, (December 1897), ISSN 0364-5134

Lewinn, E.B. The coma arousal team. *Royal Society of Health Journal,* (May 1980) Vol. 1, No 4, pp. 19-21, ISSN 1477-6006

Luautè, J.; Maucort-Boulch, D. & Tell, L. Long-term outcomes of chronic minimally conscious and vegetative states. *Neurology,* (June 2010), Vol. 75, No. 3, pp. 246-252, ISSN 0028-3878

Maquet, P. Functional neuroimaging of normal human sleep by positron emission tomography. *Journal of Sleep Research,* (April 2000), Vol. 9, No. 3 pp. 207-231, ISSN 0962-1105

Marino, S.; Zei, E.; Battaglini, M.; Vittori, C.; Buscalferri, A. et al. Acute metabolic brain changes following traumatic brain injury and their relevance to clinical severity and outcome. *Journal of Neurology, Neurosurgery and Psychiatry,* Vol.78, No.5, (May 2007), pp. 501-507, ISSN 0022-3050

Mazzini, L.; Pisano, F.; Zaccala, M.; Miscio, G.; Gareri, F. et al. Somatosensory and motor evoked potentials at different stages of recovery from severe traumatic brain injury.

Archives of Physical Medicine and Rehabilitation, Vol. 80, No. 1, (January 1999), pp. 33-39, ISSN 0003-9993

Medical aspects of the persistent vegetative state (1). The Multi-Society Task Force on PVS. *New England Journal Medicine,* Vol.330, No21, (May 1994), pp. 1499-508, ISSN 0028-4793

Mizrahi, E.M.; Pollack, M.A. & Kellaway, P. Neocortical death in infants: behavioral, neurologic, and electroencephalographic characteristics. *Pediatric Neurology,* Vol. 1, No.5, (Sep-Oct 1985), pp.302-305, ISSN 0887-8994

Moosavi, S.H.; Ellaway, P.H.; Catley, M.; Stokes, M.J. & Haque, N. Corticospinal function in severe brain injury assessed using magnetic stimulation of the motor cortex in man. *Journal of the Neurological Sciences,* Vol. 164, No. 2, (April 1999), pp. 179-186, ISSN 0022-510X

Neumann, N., & Kotchoubey, B. Assessment of cognitive functions in severely paralysed and severely brain-damged patients: neuropsychological and electrophysiological methods. *Brain Research Protocols,* Vol. 14, No. 1, (November 2004), pp. 25-36, ISSN 1385-299X

Ogawa, S.; Lee, T.M.; Nayak, A. S. & Glynn, P. Oxygenation-sensitive contrast in magnetic resonance image of rodent brain at high magnetic fields. *Magnetic Resonance in Medicine,* Vol.14, No1, (April 1990) pp.68-78, ISSN 0740-3194

Oksenberg A.; Gordon C.; Arons E. & Sazbon L. Phasic activities of rapid eye movement sleep in vegetative state patients. *Sleep,* Vol. 24, No. 6, (February 2001), pp. 703-706, ISSN 1550-9109

O'Sullivan, M.; Singhal, S.; Charlton, R. & Markus H.S. Diffusion tensor imaging of thalamus correlates with cognition in CADASIL without dementia. *Neurology,* Vol.62, No.5, (March 2004), pp. 702-707, ISSN 0028-3878

Owen, A.M.; Menon, D.K.; Johnsrude, I.S.; Bor, D.; Scott, S.K.; et al. Detecting residual cognitive function in persistent vegetative state. *Neurocase,* Vol. 8, No. 5, (2002), pp. 394-403, ISSN 1355-4794

Owen, A.M. & Coleman, M.R. Functional neuroimaging of vegetative state. *Nature Reviews Neuroscience,* (March 2008), Vol. 9, No. 9, pp.235-243, ISSN 1471-003X

Perlbarg, V.; Puybasset, L.; Tollard, E.; Lehericy, S.; Benali, H. et al. Relation between brain lesion location and clinical outcome in patients with severe traumatic brain injury: A diffusion tensor imaging study using voxel-based approaches. *Human Brain Mapping,* Vol.30, No.12, (December 2009), pp: 3924-3933, ISSN 1097-0193

Rader, M.A.; Alston, J.B. & Ellis, D.W. Sensory stimulation of severely brain-injured patients. *Brain Injury,* (August 1988), Vol. 3, No. 6, pp.141-147, ISSN 0269-9052

Ricci, R.; Barbarella, G.; Musi, P.; Boldrini, P.; Trevisan, C. et al. Localised proton MR spectroscopy of brain metabolism changes in vegetative patients. *Neuroradiology,* Vol.39, No.5, (May 1997), pp. 313-319, ISSN 0028-3940

Ringman, J.M.; O'Neill, J.; Geschwind, D.; Medina, L.; Apostolova, L.G. et al. Diffusion tensor imaging in preclinical and presymptomatic carriers of familial Alzheimer's disease mutations. *Brain,* Vol.130, No.7 (July 2007), pp. 1767-1776, ISSN 0006-8950

Ross, B.D.; Ernst, T.; Kreis, R.; Haseler, L.J.; Bayer, S. et al. ^{1}H MRS in acute traumatic brain injury. *Journal of Magnetic Resonance Imaging,* Vol.8, No.4, (August 1998), pp. 829-840, ISSN 0028-3878

Roy, C. & Sherrington, C. On the regulation of the blood-supply of the brain. *The Journal of Physiology,* Vol.11, No1-2, (January 1980), pp.85-108, ISSN 1469-7793

Salek-Haddadi, A.; Lemieux, L.; Merschhemke, M.; Friston, K.J.; Duncan, J.S. et al. Functional magnetic resonance imaging of human absence seizures. *Annals of Neurology*, (April 2003), Vol. 53, No. 10, pp. 663-667, ISSN 0364-5134

Salmond, C. H.; Menon, D. K.; Chatfield, D. A.; Williams, G.B.; Pena, A. et al. Diffusion tensor imaging in chronic head injury survivors: Correlations with learning and memory indices. *Neuroimage*, Vol.29, No.1, (January 2006), pp. 117-124, ISSN 1053-8119

Schiff, N.D.; Ribary, U.; Moreno, D.R.; Beattie, B.; Kronberg, E. et al. Residual cerebral activity and behavioural fragments can remain in the persistently vegetative brain. *Brain*, Vol.125, No6, (Jun 2002), pp.1210-1234, ISSN 0006- 8950

Schiff, N.D.; Rodriguez-Moreno, D.; Kamal, A.; Kim, K.H.S.; Giacino, J.T. et al. fMRI reveals large-scale network activation in minimally conscious patients. *Neurology*, Vol.64, No11, (December 2005), pp. 1843-1843-a, ISSN 0028-3878

Schneider, W.; Noll, D.C. & Cohen, J.D. Functional topographic mapping of the cortical ribbon in human vision with conventional MRI scanners. *Nature*, Vol.365, No6442, (September 1993), pp. 150-152, ISSN 0028-0836

Scholz, J.; Klein, M.C.; Behrens, T.E. & Johansen-Berg H. Training induces changes in white-matter architecture. *Nature Neuroscience*, Vol. 12, No.11, (November 2009), pp. 1370-1371, ISSN 1097-6256

Shutter, L.; Tong, K.A. & Holshouser B.A. Proton MRS in acute traumatic brain injury: Role for glutamate/glutamine and choline for outcome prediction. *Journal of Neurotrauma*, Vol.21, No.12, (December 2004), pp. 1693-1705, ISSN 0897-7151

Shutter, L.; Tong, K.A.; Lee, A. & Holshouser, B.A. Prognostic role of proton magnetic resonance spectroscopy in acute traumatic brain injury. *Journal of Head Trauma Rehabilitation*, Vol.21, No.4, (August 2006), pp. 334-349, ISSN 1550-509X

Signoretti, S.; Marmarou, A.; Aygok, G.A.; Fatouros. P.P.; Portella, G. et al. Assessment of mitochondrial impairment in traumatic brain injury using high-resolution proton magnetic resonance spectroscopy. *Journal of Neurosurgery*, Vol.108, No.1, (January 2008), pp. 42-52, ISSN 0022-3085

Signoretti, S.; Marmarou, A.; Fatouros, P.; Hoyle, R.; Beaumont, A. et al. Application of chemical shift imaging for measurement of NAA in head injured patients. *Acta Neurochirurgica. Supplement*, Vol.81, (2002), pp. 373-375, ISSN 0065-1419

Sinson, G.; Bagley, L.J.; Cecil, K.M.; Torchia, M.; McGowan, J.C. et al. Magnetization transfer imaging and proton MR spectroscopy in the evaluation of axonal injury: Correlation with clinical outcome after traumatic brain injury. *American Journal of Neuroradiology*, Vol.22, No.1, (January 2001), pp. 143-151, ISSN 1936-959X

Steriade, M. Active neocortical processes during quiescent sleep. *Archives Italiennes Biologie*, (September 2001), Vol.139, no. 1/2, pp. 37-51, ISSN 0003-9829

The Multi-Society Task Force on Persistent Vegetative State. Medical aspects of the persistent vegetative state (1). *The New England Journal of Medicine*, Vol. 330 , No. 21 , (May 1994), pp. 1499–508, ISSN 0028-4793

Tollard, E.; Galanaud, D.; Perlbarg, V.; Sanchez-Pena, P.; Le Fur, Y. et al. Experience of diffusion tensor imaging and ¹H spectroscopy for outcome prediction in severe traumatic brain injury: Preliminary results. *Critical Care Medicine*, Vol.37, No.4, (April 2009), pp. 1448-1455, ISSN 1364-8535

Tshibanda, L.; Vanhaudenhuyse, A.; Boly, M.; Soddu, A.; Bruno, M.A. et al. Neuroimaging after coma. *Neuroradiology*, vol. 52, N° 1, (January 2010), pp. 15-24, ISSN 0028-3940

Uzan, M.; Albayram, S.; Dashti, S.G.; Aydin, S.; Hanci, M. et al. Thalamic proton magnetic resonance spectroscopy in vegetative state induced by traumatic brain injury. *Journal of Neurolology, Neurosurgery and Psychiatry*, Vol.74, No.1, (January 2003), pp. 33-38, ISSN 0022-3050

Vanhaudenhuyse, A.; Laureys, S. & Perrin, F. Cognitive Event-Related Potentials in Comatose and Post-comatose States. *Neurocritical Care*, Vol. 8, No. 2, (2008), pp. 262–270, ISSN 1541-6933

Voss, H.U.; Uluc, A.M.; Dyke, J.P.; Watts, R.; Kobylarz, R.J. et al. Possible axonal regrowth in late recovery from the minimally conscious state. *The Journal of Clinical Investigation*, Vol. 116, No. 7, (July 2006), pp. 2005-2011, ISSN 0021-9738

Wilson, F.C.; Harpur, J.; Watson, T. & Morrow, J.I. Vegetative state and minimally responsive patients-regional survey, long-term case outcomes and service recommendations. *Neurorehabilitation*, Vol. 17, No. 3, (January 2002), pp. 231-236, ISSN 1053-8135

Wilson, S.L. & Graham E. Powell, Karen Elliott, and Helen Thwaites .Sensory stimulation in prolonged coma: four single case studies. *Brain Injury*, Vol.5,No.4, (Oct-Dec 1991),pp.393-400,ISSN 0269-9052

Wilson, S.L. & Mc Millan, T.M. A review of the evidence for the effectiveness of sensory stimulation treatment for coma and vegetative states. *Neuropsychological Rehabilitation*, (May 1993) Vol. 3, No 8, pp. 149-160 ISSN 0960-2011

Wood, R.L. Critical analysis of the concept of sensory stimulation for patients in vegetative states. *Brain* Injury, (September 1991), Vol. 5, No. 5, pp. 401-409, ISSN 0006-8950

Xu, J.; Rasmussen, I.A.; Lagopoulos, J. & Håberg, A. Diffuse axonal injury in severe traumatic brain injury visualized using high-resolution diffusion tensor imaging. *Journal of Neurotrauma*, Vol.24, No. 5, (May 2007), pp, 753-765, ISSN 0897-7151

Yamamoto, T.; Katayama, Y.; Kobayashi, K.; Oshima, H.; Fukaya, C. et al. Deep brain stimulation for the treatment of vegetative state. *European Journal of Neuroscience*, Vol. 32, No. 7, (October 2010), pp. 1145-1151, ISSN 1460-9568

Yoon, S.J.; Lee, J.H.; Kim, S.T. & Chun M.H. Evaluation of traumatic brain injured patients in correlation with functional status by localized ^{1}H MR spectroscopy. *Clinical Rehabilitation*, Vol.19, No.2, (February 2005), pp. 209-215, ISSN 1477-0873

10

Functional and Structural MRI Studies on Impulsiveness: Attention-Deficit/Hyperactive Disorder and Borderline Personality Disorders

Trevor Archer[1,*] and Peter Bright[2]
[1]Department of Psychology, University of Gothenburg, Gothenburg
[2]Department of Psychology, Anglia Ruskin University, East Road, Cambridge,
[1]Sweden
[2]UK

1. Introduction

Impulsive behavior is characterized a tendency to initiate behavior without sufficient/adequate consideration of consequences. It typically refers to ill-conceived, premature or inappropriate behavior that may be self-destructive or harmful to other individuals (Chamberlain and Sahakian, 2007). Pathological impulsiveness is associated with impaired performance on neuropsychological tests of attention and executive function and with neuroimaging evidence for structural and/or functional correlates, particular in frontal lobe regions (Congdon and Canli, 2005; Crews and Boettiger, 2009; Rubia et al., 2007). Impulsive behavior is a major component of several neuropsychiatric disorders, including schizophrenia, ADHD, substance abuse, bipolar disorder, and borderline and antisocial personality disorders. The notion of impulsiveness incorporates a multidimensional construct consisting of a range of inter-related factors including novelty-seeking and reckless behavior, lack of planning ability and self-control whereby mechanistic relations evolve from its role in initiating action (Barratt and Patton, 1983; Moeller et al., 2001). The construct incorporates motor impulsiveness, inability to tolerate delays, lack of planning and an incapacity for self-control.

Impulsiveness, with or without aggressiveness, has been associated with a range of personality disorders and other psychopathologies (Haden and Shiva, 2008; Krishnan-Sarin et al., 2007; Palomo et al., 2007a; Reynolds, 2006; Shiva et al., 2009), with impulse control difficulties often of primary diagnostic importance (e.g., Pfefferbaum & Wood, 1994; Quirk and McCormick, 1998). A variety of linear regression analyses based upon several self-report questionnaire studies including a range of cognitive-emotional personal attributes have indicated that impulsiveness is predicted by negative affect, amotivation and depressiveness and counterpredicted by positive affect and internal locus of control in healthy volunteers (Palomo et al., 2008a, b; but see also Miller et al., 2009). Cyders et al. have discussed the influence of positive urgency, acting rashly under extreme positive affect, and negative urgency as central risk factors for impulsive and maladaptive behavior (see also Cyders and Smith, 2008a, b; Cyders et al., 2009, 2010; Zapolsky et al., 2009).

---

* Corresponding Author

The inability to formulate decisions and plan actions presents a critical component of impulsiveness expressed in male offenders classified as both non-psychopathic and psychopathic (Dolan et al., 2001), euthymic and depressed bipolar patients, depressed unipolar patients and healthy controls (Peluso et al., 2007) and male forensic psychiatric in-patients facing severe criminal charges (Haden and Shiva, 2008). In a large-scale study of pathological gamblers, Ma Alvarez-Moya et al. (2010) identified four subtypes: Type I, (disorganized and emotionally unstable) showed schizotypic traits, high levels of impulsiveness, substance and alcohol abuse, and early age of onset, as well as other psychopathological disturbances;Type II (schizoid) showed high harm avoidance, social aloofness, and alcohol abuse; Type III (reward sensitive) showed high levels of sensation-seeking and impulsiveness but did not express psychopathological impairments; Type IV (high functioning)demonstrated a globally-adaptive personality profile, low levels of substance and alcohol abuse or smoking, without psychopathological disturbances but rather good general functioning. Thus, even among a broad population of pathological gamblers there exists a wide spectrum of cognitive and executive variability that requires the pathophysiological analysis of structure and function that magnetic resonance imaging may provide.

Individuals whose behavior is associated with high levels of impulsiveness frequently show general impairments over a wide range of neurocognitive tasks including tests of executive functioning (Dolan and Park, 2002; Keilp et al., 2005; Rogers, 2003), cognitive tasks demanding response control (Harrison et al., 2009; Potter and Newhouse, 2004) and cognitive flexibility [verbal fluency] (Barratt et al., 1997; Vieregge et al., 1997). The control of choice and decision-making processes seems to be modulated primarily by the eventual consequences of affective and cognitive appraisal with reinforcement/avoidance of actions directed by the underlying neural circuits (Beck et al., 2009; Frank and Claus, 2006; Koenigs and Tranel, 2007; Rustichini, 2005). Functional neuroimaging studies have implicated brain regions involved both in reinforcement and response inhibition. For example, financial rewards evoke differential patterns of recruitment in striatal and orbitofrontal cortex, as reflected in fMRI studies (Elliott and Deakin, 2005; Elliott et al., 2003). Other brain regions have been implicated in the different expressions of impulsiveness, including the inferior frontal gyrus, anterior cingulate cortex, regions of the prefrontal cortex (i.e. ventrolateral and dorsolateral), amygdala and the basal ganglia, insula and hippocampus (Love et al., 2009; Lee et al., 2009; Park et al., 2010). Gender effects have also been reported. For example, Lejuez et al. (2007) found that among 152 individuals in a residential substance-use treatment program, female subjects (37% of the sample) expressed greater use of crack/cocaine (current and lifetime heaviest) and were significantly more likely to show crack/cocaine dependence than their male counterparts. The female subjects expressed greater impulsiveness and higher levels of negative emotionality than their male counterparts, and were more likely to have suffered abuse during childhood. Impulsiveness presented a risk factor in the relationship between gender and crack/cocaine dependence and was also predictive of the quantity of drugs consumed and the duration of the dependency. These authors found no gender differences for any other forms of substance abuse (alcohol, cannabis or hallucinogens). Dysfunctional response to reinforcing stimuli, whether appetitive or aversive, appears to be a critical factor in the psychopathy of substance use and impulsiveness-related personality disorders (Petry, 2002).

Research indicates that in selecting among competing available behaviours immediate rewards are typically favoured over delayed rewards, such that with increasing delays the valuation of a future reward is reduced (known as *temporal discounting*; Ainslie, 1975).

Functional and Structural MRI Studies on Impulsiveness: Attention-Deficit/Hyperactive
Disorder and Borderline Personality Disorders

207

Recent functional neuroimaging studies have explored the neural basis of temporal discounting, indicating that different (but overlapping) distributed networks are engaged as a function of the delay between decision and reward. Making choices between payoffs available at different points in time reliably engages a decision-making circuit that includes medial and/or dorsolateral prefrontal cortex (mPFC; dlPFC), posterior cingulate cortex (PCC), and ventral striatum (VS). However, evidence for specific functional roles in the decision making process across this distributed network is limited. Theoretical claims include the possibility that one or more of these regions: (1) is sensitive to the value of rewards discounted by a function of delay ('subjective value'); (2) is differentially sensitive to the availability of an immediate reward; and (3) is implicated in general/nonspecific impulsive and/or planned decision-making. Using event-related fMRI, Ballard and Knutson (2009) showed that although activation of the nucleus accumbens, mesial prefrontal cortex, and posterior cingulate cortex was correlated positively with future reward magnitude, the activation of the dorsolateral prefrontal cortex (DLPFC) and posterior parietal cortical (PCC) region was correlated negatively with future reward delay (see also Sripada et al., 2011). They found individuals expressing greater impulsiveness displayed diminished nucleus accumbens activation to the magnitude of future rewards and greater deactivations to delays of future rewards in the mesial prefrontal cortical, DLPFC, and PCC. Their observations imply that whereas the mesolimbic dopamine projection regions show greater sensitivity to the magnitude of future rewards, lateral cortical regions show greater (negative) sensitivity to the delay of future rewards, potentially reconciling different neural accounts of temporal discounting.

Motor impulsivity occurs when individuals act 'on the spur of the moment', inadequately inhibiting inappropriate response tendencies. Go/No go task performance (a measure of the ability to inhibit a prepotent response tendency) is typically impaired in neuropsychiatric patient groups for whom impulsivity is a common feature (Durston et al., 2003, 2006; Rubia et al., 1999) whereas in healthy controls the relationship between Go/No go performance and impulsiveness is not straightforward (Helmers et al., 1995; Keilp et al., 2005). In children with attention deficit hyperactivity disorder (ADHD), fMRI studies of Go/No go task performance have shown reduced activation in the ventrolateral prefrontal cortex (VLPFC), anterior cingulate cortex, mesial prefrontal cortex and/or caudate region in comparison to age-matched normally developing controls (Casey et al., 1997; Plitzka et al., 2006; Tamm et al., 2004). Activation of the VLPFC (particularly right hemisphere) is linked to response inhibition (Aron et al., 2004). The right VLPFC and DLPFC are implicated in the relationship between response inhibition and impulsivity (Asahi et al., 2004; Horn et al., 2003; Passamonti et al., 2006). Using fMRI, Goya-Maldonado et al. (2010) examined the relationship between trait impulsivity (BIS-11) and brain activation during motor response inhibition in an uncued Go/No go task. They obtained a significant positive correlation between motor impulsivity and bilateral activation of the VLPFC, suggesting that individuals expressing high levels of motor impulsivity show stronger recruitment of the VLPFC in order to maintain task performance. In an fMRI study examining neural activation during a food specific Go/No go task in adolescent girls, Batterink et al. (2010) required subjects to inhibit prepotent responses to appetizing foods. It was found that body mass index correlated with response inhibition at both behavioural and neural levels: greater weight was positively correlated with impulsiveness and negatively correlated with activation in frontal regions associated with inhibitory control (including superior and middle frontal gyrus, VLPFC, mPFC, and orbitofrontal cortex). It should be noted also that bulimia nervosa is associated with response inhibition deficits and higher impulsiveness (BIS-11) scores (Kemps and Wilsdon, 2010).

Comorbid aspects of clinical impulsiveness remain an issue in the pathophysiology of neuropsychiatric disorders (Palomo et al. 2007b). Both ADHD and pediatric bipolar disorder (PBD) are characterized by inattention, impulsiveness, lack of behavioural inhibition and deficits in cognitive flexibility and sustained attention (Galanter and Leibenluft, 2008; Pavuluri et al., 2006), the latter generally associated with emotional dysregulation, elated mood, irritability, increased energy and disinhibition (Pavuluri et al., 2007, 2008; Pavuluri and Passarotti, 2008). Children with PBD were found to show less activation in the VLPFC in a response inhibition stop-signal task (Leibenluft et al., 2007). In a color-naming Stroop task, PBD patients demonstrated elevated activation in the putamen and thalamus compared with healthy controls (Blumberg et al., 2003). A recent fMRI study of response inhibition in PBD patients, ADHD patients and healthy controls implicated (in the context of similarly impaired behavioral performance in both patient groups) a more focal role for VLPFC and anterior cingulate involvement in PBD (as indicated by *reduced* activation in these regions). The inhibitory impairment in ADHD was associated with more extensive prefrontal and temporal involvement. A distributed network of brain regions, within which the prefrontal cortex is of particular importance, is therefore likely to drive observed response inhibition impairments observed both in PBD and ADHD patients.

A central aspect of adaptive, as opposed to maladaptive, risky decision-making requires monitoring the value of behavioural options, possibly mediated through a 'teaching signal' expressed as a reward prediction error (PE) in the striatum. The involvement of higher level cognitive control associated with PFC might be necessary for mobilization of executive processes. Park et al. (2010) employed fMRI and a reinforcement learning task to investigate the neural mechanisms underlying maladaptive behavior in human male alcohol-dependent patients. They observed that in these patients the expression of striatal PEs was intact. Nevertheless, an abnormal functional connectivity between striatum and DLPFC predicted impairments in learning and in the magnitude of alcohol craving shown by the patients. Their findings confirm the structural abnormalities in the DLPFC that are associated with substance abuse. It is evident that frontostriatal connectivity exerts a pivotal role in the adaptive updating of action values and that impaired behavioural regulation in alcoholism may be associated with deficient interactive functionality of this system.

Definitions of impulsiveness vary from considerations of lack of persistence, patience and resistence to delayed rewards, boredom-thresholds, risk-taking behaviors and sensation-seeking behaviors to impaired understanding of the future implications of a given behavior (Barratt, 1994; Buss and Plomin, 1975; Eysenck, 1993; Logue, 1995). The intimate role of faulty timing behavior/time estimation as a non-specific factor in impulsiveness has been established in laboratory settings (cf. Evenden and Ko, 2005; Rivalan et al., 2007), with particular relevance in ADHD (Barkley et al., 1997, 2001; Meaux and Chelonis, 2003; Sonuga-Barke et al., 1992; Toplak et al., 2006). In healthy adults, the frontal cortex, basal ganglia and cerebellum are linked generally to timing functions with long or short delay intervals (Ivry and Spencer, 2004; Meck and Benson, 2002; Wiener et al., 2010). Various aspects of time processing have been addressed in individuals afflicted with ADHD, whether children/adolescents (McInerney and Kerns, 2003; Radonovitch, 2004; Smith et al., 2008) or adults (Gilden and Marusich, 2009; Marx et al., 2019; Seri et al., 2002).

Developmental trajectories of impulsive behavior bear essential outcome-expectancies for eventual disorder pathophysiology (cf. Grall-Bronnec et al., 2010). Valko et al. (2010) studied

Functional and Structural MRI Studies on Impulsiveness: Attention-Deficit/Hyperactive
Disorder and Borderline Personality Disorders

209

the developmental trajectory of the time-processing deficit that has been postulated as a neuropsychological candidate endophenotype for ADHD in 33 children and 22 adults with ADHD. They found that the children and adults displayed different patterns of deficit in the discrimination of brief intervals (600 – 1,500 msecs) in Go/No go and continuous performance tasks and concluded that time-processing deficits, though expressing different age-related forms, were present in adulthood. It is likely that the manifestation of the time-processing deficit in adult ADHDs may be more closely related to the fundamental processes of arousal and/or time perception with a peripheral role of executive function and response inhibition.

Recent research on the role of excessive alcohol consumption in the development of impulsive behaviors indicates that premorbid/baseline levels of impulsivity can predict the likelihood of increased impulsive behaviours following heavy drinking (White at al., 2011). This longitudinal study of boys assessed annually for 10 years until age 18 and again in their mid twenties indicated that a "moderate" (rather than "high" or "low") level of premorbid impulsiveness was the greatest risk factor for eliciting increased impulsive behaviors following heavy drinking. Basal levels of positive affect, a characteristic invariably counter-predictive for impulsiveness, appear related to outcomes of risk perception (drinking, getting into fights) in adolescents and young adults (Haase and Silbereisen, 2010). The notion of disturbed functional connectivity (see above) in frontal-striatal circuits bears consideration. Konrad et al. (2010) observed reduced fractional anisotropy (FA) and elevated mean diffusion bilaterally in orbitomedial prefrontal and right anterior cingulate cortex using voxel-based analyses in adult patients with ADHD compared with healthy controls. Impulsiveness was associated with FA in right orbitofrontal fibre tracts whereas attention was associated with DTI parameters in the right superior longitudinal fasciculus.

Rubia et al. (2009b) have argued that impulsive behavior is distinguished on the basis of a timing disturbance, with suboptimal recruitment of prefrontal, cingulate, striatal and cerebellar regions during temporal processing. They present the case that impulsiveness in ADHD is a dysfunction in temporal processing that may be reversed by acute treatment with a dopamine (DA) reuptake inhibitor. Valera et al. (2010) used fMRI to study paced and unpaced finger-tapping in a sample of 20 unmedicated adult ADHD patients and 19 healthy controls, matched for age, gender and IQ. They found that the ADHD adults expressed greater 'clock' (paced/unpaced tapping variation linked to a central clock rather than motor implementation) rather than motor variability that was consistent with a central timing locus for the atypical movements. Relative to healthy controls, the ADHD patients demonstrated reduced activity in several regions associated with sensorimotor timing, i.e. prefrontal and precentral gyri, basal ganglia, cerebellum, inferior parietal lobule, superior temporal gyri and insula. They concluded that (i) the ADHD abnormalities persisted into adulthood, and (ii) these abnormalities arose from the atypical functioning of corticocerebellar and corticostriatal timing circuits (see also Coull and Nobre, 2008; Smith et al., 2008; Terry et al., 2009).

A plethora of neuropsychological evidence indicates that abnormalities in executive functioning, particularly with regard to behavioural inhibition, are dysfunctional in in ADHD (Barkley, 1997; Chamberlain et al., 2010; Lambek et al., 2011; Mattison and Mayes, 2012). Arendts et al. (2010) have presented evidence of visual cortex abnormalities in adults with ADHD, using voxel-based morphometry of high resolution MRI scans, that may be related to impairments in early-stage, "subexecutive" attentional mechanisms. Accordingly, a neurocognitive model of ADHD presents the disorder as executive dysfunction originating from disturbances in the fronto-dorsal striatal circuit and associated dopaminergic branches (e.g. the mesocortical pathway). Nevertheless, a motivation-based account of altered reward processing, consisting of fronto-ventral striatal reward circuits and those meso-limbic branches that terminate in the ventral striatum and nucleus accumbens, implicates the avoidance of delay due to disturbances in the reward centres (Dalen et al., 2004; Sonuga-Barke, 2002, 2003; Sonuga-Barke et al., 2003). Sonuga-Barke et al. (2008) have argued that while executive dysfunction and delay aversion are implicated in ADHD neither is necessary for ADHD nor specific to the disorder. Several studies focused on the neural basis of individual differences in reward sensitivity have implicated the ventral striatum as a core component of the human reward system (Sescousse et al., 2010).

Adaptive, planned decision-making involves the selection of a particular behavior from several available options on the basis of a valuation of potential costs and benefits. Neuroimaging studies of delay and effort discounting suggest that there may be distinct valuation subsystems involved in the assessment of different types of costs (Prevost et al., 2010). The ventral striatum and the ventromedial prefrontal cortex represent the increasing subjective value of delayed rewards, whereas a distinct network comprised of the anterior cingulate cortex and the anterior insula, represent the decreasing value of an effortful option. Hahn et al. (2010) have shown that dopamine transporter variation (i.e., differences in DA availability affecting synaptic plasticity within the ventral striatum) moderates the association between ventral striatum-reactivity and trait reward sensitivity. In order to analyse further the contribution of reward processes, Carmona et al. (2009) applied a manual region-of-interest approach to assay for ventral striatum volumetric (MRIcro) alterations in 42 ADHD children/adolescents (age range: 6-18 years) compared to 42 healthy controls matched for age, gender and handedness. ADHD children/adolescents displayed marked reductions in both right and left ventro-striatal volume. Furthermore, the volume of the right ventral striatum was correlated negatively with the hyperactivity/impulsivity rating given by the mothers of the ADHD children/adolescents. Reduced volume of the ventral striatum is also associated with cognitive decline in the elderly (de Jong et al., 2012; see also Sripada et al., 2011).

The notion that ADHD symptoms are linked to altered reinforcement sensitivity has gathered momentum (cf. Luman et al., 2010). In an fMRI study comparing neural activity within the striatum in ADHD adolescent individuals and healthy controls, Scheres et al. (2007) observed reduced ventral striatal activation during reward anticipation in the ADHD group. Consistent with other studies, ventral striatal activation was negatively correlated with parent-rated hyperactive/impulsive symptoms across the entire sample. Both frontal-striatal and fronto-cerebellar circuits, necessary for the prediction of occurrence and timing of behaviourally-relevant are also implicated in expectancy violations. For example, Durston et al. (2007) have found fMRI evidence that individuals with ADHD have diminished cerebellar activity in response to violations of stimulus timing and diminished ventral prefrontal and anterior cingulate activity to violations in stimulus timing and identity (relative to healthy age matched controls).

The dysfunctional processing of reward, in combination with a limited capacity to tolerate delay in reward, may offer an important feature of ADHD. Reinforcement Sensitivity Theory, as a conceptual notion, involves three basic brain systems: the Behavioral Approach System and the Behavioral Inhibition System (both of which activate in response to stimulus signalling events), and the fight-fright-freeze system (which responds to actual aversive stimuli; Gray, 1982; Gray and McNaughton, 2000). Gray's impulsivity notion, reflecting trait

Functional and Structural MRI Studies on Impulsiveness: Attention-Deficit/Hyperactive
Disorder and Borderline Personality Disorders

211

reward sensitivity, deals with the extent to which environmental stimuli activate the Behavioral Approach System (Gray, 1991). Higher Behavioral Approach System activation due to increased trait reward sensitivity is implicated in 'disinhibitory' disorders, including ADHD and alcoholism (Franken et al., 2006; Mitchell and Nelson-Gray, 2006; Sher and Trull, 1994). Using fMRI in an appetitive task, Beaver et al. (2006) showed that the tendency to pursue Behavioral Approach System rewards was linked to a fronto-striatal-amygdala-midbrain network activation whereas Barros-Loscertales et al. (2006) describe a negative correlation between dorsal striatum/prefrontal cortex volumes and trait reward sensitivity using voxel-based morphometry. Hahn et al. (2009) studied the relationship, in 20 healthy subjects, between impulsiveness, according to Gray's notions, and event-related fMRI BOLD-response to reward anticipation in brain regions associated with reward processing. Higher trait reward sensitivity was related to cues for potential reward. Thus, the anticipation of reward during a monetary incentive delay task elicited activation in key components of the human reward circuitry, including the ventral striatum, orbitofrontal cortex and amygdala. Plichta et al. (2009) examined brain activation, with fMRI, in 14 adults with ADHD and 12 healthy controls in a task which required choosing between two monetary reward options based on immediate versus delayed reward conditions. For both immediate and delayed rewards, ADHD patients showed hyporesponsiveness of the ventral-striatum reward system compared with healthy controls. In the ADHD individuals, delayed rewards also elicited hyperresponsiveness in the dorsal caudate nucleus and the amygdala: in both structures neural activity correlated significantly with self-rated ADHD symptom severity. The authors concluded that hyperactivation, incremental along the ventral-dorsal caudate nucleus extension and amygdala, substantiates the delay aversion hypothesis. The spectre of temporal discounting (see above), in one form or another, emerges as a plausible mediating factor in the expression, both neural and functional, of impulsiveness in ADHD (see also, Rogers et al., 1999).

Given the cross-national prevalence of 3.4 % for adult ADHD (Fayyad et al., 2007), the potential and current problems associated with the disorder pose a bleak clinical reality. Functional imaging studies of children and adolescents with ADHD have implicated dysfunction of the VLPFC and DLPFC, anterior cingulate, insula, amygdala, hippocampus and ventral striatum (e.g. Amico et al., 2011; Kobel et al., 2010; Rogers et al., 1999; Sasayama et al., 2010; Sheridan et al., 2010); in adult ADHD similar regions are implicated (e.g. Depue et al., 2010a, b; Dillo et al., 2010; Schneider et al., 2010). For example, Schneider et al. (2010) observed (during a continuous performance Go/Nogo test) reduced activity in the caudate nuclei, anterior cingulate cortex and parietal cortical structures in ADHD, together with increased activity in the insular cortex, and that this was associated with the symptoms of impulsiveness and inattention. This widespread regional dysfunction was linked to symptom-profile severity in adults with a history of childhood ADHD, whether or not they qualified for a full ADHD diagnosis in adulthood. Such findings illustrate an important role for MRI in the characterization of neurodevelopmental trajectories (see also, Giedd and Rapoport, 2010; Wilens and Spencer, 2010).

Structural MRI studies indicate broad pathological heterogeneity in ADHD (e.g., Filipek et al., 1997; Mostofsky et al., 2002; Overmeyer et al., 2001; Semrud-Clikeman et al., 2006). Qiu et al. (2009) have published evidence that ADHD in boys may be associated with reduced basal ganglia volumes compared with boys with normal development. Large deformation diffeomorphic metric mapping (LDDMM) indicated that the two groups differed markedly with regard to basal ganglia morphology: bilateral volumetric compression was observed in the caudate head and body and anterior putamen, as well as in the left anterior globus pallidus and right ventral putamen. Coversely, volumetric expansion was observed in the posterior putamen. The authors concluded that the observed deviations from normal brain development involved multiple frontal-subcortical control loops that included circuits with premotor, oculomotor and prefrontal cortex regions. The relevance of developmental trajectories in impulsive disorders was illustrated further by Christakou et al. (2010) who demonstrated that age-related reductions in choice impulsivity were associated with changes in activation in the VLPFC, ACC, ventral striatum, insula, inferior temporal gyrus and posterior parietal cortex. They indicate that the maturational pattern of functional connectivity incorporates activation-coupling between the VLPFC and DLPFC, and the parietal and insular cortices during selection between delayed options, and between the ventromedial PFC and the ventral striatum. Maturational mechanisms within limbic frontostriatal circuitry form the basis of post-pubertal reductions in impulsive choice with age increments linked to activation coherence in networks modulating inter-temporal decision-making (Christakou et al., 2010).

Borderline Personality Disorder (BPD), the most common personality disorder clinically, is characterized by severe and persistent emotional, cognitive, behavioural and interpersonal impairments (American Psychiatry Association, 2000); a pervasive pattern of instability in affect regulation, impulse control, interpersonal relationships, and self-image are linked to the clinical signs of emotional dysregulation, impulsive aggression, repeated self-injury, and chronic suicidal tendencies (Lieb et al., 2004). Some patients are able to sustain a certain level of social and occupational functioning, while others experience a very high level of emotional distress (cf. Jordanova and Rossin, 2010). There is often rapid fluctuation from periods of confidence to despair. Early-life stress exerts damaging effects on brain development (Archer, 2010a, b; Archer et al., 2010b) and neuroimaging studies (e.g. Koenigsberg et al., 2009) have yielded important insight into the role of the hypothalamic-pituitary-adrenal (HPA) axis in BPD (see Wingenfeld et al., 2010 for review).

Patients with BPD have shown volumetric reductions of the hippocampal and (in some cases) amygdala regions in structural MRI studies (Brambilla et al., 2004; Driessen et al., 2000; Schmahl et al., 2003), with or without comorbid aggression or depression (Zetzsche et al., 2006, 2007). Krull et al. (2010) reviewed the multi-dimensional aspect of BPD from phenotypic, genetic, and endophenotypic perspectives. One major feature is the comorbid expression of the disorder with posttraumatic stress disorder which occurs in 50%-70% of patient populations (Zanarini et al., 1998b; Zimmermann and Mattia, 1999) with marked hippocampal volume reductions (Bremner et al., 1997, 2003; Stein et al., 1997; Zlotnick et al., 2003). Both BPD and PTSD share etiologic factors, e. g., trauma, symptom profiles (such as hyperarousal or dissociation states), and neurobiological factors (such as aberrant patterns of neural activation in prefrontal cortex and limbic regions; Schmahl and Bremner, 2006). Amygdala-deactivation has been indicated in BPD patients comorbid for PTSD but not those without PTSD (Kraus et al., 2009). Schmahl et al. (2009) compared a group of BPD with PTSD (n = 10) and a group of BPD without PTSD (n = 15) with 25 healthy female controls applying T1- and T2-weighted MRIs for manual tracing and 3-dimensional reconstruction of the hippocampus and amygdala. They found that the hippocampal volumes of BPD patients with PTSD were lower than those of the healthy female controls concomitant with significant correlations between impulsiveness and hippocampal volumes in these patients. These results and similar observations underlie the necessity of comorbidity considerations in BPD (Bahorik and Eack, 2010; Joshi et al., 2012; Rösch et al., 2010).

BPD and antisocial personality disorders (ASPD) present common characteristics such as high levels of impulsiveness (Becker et al., 2005; Paris, 1997) and marked comorbidity (Chabrol and Leichsenring, 2006; Zanarini et al., 1998). Nevertheless, Völlm et al. (2004) have provided fMRI evidence that ASPD and BPD patients recruit different brain regions when successfully inhibiting pre-potent responses. Employing a Go/No Go task, they found that for healthy controls the main focus of activation during response inhibition was in the prefrontal cortex, in particular the right dorsolateral and the left orbitofrontal cortex. For ASPD and BDP patients, the active regions expressed a more bilateral and extended pattern of activation across the medial, superior and inferior frontal gyri extending to the anterior cingulate cortex. Völlm et al. (2009) studied the effects of positive (financial reward) and negative (financial loss) outcomes on blood-oxygen-level dependence (BOLD) responses in Cluster B (ASPD and BPD) patients (n = 8) and healthy controls (n = 14). They observed that: (i) there was an absence of prefrontal responses and reduced BOLD signal in the subcortical reward system of the patient group but not the control group, and (ii) for the patient group, but not control group, impulsiveness scores were correlated negatively with prefrontal responses during both reward and loss. The authors concluded that the response system to reward/loss in Cluster B was dysfunctional.

One prevailing notion is that emotional instability in BPD stems from an interaction of emotional vulnerability and an invalidating environment mediated hypersensitivity and hyperreactivity to emotional stimuli together with delayed return to baseline arousal level (Linehan, 1993; Linehan et al., 1999; Reeves et al., 2010). Niedtfeld et al. (2010) have found that both negative and neutral picture-presentations can lead to stronger activation of the amygdala, insula, and anterior cingulate cortex in patients with BPD compared with healthy controls. Structurally, a significant 24% reduction of the left orbitofrontal and a 26% reduction of the right anterior cingulate cortex in BPD in comparison to controls has been observed (Tebartz van Elst et al., 2003). Other studies show volumetric reductions of the hippocampus, orbitofrontal cortex and amygdala in BPD (Domes et al., 2009; Lis et al., 2007) and „ enhanced emotional-cue related activation in the amygdala (Donegan et al., 2003; Minzenberg et al., 2007), and middle and inferior temporal regions (Guitart-Masip et al., 2009) known to be involved in the processing of facial features carrying emotional content. Dyck et al. (2009) suggest that a selective deficit of BPD patients in rapid and direct discrimination of negative and neutral emotional expressions may in large part underlie their difficulties in social interactions.

In BPD, fronto-limbic neural dysfunction has been implicated in the expressions of emotional dysregulation and impulsivity. Using structural MRI and impulsiveness instrument, Takahashi et al (2009), examined the insular cortex volume and its relationship to clinical characteristics in a first-presentation teenage BPD sample of 20 BPD (5 male participants) and 20 healthy controls (5 male participants). They found no association between the insular volume and parasuicidal episodes, trauma exposure, or comorbid Axis I disorders; nevertheless, the BPD participants with a history of violent episodes during the previous 6 months showed a smaller insular volume bilaterally compared with those without such episodes. In addition, the right anterior insular volume in the BPD participants correlated negatively with the impulsiveness score. The potential relationship between the insular cortex volume and impulsiveness expression seems specific to BPD. Whittle et al. (2009) investigated anterior cingulate cortex volume in a first-presentation teenage BPD population with minimal exposure to treatment. Fifteen female BPD patients and 15 healthy female control participants underwent MRI scanning. Anterior cingulate cortex volumes were estimated with a method that accounts for inter-individual variation in sulcal morphology with measurements between the two groups compared. ANOVA revealed a decrease in volume of the left anterior cingulate cortex in BPD patients compared with control participants that correlated with parasuicidal behavior and impulsivity. Anterior cingulate cortex volumetric asymmetry correlated also with fear of abandonment symptoms, implying that these volumetric abnormalities early in the course of BPD may relate to the clinical correlates of the disorder. Krause et al. (2010) explored the neural correlates of script-driven imagery of self-injurious behavior in female BPD patients and healthy controls. When imagining the reactions to a situation triggering self-injurious behavior, BPD patients showed significantly less activation in the orbitofrontal cortex but increased activity in the DLPFC. Imagining the self-injurious act itself was associated with a decrease in the mid-cingulate in the patient group. Together, these structural and functional neuroimaging findings suggest that frontal, insular, mid- and anterior cingulate regions and medial temporal lobe structures may be critically involved in the impaired regulation of impulse and affect observed in BPD (e.g., Soloff et al., 2008).

In conclusion, the notions of aberrant reward learning, dysregulated response inhibition and pathological hypersensitivity to temporal delays in reinforcement form the essential behavioural endophenotype of impulsiveness that is witnessed in ADHD and BPD, as well as in compulsive gambling, addictive disorders and dopamine dysregulation syndrome. Developmental trajectories of impulsive behaviors and the damaging effects of early-life trauma on brain development bear essential outcome-expectancies for eventual understanding of etiopathogenesis. Structural and functional resonance imaging has served to provide a point of convergence for the resolution of neurobehavioural, epigenetic and neurodevelopmental factors.

2. References

Ahrendts J, Rüsch N, Wilke M, Philipsen A, Eickhoff SB, Glauche V, Perlov E, Ebert D, Hennig J, Tebartz van Elst L (2010) Visual cortex abnormalities in adults with ADHD: A structural MRI study. *World J Biol Psychiatry* 12, 260-270.

Ainslie, G. (1975). Specious reward: a behavioral theory of impulsiveness and impulse control. *Psychol Bull* 82, 463-496.

American Psychiatry Association (2000) Diagnostic and Statistical Manual of Mental Disorders. 4th Edition, Washington, DC: American Psychiatric Press.

Amico F, Stauber J, Koutsouleris N, Frodl T (2011) Anterior cingulate cortex gray matter abnormalities in adults with attention deficit hyperactivity disorder: A voxel-based morphometry study. *Psychiatry Res: Neuroimaging* 191, 31-35.

Archer T (2010a) Neurodegeneration in schizophrenia. Expert Rev Neurother 10, 1131-1141.

Archer T (2010b) Effects of exogenous agents on brain development: Stress, abuse and therapeutic compounds. *CNS Neurosci Ther* 17, 470-489.

Archer T, Kostrzewa RM, Beninger RJ, Palomo T (2010b) Staging perspectives in neurodevelopmental aspects of neuropsychiatry: agents, phases and ages at expression. *Neurotox Res* 18, 287-305.

Archer T, Beninger RJ, Palomo T and Kostrzewa RM (2010a) Epigenetics and biomarkers in the etiopathogenesis of neuropsychiatric disorders. *Neurotoxicity Res* 18 347-366.

Aron AR, Robbins TW, Poldrack RA (2004) Inhibition and the right inferior frontalcortex. *Tr Cogn Sci* 8 170-177.

Functional and Structural MRI Studies on Impulsiveness: Attention-Deficit/Hyperactive
Disorder and Borderline Personality Disorders

215

Asahi S, Okamoto Y, Okada G, Yamawaki S, Yokota N (2004) Negative correlation between right prefrontal activity during response inhibition and impulsiveness: a fMRI study. *Eur Arch Psychiatr Clin Sci* 254, 245-251.

Bahorik AL, Eack SM (2010) Examining the course and outcome of individuals diagnosed with schizophrenia and comorbid borderline personality disorder. *Schizophr Res* 124, 29-35.

Ballard K, Knutson B (2009) Dissociable neural representations of future reward magnitude and delay during temporal discounting. *Neuroimage* 45 143-150.

Barratt ES, Patton JH (1983) Impulsivity: cognitive, behavioural, and psychophysiological correlates. In: Biological Basis of Sensation-seeking, Impulsivity and Anxiety (Zuckerman M, Ed), LEA: Hillsdale, NJ, pp. 77-116.

Barratt ES, Stanford MS, Kent TA, Felthous A (1997) Neuropsychological and psychophysiological substrates of impulsive aggression. *Biol Psychiatr* 41, 1045-1061.

Barkley RA (1997) Behavioural inhibition, sustained attention, and executive functions: constructing a unified theory of ADHD. *Psychol Bull* 121, 65-94.

Barkley RA, Fischer M (2010) The unique contribution of emotional impulsiveness to impairment in major life activities in hyperactive children as adults. *J Am Acad Child Adolesc Psychiatr* 49, 503-513.

Barkley RA, Koplowitz S, Anderson T, McMurray MB (1997) Sense of time in children with ADHD: effects of duration, distraction and stimulant medication. *J Int Neuropsychol Soc* 3, 359-369.

Barkley RA, Murphy KR, Bush T (2001) Time perception and reproduction in young adults with attention deficit hyperactivity disorder. *Neuropsychology* 15, 351-360.

Barratt ES (1994) Impulsiveness and aggression. In: *Violence and Mental Disorder* (Monahan J, Steadman HJ, eds) Chicago, Il: University of Chicago Press, pp. 61-79.

Barros-Loscertales A, Meseguer V, Sanjuan A, Belloch V, Parcet MA, Torrubia R, Avila C (2006) Striatum grey matter reduction in males with an overactive behavioural activation system. *Eur J Neurosci* 24, 1943-1961.

Batterink L, Yokum S, Stice E (2010) Body mass correlates inversely with inhibitory control in response to food among adolescent girls: an fMRI study. *Neuroimage* 52, 1696-1703.

Beaver JD, Lawrence AD, van Ditzhuizen J, Davis MH, Woods A, Calder AJ (2006) Individual differences in reward drive predict neural response to images of food. *J Neurosci* 26, 5160-5166.

Beck A, Schlagenhauf F, Wüstenberg T, Hein J, Kienast T, Kahnt T, Schmack K, Hägele C, Knutson B, Heinz A, Wrase J (2009) Ventral striatal activation during reward anticipation correlates with impulsivity in alcoholics. *Biol Psychiatr* 66,734-742.

Becker DF, Grilo CM, Anez LM, Paris M, McGlashan TH (2005) Discriminant efficiency of antisocial and borderline personality disorder criteria in Hispanic men with substance abuse disorders. *Comprehen Psychiatr* 46, 140-146.

Bickel WK, Odum AL, Madden GJ (1999) Impulsivity and cigarette smoking: delay discounting in current, never, and ex-smokers. *Psychopharmacology (Berl)* 146, 447-454.

Blakemore SJ (2008) The social brain in adolescence. *Nat Rev Neurosci* 9, 267-277.

Blumberg HP, Martin A, Kaufman J, Leung HC, Skudlarski P, Lacadie C, Fulbright RK, Gore JC, Charney DS, Krystal JH, Peterson BS (2003) Frontostriatal abnormalities in adolescents with bipolar disorder: preliminary observations from functional MRI. *Am J Psychiatr* 160, 1345-1347.

Brambilla P, Soloff PH, Sala M, Nicoletti MA, Keshavan MS, Soares JC (2004) Anatomical MRI study of borderline personality disorder patients. *Psychiatry Res* 131, 125-133.

Bremner JD, Randall P, Vermetten E, Staib L, Bronen RA, Mazure C, Capelli S, McCarthy G, Innis RB, Charney DS (1997) Magnetic resonance imaging-based measurement of hippocampal volume in posttraumatic stress disorder related to childhood physical and sexual abuse--a preliminary report. *Biol Psychiatry* 41, 23-32.

Bremner JD, Vythilingam M, Vermetten E, Southwick SM, McGlashan T, Nazeer A, Khan S, Vaccarino LV, Soufer R, Garg PK, Ng CK, Staib LH, Duncan JS, Charney DS (2003) MRI and PET study of deficits in hippocampal structure and function in women with childhood sexual abuse and posttraumatic stress disorder. *Am J Psychiatry* 160, 924-932.

Buss AH, Plomin R (1975) *A Temperament Theory of Personality Development*. New York, NY: Wiley.

Calvert AL, Green L, Myerson J (2010) Delay discounting of qualitatively different reinforcers in rats. *J Exp Anal Behav* 93, 171-184.

Carmona S, Proal E, Hoekzema EA, Gispert J-D, Picado M, Moreno I, Soliva JC, Bielsa A, Rovira M, Hilferty J, Bulbena A, Casas M, Tobena A, Vilarroya O (2009) Ventro-striatal reductions underpin symptoms of hyperactivity and impulsivity in attention-deficit/hyperactivity disorder. *Biol Psychiatr* 66, 972-977.

Casey BJ, Castellanos FX, Giedd JN, Marsh WL, Hamburger SD, Schubert AB, Vauss YC, Vaituzis AC, Dickstein DP, Sarfatti SE, Rapaport JL (1997) Implication of right frontostriatal circuitry in response inhibition and attention-deficit/hyperactivity disorder. *J Am Acad Child Adolesc Psychiatr* 36, 374-383.

Castellanos FX, Sharp WS, Gottesman RF, Greenstein DK, Giedd JN, Rapoport JL (2003) Anatomic brain abnormalities in monozygotic twins discordant for attention deficit hyperactivity disorder. *Am J Psychiatr* 160, 1693-1696.

Celikel FC, Kose S, Cumurcu BE, Erkorkmaz U, Sayar K, Borckardt JJ, Cloninger CR (2009) Cloninger's temperament and character dimensions of personality in patients with major depressive disorder. *Compr Psychiatry* 50, 556-561.

Chabrol H, Leichsenring F (2006) Borderline personality organization and psychopathic traits in nonclinical adolescents: relationships of identity diffusion, primitive defense mechanisms and reality testing with callousness and impulsivity traits. *Bull Menninger Clin* 70, 160-170.

Chamberlain SR, Sahakian BJ (2007) The neuropsychiatry of impulsivity. *Curr Opin Psychiatr* 20, 255-261.

Chamberlain SR, Robbins TW, Winder-Rhodes S, Müller U, Sahakian BJ, Blackwell AD, Barnett JH (2010) Translational approaches to frontostriatal dysfunction in attention-deficit/hyperactivity disorder using a computerized neuropsychological battery. *Biol Psychiatry* 69, 1192-203.

Christakou A, Brammer M, Rubia K (2010) Maturation of limbic corticostriatal activation and connectivity associated with developmental changes in temporal discounting. *Neuroimage* 54, 1344-1354.

Cloninger CR, Zohar AH (2011) Personality and the perception of health and happiness. *J Affect Disord* 128, 24-32.

Congdon E, Canli T (2005) The endophenotype of impulsivity: reaching consilience through behavioural, genetic, and neuroimaging approaches. *Behav Cogn Neurosci Rev* 4, 262-281.

Coull J, Nobre A (2008) Dissociating explicit timing from temporal expectation with fMRI. *Curr Opinion Neurobiol* 18, 137-144.

Crews FT, Boettiger CA (2009) Impulsivity, frontal lobes and risk for addiction. *Pharmacol Biochem Behav* 93, 237-247.

Cyders MA, Flory K, Rainer S, Smith G (2009) The role of personality dispositions to risky behaviour in predicting first-year college drinking. *Addiction* 104, 193-202.

Cyders MA, Smith GT (2008a) Emotion-based dispositions to rash action: positive and negative urgency. *Psychol Bull* 134, 807-828.

Cyders MA, Smith GT (2008b) Clarifying the role of personality dispositions in risk for increased gambling behaviour. Pers Individ Diff 45, 503-508.

Cyders MA, Smith GT (2009) Longitudinal validation of the urgency traits over the first year of college. *J Pers Assess* 92, 63-9.

Cyders MA, Zapolski TC, Combs JL, Settles RF, Fillmore MT, Smith GT (2010) Experimental effect of positive urgency on negative outcomes from risk taking and on increased alcohol consumption. *Psychol Addict Behav* 24, 367-375.

Dalen L, Sonuga-Barke EJ, Hall M, Remington B (2004) Inhibitory deficits, delay aversion and preschool AD/HD: implications for the dual pathway model. *Neural Plast* 11, 1-11.

de Jong LW, Wang Y, White LR, Yu B, Buchem MA, Launer LJ (2012) Ventral striatal volume is associated with cognitive decline in older people: A population based MR-study. *Neurobiol Aging* 33, 424.e1-10.

de Wit H (2009) Impulsivity as a determinant and consequence of drug use: a review of underlying processes. *Addict Biol* 14, 22-31.

Depue BE, Burgess GC, Bidwell LC, Willcutt EG, Banich MT (2010a) Behavioural performance predicts grey matter reductions in the right inferior frontal gyrus in young adults with combined type ADHD. *Psychiatry Res* 182, 231-237.

Depue BE, Burgess GC, Willcutt EG, Bidwell LC, Ruzic L, Banich MT (2010) Symptom-correlated brain regions in young adults with combined-type ADHD: their organization, variability, and relation to behavioural performance. *Psychiatry Res* 182, 96-102.

Dillo W, Göke A, Prox-Vagedes V, Szycik GR, Roy M, Donnerstag F, Emrich HM, Ohlmeier MD (2010) Neuronal correlates of ADHD in adults with evidence for compensation strategies--a functional MRI study with a Go/No-Go paradigm. *Ger Med Sci* 8, Doc09.

Dolan MC, Deakin JFW, Roberts N, Anderson IM (2002) Serotonergic and cognitive impairment in impulsive aggressive personality disorders offenders: are there implications for treatment? *Psychol Med* 32, 105-117.

Dolan M, Park I (2002) The neuropsychology of antisocial personality disorder. *Psychol Med* 32, 417-27.

Domes G, Schulze L, Herpertz SC (2009) Emotion recognition in borderline personality disorder – a review of the literature. *J Personal Disord* 23, 6-19.

Donegan NH, Sanislow CA, Blumberg HP, Fulbright RK, Lacadie C, Scudlarski P et al (2003) Amygdala hyperreactivity in borderline personality disorder: implications for emotional dysregulation. *Biol Psychiatry* 54, 1284-1293.

Driessen M, Herrmann J, Zwaan M, Meier S, Hill A, Osterheider M, Petersen D (2000) Magnetic resonance imaging volumes of the hippocampus and amygdala in women with borderline personality disorder and early traumatization. *Arch Gen Psychiatr* 57, 1115-1122.

Durston S, Davidson MC, Mulder MJ, Spicer JA, Galvan A, Tottenham N, Scheres A, Xavier Castellanos F, van Engeland H, Casey BJ (2007) Neural and behavioural correlates of expectancy violations in attention-deficit hyperactivity disorder. *J Child Psychol Psychiatry* 48, 881-9.

Durston S, Mulder M, Casey BJ, Ziermans T, van Engeland H (2006) Activation in ventral prefrontal cortex is sensitive to genetic vulnerability for attention deficit hyperactivity disorder. *Biol Psychiatr* 60, 1062-1070.

Durston S, Tottenham NT, Thomas KM, Davidson MC, Eigsti IM, Yang Y, Ulug AM, Casey BJ (2003) Differential patterns of striatal activation in young children with and without ADHD. *Biol Psychiatr* 53, 871-878.

Dyck M, Habel U, Slodczyk J, Schlummer J, Backes V, Schneider F, Reske M (2009) Negative bias in fast emotion discrimination in borderline personality disorder. *Psychol Med* 39, 855-864.

Elliott R, Deakin B (2005) Role of the orbitofrontal cortex in reinforcement processing and inhibitory control: evidence from functional magnetic resonance imaging studies in healthy human subjects. *Int Rev Neurobiol* 65, 89-116.

Elliott R, Newman JL, Longe OA, Deakin JF (2003) Differential response patterns in the striatum and orbitofrontal cortex to financial reward in humans: a parametric functional magnetic resonance imaging study. *J Neurosci* 23, 303-307.

Estle SJ, Green L, Myerson J, Holt DD (2006) Differential effects of amount on temporal and probability discounting of gains and losses. *Mem Cognit* 34, 914-28.

Evenden J, Ko T (2005) The psychopharmacology of impulsive behaviour in rats VIII: effects of amphetamine, methylphenidate, and other drugs on responding maintained by a fixed consecutive number avoidance schedule. *Psychopharmacology* 180, 294-305.

Eysenck SGB (1993) The nature of Impulsivity. In: *The Impulsive Client: Theory, Research and Treatment* (McCown WG, Johnson AL, Shure MB, eds) Washington, DC: American Psychological Association.

Fayyad J, De Graaf R, Alonso J, Angermeyer M, Demyttenaere K, De Girolamo G, Haro JM, Karam EG, Lara C, Lépine JP, Ormel J, Posada-Villa J, Zaslavsky AM (2007). Cross-national prevalence and correlates of adult attention-deficit hyperactivity disorder. *Brit J Psychi* 190, 402-409.

Filipek PA, Semrud-Clikeman M, Steingard RJ, Renshaw PF, Kennedy DN, Biederman J (1997) Volumetric MRI analysis comparing subjects having attention-deficit hyperactivity disorder with normal controls. *Neurology* 48, 589-601.

Frank MJ, Claus ED (2006) Anatomy of a decision: striato-orbitofrontal interactions in reinforcement learning, decision making and reward. Psychol Rev 113, 300-326.

Franken IH, Muris P, Georgieva I (2006) Gray's model of personality and addiction. *Addict Behav* 31, 399-403.

Galenter CA and Leibenluft E (2008) Frontiers between attention deficit hyperactivity disorder and bipolar disorder. *Child Adolesc Psychiatr Clin N Am* 17, 325- 346.

Giedd JN, Rapoport JL (2010) Structural MRI of pediatric brain development: what have we learned and where are we going? *Neuron* 67, 728-734.

Gilden DL, Marusich LR (2009) Contraction of time in attention-deficit hyperactivity disorder. *Neuropsychology* 23, 265-269.

Goya-Maldonado R, Walther S, Simon J, Stippich C, Weisbrod M, Kaiser S (2010) Motor impulsivity and the ventrolateral prefrontal cortex. *Psychiatr Res Neuroimaging* 183, 89-91.

Grall-Bronnec M, Bouju G, Landréat-Guillou M, Vénisse JL (2010) [Socio-demographic and clinical assessment, and trajectory of a sample of French pathological gamblers.] *Encephale* 36, 452-460.

Gray JA (1982) *The Neuropsychology of Anxiety: An Enquiry into the Functions of the Septo-hippocampal system*. Oxford University Press, Oxford.

Gray JA (1991) The neuropsychology of temperament. In: Strelau J, Angleitner A (eds.), *Explorations in Temperament*. Plenum Press, New York, pp. 105-128.

Gray JA, McNaughton N (2000) *The Neuropsychology of Anxiety: An Enquiry into the Functions of the Septo-hippocampal system*. 2nd Edition, Oxford University Press, Oxford.

Green L, Myerson J (2004) A discounting framework for choice with delayed and probabilistic rewards. *Psychol Bull* 130, 769-792.

Guitart-Masip M, Pascual JC, Carmona S, Hoekzema E, Bergé D, Pérez V, Soler J, Soliva JC, Rovira M, Bulbena A, Vilarroya O (2009) Neural correlates of impaired emotional discrimination in borderline personality disorder: an fMRI study. *Prog Neuropsychopharmacol Biol Psychiatry* 33, 1537-1345.

Ha RY, Namkoong K, Kang JI, Kim YT, Kim SJ (2010) Interaction between serotonin transporter promoter and dopamine receptor D4 polymorphisms on decision making. *Prog Neuropsychopharmacol Biol Psychiatry* 33, 1217-1222.

Haase CM, Silbereisen RK (2010) Effects of positive affect on risk perceptions in adolescence and young adulthood. *J Adolesc* 34, 29-37.

Haden SC, Shiva A (2008) Trait impulsivity in a forensic inpatient sample: an evaluation of the Barratt impulsiveness scale. *Behav Sci Law* 26, 675-690.

Hahn T, Dresler T, Ehlis A-C, Plichta MM, Heinzel S, Polak T, Lesch K-P, Breuer F, Jakob PM, Fallgatter AJ (2009) Neuralresponse to reward anticipation is modulated by Gray's impulsivity. *Neuroimage* 46, 1148-1153.

Hahn T, Heinzel S, Dresler T, Plichta MM, Renner TJ, Markulin F, Jakob PM, Lesch KP, Fallgatter AJ (2010) Association between reward-related activation in the ventral striatum and trait reward sensitivity is moderated by dopamine transporter genotype. *Hum Brain Mapp* 32, 1557-65.

Halperin JM, Schulz KP (2006) Revisiting the role of prefrontal cortex in the pathophysiology of attention-deficit/hyperactivity disorder. *Psychol Bull* 132, 560-581.

Harrison EL, Coppola S, McKee SA (2009) Nicotine deprivation and trait impulsivity affect smokers' performance on cognitive tasks of inhibition and attention. *Exp Clin Psychopharmacol* 17, 91-98.

Helmers KF, Young SN, Pihl RO (1995) Assessment of measures of impulsivity in healthy male volunteers. *Pers Individ Diff* 19, 927-935.

Hooley JM, Gruber SA, Parker HA, Guillaumot J, Rogowska J, Yurgelun-Todd DA (2010) Neural processing of emotional overinvolvement in borderline personality disorder. *J Clin Psychiatry* 71, 1017-1024.

Horn NR, Dolan M, Elliott R, Deakin JF, Woodruff PW (2003) Response inhibition and impulsivity: an fMRI study. *Neuropsychologia* 41, 1959-1966.

Ivry RB, Spencer RM (2004) The neural representation of time. *Curr Opin Neurobiol* 14, 225-232.

Jordanova V, Rossin P. (2010). Borderline personality disorder often goes undetected. *Practitioner* 254(1729), 23-6.

Joshi G, Biederman J, Wozniak J, Doyle R, Hammerness P, Galdo M, Sullivan N, Williams C, Brethel K, Woodworth KY, Mick E (2012) Response to Second Generation Antipsychotics in Youth with Comorbid Bipolar Disorder and Autism Spectrum Disorder. *CNS Neurosci Ther* 18, 28-33.

Kalia M (2008) Brain development: anatomy, connectivity, adaptive plasticity, and toxicity. *Metabolism* 57 [Suppl 2], S2-S5.

Keilp JG, Sackeim HA, Mann JJ (2005) Correlates of trait impulsiveness in performance measures and neuropsychological tests. *Psychiatr Res* 135, 191-201.

Kemps E, Wilsdon A (2010) Preliminary evidence for a role for impulsivity in cognitive disinhibition in bulimia nervosa. *J Clin Exp Neuropsychol* 32, 515-521.

Kobel M, Bechtel N, Specht K, Klarhöfer M, Weber P, Scheffler K, Opwis K, Penner IK (2010) Structural and functional imaging approaches in attention deficit/hyperactivity disorder: does the temporal lobe play a key role? *Psychiatry Res* 183, 230-236.

Koenigs M, Tranel D (2007) Irrational economic decision-making after ventromedial prefrontal damge: evidence from the Ultimate game. *J Neurosci* 27, 951-956.

Koenigsberg HW, Fan J, Ochsner KN, Liu X, Guise KG, Pizzarello S, Dorantes C, Guerreri S, Tecuta L, Goodman M, New A, Siever LJ (2009) Neural correlates of the use of psychological distancing to regulate responses to negative social cues: a study of patients with borderline personality disorder. *Biol Psychiatry* 66, 854-863.

Konrad A, Dielentheis TF, El Masri D, Bayerl M, Fehr C, Gesierich T, Vucurevic G, Stoeter P, Winterer G (2010) Disturbed structural connectivity is related to inattention and impulsivity in adult attention deficit hyperactivity disorder. *Eur J Neurosci* 31, 912-919.

Kraus A, Esposito F, Seifritz E, Di Salle F, Ruf M, Valerius G, Ludaescher P, Bohus M, Schmahl C (2009) Amygdala deactivation as a neural correlate of pain processing in patients with borderline personality disorder and co-occurrent posttraumatic stress disorder. *Biol Psychiatry* 65, 819-822.

Kraus A, Valerius G, Seifritz E, Ruf M, Bremner JD, Bohus M, Schmahl C (2010) Script-driven imagery of self-injurious behavior in patients with borderline personality disorder: a pilot fMRI study. *Acta Psychiatrica Scandinavica* 121, 41-51

Krishnan-Sarin S, Reynolds B, Duhig AM, Smith A, Liss T, McFetridge A, Cavallo DA, Carroll KM, Potenza MN (2007) Behavioural impulsivity predicts treatment outcome in a smoking cessation program for adolescent smokers. *Drug Alcohol Depend* 88, 79-82.

Kurian JR, Bychowski ME, Forbes-Lorman RM, Auger CJ and Auger AP (2008) Mecp2 organizes juvenile social behaviour in a sex-specific manner. *J Neurosci* 28, 7137-7142.

Kwok SL, Shek DT (2010) Cognitive, emotive, and cognitive-behavioural correlates of suicidal ideation among Chinese adolescents in Hong Kong. *ScientificWorld Journal* 5, 366-379.

Lach LM, Kohen DE, Garner RE, Brehaut JC, Miller AR, Klassen AF and Rosenbaum PL (2009) The health and psychosocial functioning of caregivers of children with neurodevelopmental disorders. *Disabil Rehabil* 31, 741-752.

Lambek R, Tannock R, Dalsgaard S, Trillingsgaard A, Damm D, Thomsen PH (2011) Executive Dysfunction in School-Age Children With ADHD. *J Atten Disord* 15, 646-655.

Functional and Structural MRI Studies on Impulsiveness: Attention-Deficit/Hyperactive
Disorder and Borderline Personality Disorders

221

Lee TMY, Guo L, Shi H, Li Y, Luo Y, Sung CYY, Chan CCH, Lee TMC (2009) Neural correlates of Traditional Chinese Medicine induced advantageous risk-taking decision-making. *Brain Cogn* 71, 354-361.

Leibenluft E, Rich BA, Vinton DE, Nelson EE, Fromm SJ, Berghorst LH, Joshi P, Robb A, Schachar RJ, Dickstein DP, McClure EB, Pine DS (2007) Neural circuitry engaged during unsuccessful motor inhibition in pediatric bipolar disorder. *Am J Psychiatr* 164, 52-60.

Lejuez CW, Bornovalova MA, Reynolds EK, Daughters SB, Curtin JJ (2007) Risk factors in the relationship between gender and crack/cocaine. *Exp Clin Psychopharmacol* 15, 165-175.

Lieb K, Zanarini MC, Schmahl C, Linehan MM, Bohus M (2004) Borderline personality disorder. *Lancet* 364, 453-461.

Linehan MM, Schmidt H 3rd, Dimeff LA, Craft JC, Kanter J, Comtois KA (1999) Dialectical behaviour therapy for patients with borderline personality disorder and drug-dependence. *Am J Addict* 8, 279-292.

Logue AW (1975) *Self-control*. Englewood Cliffs, NJ: Prentice-Hall.

Love TM, Stohler CS, Zubieta JK (2009) Positron emission tomography measures of endogenous opioid neurotransmissions and impulsiveness traits in humans. *Arch Gen Psychiatr* 66, 1124-1134.

Luman M, Tripp G, Scheres A (2010) Identifying the neurobiology of altered reinforcement sensitivity in ADHD: a review and research agenda. *Neurosci Biobehav Rev* 34, 744-754.

Luna B, Sweeney JA (2004) The emergence of collaborative brain function: fMRI studies of the development of response inhibition. *Ann NY Acad Sci* 1021, 296-309.

Ma Alvarez-Moya E, Jiménez-Murcia S, Aymamí MN, Gómez-Peña M, Granero R, Santamaría J, Menchón JM, Fernández-Aranda F (2010) Subtyping study of a pathological gamblers sample. *Can J Psychiatry* 55, 498-506.

Makris N, Biederman J, Valera EM, Bush G, Kaiser J, Kennedy DN, Caviness VS, Faraone SV, Seidman LJ (2007) Cortical thinning of the attention and executive function networks in adults with attention-deficit/hyperactivity disorder. *Cereb Cortex* 17, 1364-1375.

Martinotti G, Mandelli L, Di Nicola M, Serretti A, Fossati A, Borroni S, Cloninger CR, Janiri L (2008) Psychometric characteristic of the Italian version of the Temperament and Character Inventory--revised, personality, psychopathology, and attachment styles. *Compr Psychiatry* 49, 514-522.

Mattison RE, Mayes SD (2012) Relationships between learning disability, executive function, and psychopathology in children with ADHD. *J Atten Disord* 16, 138-146.

Marx I, Hübner T, Herpertz SC, Berger C, Reuter E, Kircher T, Herpertz-Dahlmann B, Konrad K (2010) Cross-sectional evaluation of cognitive functioning in children, adolescents and young adults with ADHD. *J Neural Transm* 117, 403-419.

McInerney RJ, Kerns KA (2003) Time reproduction in children with ADHD: motivation matters. *Child Neuropsychol* 9, 91-108.

Meaux JB, Chelonis JJ (2003) Time perception differences in children with and without ADHD. *J Pediatr Health Care* 17, 64-71.

Meck WH, Benson AM (2002) Dissecting the brain's internal clock: How frontal-striatal circuitry keeps time and shifts attention. *Brain Cogn* 48, 195-211.

Miller DJ, Vachon DD, Lynam DR (2009) Neuroticism, Negative Affect, and Negative Affect
    Instability: Establishing Convergent and Discriminant Validity Using Ecological
    Momentary Assessment. *Pers Individ Diff* 47, 873-877.
Mitchell JT, Nelson-Gray RO (2006) Attention-deficit/hyperactivity disorder symptoms in
    adults: relationship to Gray's behavioural approach system. *Pers Individ Differ* 40,
    749-760.
Moeller FG, Barratt ES, Dougherty DM, Schmitz JM, Swann AC (2001) Psychiatric aspects of
    impulsivity. *Am J Psychiatry* 158, 1783-1793.
Mostofsky SH, Cooper KL, Kates WR, Denckla MB, Kaufmann WE (2002) Smaller prefrontal
    and premotor volumes in boys with ADHD. *Biol Psychiatr* 52, 785-794.
Niedtfeld I, Schulze L, Kirsch P, Herpertz SC, Bohus M, Schmahl C (2010) Affect regulation
    and pain in borderline personality disorder: a possible link to the understanding of
    self-injury. *Biol Psychiatry* 68, 383-391.
Overmeyer S, Bullmore ET, Suckling J, Simmons A, Williams SC, Santosh PJ, Taylor E (2001)
    Distributed grey and white matter deficits in hyperkinetic disorder: MRI evidence
    for anatomical abnormality in an attentional network. *Psychol Med* 31, 1425-1435.
Palijan TZ, Radeljak S, Kovac M, Kovacević D (2010) Relationship between comorbidity and
    violence risk assessment in forensic psychiatry - the implication of neuroimaging
    studies. *Psychiatr Danub* 22, 253-256.
Palomo T, Beninger RJ, Kostrzewa RM, Archer T (2007a) Treatment consideration and manifest
    complexity in comorbid neuropsychiatric disorders. *Neurotoxicity Res* 12, 43-60.
Palomo T, Beninger RJ, Kostrzewa RM, Archer T (2007b) Comorbidity implications in brain
    disease: neuronal substrates of symptom profiles. *Neurotox Res* 12, 1-15.
Palomo T, Beninger RJ, Kostrzewa RM, Archer T (2008a) Focusing on symptoms rather than
    diagnoses in brain dysfunction: conscious and nonconscious expression in
    impulsiveness and decision-making. *Neurotoxicity Res* 14, 1-20.
Palomo T, Beninger RJ, Kostrzewa RM, Archer T (2008b) Affective status in relation to
    impulsive, motor and motivational symptoms: personality, development and
    physical exercise. *Neurotoxicity Res* 14, 151-168.
Paris J (1997) Antisocial and borderline personality disorders: two separate diagnoses or two
    aspects of the same psychopathology? *Comprehen Psychiatr* 38, 237-242.
Park HS, Kim SH, Bang SA, Yoon EJ, Cho SS, Kim SE (2010) Altered regional cerebral
    glucose metabolism in internet game overusers: a 18F-fluorodeoxyglucose positron
    emission tomography study. *CNS Spectr* 15, 159-166.
Park SQ, Kahnt T, Beck A, Cohen MX, Dolan RJ, Wrase J, Heinz A (2010) Prefrontal cortex
    fails to learn from reward prediction errors in alcohol dependence. *J Neurosci* 30,
    7749-7753.
Passamonti I, Fera F, Magariello A, Cerasa A, Gioia MC, Muglia M, Nicoletti G, Gallo O,
    Provincialli L, Quattrone A (2006) Monoamine oxidase-A genetic variations
    influence brain activity associated with inhibitory control: new insight into the
    neural correlates of impulsivity. *Biol Psychiatr* 59, 334-340.
Passarotti AM, Sweeney JA, Pavuluri MN (2010) Neural correlates of response inhibition in
    pediatric bipolar disorder and attention deficit hyperactivity disorder. *Psychiatr Res
    Neuroimaging* 181, 36-43.
Paus T, Keshavan M, Giedd JN (2008) Why do many psychiatric disorders emerge during
    adolescence? *Nat Rev Neurosci* 9, 947-957.

Pavuluri MN, Passarotti AM (2008) Neural bases of emotional processing in pediatric bipolar disorder. *Expert Rev Neurotherap* 8, 1381-1387.

Pavuluri MN, Shenkel LS, Aryal S, Harral E, Hill K, Herbener ES, Sweeney JA (2006) Neurocognitive function in unmedicated manic and medicated euthymic pediatric bipolar patients. *Am J Psychiatr* 163, 286-293.

Pavuluri MN, O'Connor MM, Harral EM, Sweeney JA (2007) Affective neural circuitry during facial emotion processing in pediatric bipolar disorder. *Biol Psychiatr* 62, 158-167.

Pavuluri MN, O'Connor MM, Harral EM, Sweeney JA (2008) An fMRI study of the interface between affective and cognitive neural circuitry in pediatric bipolar disorder. *Psychiatr Res* 162, 244-245.

Peluso MA, Hatch JP, Glahn DC, Monkul ES, Sanches M, Najt P, Bowden CL, Barratt ES, Soares JC (2007) Trait impulsivity in patients with mood disorders. *J Affect Disord* 100, 227-231.

Petry NM (2002) Discounting of delayed rewards in substance abusers: relationship to antisocial personality disorder. *Psychopharmacology* 162, 425-432.

Pfefferbaum B, Wood PB (1994) Self-report study of impulsive and delinquent behaviour in college students. *J Adolesc Health* 15, 295-302.

Pierò A (2010) Personality correlates of impulsivity in subjects with generalized anxiety disorders. *Compr Psychiatry* 51, 538-545.

Pine A, Shiner T, Seymour B, Dolan RJ (2010) Dopamine, time, and impulsivity in humans. *J Neurosci* 30, 8888-8896.

Plichta MM, Vasic N, Wolf RC, Lesch KP, Brummer D, Jacob C, Fallgatter AJ, Grön G (2009) Neural hyporesponsiveness and hyperresponsiveness during immediate and delayed reward processing in adult attention-deficit/hyperactivity disorder. *Biol Psychiatr* 65, 7-14.

Plitzka SR, Glahn DC, Semrud-Clikeman M, Franklin C, Perez R, Xiong J, Liotti M (2006) Neuroimaging of inhibitory control areas in children with attention deficit hyperactivity disorder who were treatment naïve or in long-term treatment. *Am J Psychiatr* 163, 1052-1060.

Potter AS, Newhouse PA (2004) Effects of acute nicotine administration on behavioural inhibition in adolescents with attention-deficit/hyperactivity disorder. *Psychopharmacology* 176, 182-194.

Powell J, Dawkins L, West R, Powell J, Pickering A (2010) Relapse to smoking during unaided cessation: clinical, cognitive and motivational predictors. *Psychopharmacology* 212, 537-549.

Prévost C, Pessiglione M, Météreau E, Cléry-Melin ML, Dreher JC (2010) Separate valuation subsystems for delay and effort decision costs. *J Neurosci* 30, 14080-14090.

Qiu A, Crocetti D, Adler M, Mahone EM, Denckla MB, Miller MI, Mostofsky SH (2009) Basal ganglia volume and shape in children with attention deficit hyperactivity disorder. *Am J Psychiatr* 166, 74-82.

Quirk SW, McCormick RA (1998) Personality subtypes, coping styles, symptom correlates, and substances of choice among a cohort of substance abusers. *Assessment* 5, 157-169.

Radonovich KJ, Mostofsky SH (2004) Duration judgements in children with ADHD suggest deficit utilization of temporal information rather than general impairment in timing. *Child Neuropsychol* 10, 162-172.

Raine A, Dodge K, Loeber R, Gatzke-Kopp L, Lynam D, Reynolds C, Stouthamer-Loeber M, Liu J (2006) The Reactive-Proactive Aggression Questionnaire: Differential Correlates of Reactive and Proactive Aggression in Adolescent Boys. *Aggress Behav* 32, 159-171.

Reynolds B (2006) A review of delay-discounting research with humans: relations to drug use and gambling. *Behav Pharmacol* 17, 651-667.

Reynolds WM, Stark KD (1986) Self-control in children: a multimethod examination of treatment outcome measures. *J Abnorm Child Psychol* 14, 13-23.

Rivalan M, Gregoire S, dellu-Hagedorn F (2007) Reduction of impulsivity with amphetamine in an appetitive fixed consecutive number schedule with cue for optimal performance in rats. *Psychopharmacology* 192, 171-182.

Rogers RD (2003) Neuropsychological investigations of the impulsive personality disorders. *Psychol Med* 33, 1335-1340.

Rogers RD, Owen AM, Middleton HC, Williams EJ, Pickard JD,Sahakian BJ, Robbins TW (1999) Choosing between small, likely rewards and large, unlikely rewards activates inferior and orbital prefrontal cortex. *J Neurosci* 19, 9029-9038.

Rubia K (2002) The dynamic approach to developmental psychiatric disorders: use of fMRI combined with neuropsychology to elucidate the dynamics of psychiatricdisorders, exemplified in ADHD and Schizophrenia. *Behav Brain Res* 130, 47-56.

Rubia K, Smith AB, Oksannan H, Fumie MM, Taylor E, Brammer MJ (2009a) Disorder-specific dissociation of orbitofrontal dysfunction in boys with pure conduct disorder during reward and ventrolateral prefrontal dysfunction in boys with pure ADHD during sustained attention. *Am J Psychiatr* 166, 83-94.

Rubia K, Halari R, Christakou A, Taylor E (2009b) Impulsiveness as a timing disturbance: neurocognitive abnormalities in attention-deficit hyperactivity disorder during temporal processes and normalization with methylphenidate. *Phil Transac R Soc* 364, 1919-1931.

Rubia K, Overmeyer S, Taylor E, Brammer M, Williams SC, Simmons A, Andrews C, Bullmore ET (1999) Hypofrontality in attention deficit hyperactivity disorder during higher-order motor control: a study with functional MRI. *Am J Psychiatr* 156, 891-896.

Rubia K, Smith AB, Taylor E, Brammer MJ (2007) Linear age-correlated functional development of right inferior fronto-striato-cerebellar networks during response inhibition and anterior cingulate during error-related processes. *Hum Brain Mapp* 28, 1163-1177.

Rubia K, Taylor E, Smith H, OksannenH, Overmeyer S, Newman S (2001) Neuropsychological analyses of impulsiveness in childhood hyperactivity. *Br J Psychiatr* 179, 138-143.

Rubia K, Smith A (2004) The neural correlates of cognitive time managament. *Acta Neurobiol Exp* 64, 329-340.

Ruchsow M, Groen G, Kiefer M, Hermle L, Spitzer M, Falkenstein M (2008) Impulsiveness and ERP components in a Go/No go task. *J Neural Transm* 115, 909-915.

Rüsch N, Schulz D, Valerius G, Steil R, Bohus M, Schmahl C (2011) Disgust and implicit self-concept in women with borderline personality disorder and posttraumatic stress disorder. *Eur Arch Psychiatry Clin Neurosci* 261, 369-376.

Rustichini A (2005) Emotion and reasoning in making decisions. *Science* 310, 1624-1625.

Functional and Structural MRI Studies on Impulsiveness: Attention-Deficit/Hyperactive
Disorder and Borderline Personality Disorders

225

Sasayama D, Hayashida A, Yamasue H, Harada Y, Kaneko T, Kasai K, Washizuka S, Amano
    N (2010) Neuroanatomical correlates of attention-deficit-hyperactivity disorder
    accounting for comorbid oppositional defiant disorder and conduct disorder.
    Psychiatry Clin Neurosci 64, 394-402.
Scahill L (2009) Alpha-2 adrenergic agonists in children with inattention, hyperactivity and
    impulsiveness. *CNS Drugs* 23 Suppl 1, 43-49.
Scheres A, Hamaker EL (2010) What we can and cannot conclude about the relationship
    between steep temporal reward discounting and hyperactivity-impulsivity
    symptoms in attention-deficit/hyperactivity disorder. *Biol Psychiatry* 68, 17-18.
Scheres A, Dijkstra M, Ainslie E, Balkan J, Reynolds B, Sonuga-Barke E, Castellanos FX
    (2006) Temporal and probabilistic discounting of rewards in children and
    adolescents: effects of age and ADHD symptoms. *Neuropsychologia* 44, 2092-2103.
Scheres A, Lee A, Sumiya M (2008) Temporal reward discounting and ADHD: task and
    symptom specific effects. *J Neural Transm* 115, 221-226.
Scheres A, Milham MP, Knutson B, Castellanos FX (2007) Ventral striatal
    hyporesponsiveness during reward anticipation in attention-deficit/hyperactivity
    disorder. *Biol Psychiatry* 61, 720-724.
Scheres A, Sumiya M, Thoeny AL (2010) Studying the relation between temporal reward
    discounting tasks used in populations with ADHD: a factor analysis. *Int J Methods
    Psychiatr Res* 19, 167-176.
Scheres A, Tontsch C, Thoeny AL, Kaczkurkin A (2010) Temporal reward discounting in
    attention-deficit/hyperactivity disorder: the contribution of symptom domains,
    reward magnitude, and session length. *Biol Psychiatry* 67, 641-648.
Schmahl C, Berne K, Krause A, Kleindienst N, Valerius G, Vermetten E, Bohus M (2009)
    Hippocampus and amygdala volumes in patients with borderline personality disorder
    with or without posttraumatic stress disorder. *J Psychiatr Neurosci* 34, 289-295.
Schmahl C, Bremner JD (2006) Neuroimaging in borderline personality disorder. *J Psychiatr
    Res* 40, 419-427.
Schmahl C, Vermetten E, Elzinga BM, Bremner BJ (2003) Magnetic resonance imaging of
    hippocampal and amygdala volume in women with childhood abuse and
    borderline personality disorder. *Psychiatr Res* 122, 193-198.
Schneider MF, Krick CM, Retz W, Hengesch G, Retz-Junginger P, Reith W, Rösler M (2010)
    Impairment of fronto-striatal and parietal cerebral networks correlates with
    attention deficit hyperactivity disorder (ADHD) psychopathology in adults - a
    functional magnetic resonance imaging (fMRI) study. *Psychiatry Res* 183, 75-84.
Schumann G, Loth E, Banaschewski T, Barbot A, Barker G, Büchel C, Conrod PJ, Dalley JW,
    Flor H, et al (2010) The IMAGEN study: reinforcement-related behaviour in normal
    brain function and psychopathology. *Molec Psychiatr* 15, 1128-1139.
Semrud-Clikeman M, Pliszka SR, Lancaster J, Liotti M (2006) Volumetric MRI differences in
    treatment-naïve vschronically treated children with ADHD. *Neurology* 67, 1023-1027.
Seri Y, Kofman O, Shay L (2002) Time estimation could be impaired in male, but not female
    adults with attention deficits. *Brain Cogn* 48, 553-558.
Sescousse G, Redouté J, Dreher JC (2010) The architecture of reward value coding in the
    human orbitofrontal cortex. *J Neurosci* 30, 13095-13104.
Sher KJ, Trull TJ (1994) Personality and disinhibitory psychopathology: alcoholism and
    antisocial personality disorder. *J Abnormal Psychol* 103, 92-102.

Sheridan MA, Hinshaw S, D'Esposito M (2010) Stimulant medication and prefrontal functional connectivity during working memory in ADHD: a preliminary report. *J Atten Disord* 14, 69-78.

Shiva A, Haden SC, Brooks J (2009a) Forensic and civil psychiatric inpatients: development of the inpatient satisfaction questionnaire. *J Am Acad Psychiatry Law* 37, 201-213.

Shiva A, Haden SC, Brooks J (2009b) Psychiatric civil and forensic inpatient satisfaction with care: the impact of provider and recipient characteristics. *Soc Psychiatry Psychiatr Epidemiol* 44, 979-987.

Smith AB, Taylor E, Brammer M, Halari R, Rubia K (2008) Reduced activation in right lateral prefrontal cortex and anterior cingulate gyrus in medication-naïve adolescents with attention deficit hyperactivity disorder during time discrimination. *J Child Psychol Psychiatr* 48, 881-889.

Soloff P, Nutche J, Goradia D, Diwadkar V (2008) Structural brain abnormalities in borderline personality disorder: a voxel-based morphometry study. *Psychiatry Res* 164, 223-236.

Sonuga-Barke EJ (2002) Psychological heterogeneity in AD/HD – a dual pathway model of behaviour and cognition. *Behav Brain Res* 130, 29-36.

Sonuga-Barke EJ (2003) The dual pathway model of AD/HD: an elaboration of neuro-developmental characteristics. *Neurosci Biobehav Rev* 27, 593-604.

Sonuga-Barke EJ, Dalen L, Remington B (2003) Do executive deficits and delay aversion make independent contributions to preschool attention-deficit/hyperactivity disorder symptoms? *J Am Acad Child Adolesc Psychiatry* 42, 1335-1342.

Sonuga-Barke EJ, Taylor E, Sembi S, Smith J (1992) Hyperactivity and delay aversion – I. *J Child Psychol Psychiatr* 33, 387-398.

Sripada CS, Gonzalez R, Luan Phan K, Liberzon I (2011) The neural correlates of intertemporal decision-making: Contributions of subjective value, stimulus type, and trait impulsivity. *Hum Brain Mapp* 32, 1637-1648.

Stein MB, Koverola C, Hanna C, Torchia MG, McClarty B (1997) Hippocampal volume in women victimized by childhood sexual abuse. *Psychol Med* 27, 951-959.

Takahashi T, Chanen AM, Wood SJ, Yücel M, Tanino R, Suzuki M, Velakoulis D, Pantelis C, McGorry PD (2009) Insular cortex volume and impulsivity in teenagers with first-presentation borderline personality disorder. *Prog Neuropsychopharmacol Biol Psychiatry* 33, 1395-1400.

Tamm L, Menon V, Ringel J, Reiss AL (2004) Event-related fMRI evidence of frontotemporal involvement in aberrant response inhibition and task switching in attention-deficit/hyperactivity disorder. *J Am Acad Child Adolesc Psychiatr* 43, 1430-1440.

Tebartz van Elst L, Hesslinger B, Thiel T, Geiger E, Haegele K, Lemieux L, Lieb K, Bohus M, Hennig J, Ebert D (2003) Frontolimbic brain abnormalities in patients with borderline personality disorder: a volumetric magnetic resonance imaging study. *Biol Psychiatry* 54, 163-171.

Terry P, Doumas M, Desai RI, Wing AM (2009) Dissociations between motor timing, motor coordination, and time perception after the administration of alcohol or caffeine. *Psychopharmacology* 202, 719-729.

Toplak ME, Dockstader C, Tannock R (2006) Temporal information processing in ADHD: findings to date and new methods. *J Neurosci Methods* 151, 15-29.

Valera EM, Spencer RMC, Zeffiro TA, Makris N, Spencer TJ, Faraone SV, Biederman J, Seidman LJ (2010) Neural substrates of impaired sensorimotor timing in adult attention-deficit/hyperactivity disorder. *Biol Psychiatr* 68, 359-367.

Valko L, Schneider G, Doehnert M, Müller U, Brandels D, Steinhausen H-C, Drechsler R (2010) Time processing in children and adults with ADHD. *J Neural Transm* 117, 1213-1228.

Vieregge P, Heberlein I, Kömpf D (1997) Are neuropsychological tests useful in screening for the genetic risk of Parkinson's disease? *Parkinsonism Relat Disord* 3, 141-150.

Völlm B, Richardson P, Stirling J, Elliott R, Dolan M, Chaudhry I, Del Ben C, McKie S, Anderson I, Deakin B (2004) Neurobiological substrates of antisocial and borderline personality disorder: preliminary results of a functional fMRI study. *Crim Behav Ment Health* 14, 39-54.

Völlm B, Richardson P, McKie S, Elliott R, Dolan M, Deakin B (2007) Neuronal correlates of reward and loss in cluster B personality disorders: a functional magnetic resonance imaging study. *Psychiatr Res: Neuroimaging* 156,151-167.

Wiener M, Turkeltaub P, Coslett HB (2010) The image of time: a voxel-wise meta-analysis. *Neuroimage* 49, 1728-1740.

White HR,Marmorstein NR, Crews FT, Bates ME, Mun E-Y, Loeber R (2011) Associations between heavy drinking and changes in impulsive behaviour amongadolescent boys. *Alcohol Clin Exp Res* 35, 1-9.

Whittle S, Chanen AM, Fornito A, McGorry PD, Pantelis C, Yücel M (2009) Anterior cingulate volume in adolescents with first-presentation borderline personality disorder. *Psychiatry Res* 172, 155-160.

Wilens TE, Spencer TJ (2010) Understanding attention-deficit/hyperactivity disorder from childhood to adulthood. *Postgrad Med* 122, 97-109.

Wingenfeld K, Spitzer C, Rullkötter N, Löwe B (2010) Borderline personality disorder: hypothalamus pituitary adrenal axis and findings from neuroimaging studies. *Psychoneuroendocrinology* 35, 154-170.

Wolf RC, Plichta MM, Sambataro F, Fallgatter AJ, Jacob C, Lesch K-P, Hermann MJ, Schönfeldt-Lecuona C, Connemann BJ, Grön G, Vasic N (2009) Regional brain activation changes and abnormal functional connectivity of the ventrolateral prefrontal cortex during working memory processing in adults with attention-deficit/hyperactivity disorder. *Hum Brain Mapp* 30, 2252-2266.

Woolverton WL, Myerson J, Green L (2007) Delay discounting of cocaine by rhesus monkeys. *Exp Clin Psychopharmacol* 15, 238-244.

Zanarini MC, Frankenburg FR, Dubo ED, Sickel AE, Trikha A, Levin A, Reynolds V (1998a) Axis II comorbidity of borderline personality disorder. *Comprehen Psychiatr* 39, 296-302.

Zanarini MC, Frankenburg FR, Dubo ED, Sickel AE, Trikha A, Levin A, Reynolds V (1998b) Axis I comorbidity of borderline personality disorder. *Am J Psychiatr* 155, 1733-1739.

Zapolski TC, Cyders MA, Smith GT (2009) Positive urgency predicts illegal drug use and risky sexual behaviour. *Psychol Addict Behav* 23, 348-354.

Zetzsche T, Frodl T, Preuss UW, Schmitt G, Seifert D, Leinsinger G, Born C, Reiser M, Möller HJ, Meisenzahl EM (2006) Amygdala volume and depressive symptoms in patients with borderline personality disorder. *Biol Psychiatry* 60, 302-310.

Zetzsche T, Preuss UW, Frodl T, Schmitt G, Seifert D, Münchhausen E, Tabrizi S, Leinsinger G, Born C, Reiser M, Möller HJ, Meisenzahl EM (2007) Hippocampal volume reduction and history of aggressive behaviour in patients with borderline personality disorder. *Psychiatry Res* 154, 157-170.

Zimmermann M, Mattia JI (1999) Axis I diagnostic comorbidity and borderline personality disorder. *Compr Psychiatr* 40, 245-252.

Zlotnick C, Johnson DM, Yen S, Battle CL, Sanislow CA, Skodol AE, Grilo CM, McGlashan TH, Gunderson JG, Bender DS, Zanarini MC, Shea MT (2003) Clinical features and impairment in women with Borderline Personality Disorder (BPD) with Posttraumatic Stress Disorder (PTSD), BPD without PTSD, and other personality disorders with PTSD. *J Nerv Ment Dis* 191, 706-713.

11

MRI Techniques to Evaluate Exercise Impact on the Aging Human Brain

Bonita L. Marks and Laurence M. Katz
University of North Carolina at Chapel Hill
USA

1. Introduction

The aging human brain undergoes a variety of structural and metabolic changes, often coinciding with, or leading to, cognitive decline (Bullitt et al., 2009). Over the past decade, investigators have been searching for better methods to detect, treat, and prevent cognitive decline. This has lead to the development of a plethora of pharmaceutical approaches with limited success. Identifying non-pharmaceutical approaches for the prevention/treatment of cognitive decline is paramount. Because of its non-invasiveness, neuroimaging is fast becoming a preferred technology for evaluating brain structure and function. In addition, exercise is being recognized as a potential adjunct modality for preventing or reducing structural decline in the brain and perhaps attenuating corresponding cognitive decline. These two methodologies can work in tandem: first, for identification of subtle changes in the brain not detectable via standard cognitive testing and second, for application of appropriate exercise regimes shown to be associated with healthy brain aging. Taken together, disruptions in cognitive function may be delayed, or even halted, but only if intervention occurs "soon enough". The obvious questions to answer are: 1) What is "soon enough"? 2) What type of neuroimaging might be "best"? and, 3) What kind of exercise? Simple questions with no simple answers. This chapter will begin with common, often overlooked issues regarding the use of exercise as a research modality and then progress to incorporating exercise into neuroimaging studies.

1.1 Sedentary and unhealthy

A sedentary lifestyle, low aerobic fitness and obesity are associated with both cardiovascular and cerebrovascular diseases (Burns et al. 2008). Research over the last decade has shown that 6 months of aerobic exercise may reduce or prevent brain volume atrophy in the prefrontal brain region related to executive function and memory in the aged (Burns et al., 2008; Colcombe et al., 2006; Erickson et al.,2009). It has also been suggested that aerobic fitness and obesity may selectively impact brain regions as well as different hemispheres (Cronk et al., 2009; Gustafson et al., 2004, 2008; Marks et al., 2007, 2010; Raji et al., 2009; Soreca et al., 2009; Ward et al., 2005). For instance, greater aerobic fitness has been moderately associated with greater cerebral white matter integrity in the anterior and middle cingulum regions on the left side of the brain whereas a higher body mass index and higher abdominal girth have been significantly associated with lower cerebral white matter integrity in the posterior cingulum region on the right side of the brain (Marks et al., 2010).

This of course has implications beyond executive dysfunction; disruption of cerebral white matter integrity in the middle-posterior cingulum regions could impact motor movement, learning, and reading comprehension. Early transcranial doppler studies concluded that aerobic exercise may be beneficial for maintenance of cerebral blood flow (Marks et al., 2000; Orlandi and Murri, 1996). A decade later, cerebral blood vessel morphology studies suggested physically active older adults have younger-looking cerebral vasculature (Bullitt et al., 2009, 2010).

However, the retention and improvement of human brain plasticity via exercise is still not well understood. Despite animal studies demonstrating that exercise may promote neurogenesis, and human studies demonstrating a maintenance/increase in brain volume with exercise (Cotman et al., 2007; Ferris et al., 2007; van Praag et al., 1999), there is little information demonstrating the mechanism(s) for such changes. Furthermore, much of the evidence is equivocal as to whether these brain adaptations, presumably due to physical exercise, equates to improved cognitive function (Colcombe et al., 2003; Etnier and Nowell, 2006; Heyn et al., 2004; Kharti et al., 2001).

These aforementioned discrepancies may be due, at least in part, to the state of flux with research in this area. Numerous neuroimaging techniques are being used and the technology itself is rapidly changing. Cognitive tests commonly used for those with known cognitive deficits may not be sensitive enough to detect subtle cognitive changes in presumed healthy community dwelling elderly. Furthermore, researchers are using a variety of exercise paradigms, some of which are not reproducible due to lack of reporting standard exercise prescription procedures. Other factors such as age, gender, training status, and diet, known to be potential confounders in exercise and aging studies, are often overlooked. Finally, there is confusion in which term to use to simply identify the exercise paradigm itself. All of these factors make comparisons across studies difficult and the ability to draw definitive conclusions impossible (American College of Sports Medicine, 2010; Leasure and Jones, 2008; Lommatzsch et al., 2005).

Therefore, the aims of this chapter are threefold: 1) Clarify the use of exercise, physical activity and related terms as profiling variables versus intervention modalities, 2) Review neuroimaging techniques currently being used to study the impact of exercise and physical activity on the aging human brain structure, and 3) Highlight the pros and cons for use of such methods with exercise paradigms.

2. Is it physical activity, exercise, or fitness?

Physical activity is associated with changes in brain structure. Regular exercise improves brain function. High aerobic fitness mediates cerebral white matter integrity. Do all these statements mean the same thing, or are there subtle differences in interpretation rendering the results difficult to compare?

2.1 Defining "exercise"

The terms "physical activity", "exercise", and "fitness" are often used interchangeably. But as with any discipline, these terms have distinct connotations and therefore should not be use as mere synonyms. To add to the terminology confusion, a myriad of additional phrases are incorporated in an attempt to better clarify the exercise paradigm. Typical terms include, but are not limited to: aerobic fitness, health fitness, physical fitness, calisthenics, circuit training, core training, resistance training, stretching and toning, strength training, and weight lifting. Thus, physical activity or exercise could mean participating in a marathon or dance class, lifting a 10 kg medicine ball, raking leaves, meditating while performing yoga, or simply walking around a shopping mall.

2.2 Working definitions

Exercise scientists and physical educators continually find themselves clarifying the words that describe their work and this debate has raged for decades. For instance, the term *physical activity* is classically defined as any bodily movement that results in muscular contractions and increases energy expenditure above that which is used during rest (USDHHS/NHLBI, 2008). In contrast, the term *exercise* is defined as "*the regular or repeated use of a faculty or bodily organ*" (Meriam Webster Free Dictionary, 2011). Thus, the term physical activity is often used due to its broader utility, but the term exercise should be used whenever the researcher's intent is to demonstrate the impact of *repeated exposure* to a *specific type* of physical activity. Therefore, exercise can be considered a structured sub-category of physical activity, with specific dosing parameters that result in health maintenance and/or improvement (Caspersen et al., 1985). The term *fitness*, in biological terms, simply means the ability of an organism to survive and reproduce. This generic term is most often used to connote one's health status and is expanded as needed (i.e., health fitness, physical fitness, aerobic fitness, brain fitness). The American College of Sports Medicine (1990) suggested the following definition be used for *physical fitness*: "fitness is the ability to perform moderate to vigorous levels of physical activity without undue fatigue and the capability of maintaining such ability throughout life." Obviously, this exercise science-based definition can be applied to the neurological system as well, suggesting that *brain fitness* can be defined as *the ability to perform daily cognitive tasks without undue mental fatigue or memory impairment and the capability to maintain cognitive abilities throughout life.*

3. Acute versus chronic exercise participation

Distinctions need to be made between the *acute* versus *chronic* impact of exercise on a physiological system, in this case, the brain. While it is important to know the short-term impact exercise has on physiological systems from a biological or safe participation standpoint, the establishment of long-term health benefits attributed to exercise exposures must account for the chronic adaptations due to historical (i.e., long-term) participation in an exercise regime. It is well-established that exercise is an acute stressor, thereby resulting in (relatively) immediate elevations in blood flow, heart rate, oxygen uptake, respiration, and increased circulation/uptake of most hormones and many metabolic substrates. However, the question remains, do any of these acute exercise responses, when experienced multiple times throughout the week, over several months to many years (i.e., chronic exposure), impact the brain in such a way as to become neuro-protective and prevent or attenuate neurological degeneration and cognitive decline commonly attributed to unsuccessful brain aging?

3.1 Cross-sectional or outcome study?

Evaluating the brain at one point in time with a selection of a population is a cross-sectional study. One is able to infer relationships between brain structure/function and a host of variables, ranging from cognitive test scores to health fitness ratings. This is an excellent starting point and is where most of the exercise neurobiology literature is currently focused, likely due to time, facility limitations, and monetary constraints. However, care must be taken when reporting the results from cross-sectional studies. Regardless of the strength of the associations, results should not be reported in such a way as to infer causation. Cross-sectional research has pointed the way towards the need for more controlled, randomized longitudinal outcome studies which can take the significant associations one step further and determine causation of an intervention. While acute outcome studies are able to state how exercise stresses the brain on an immediate basis, only longitudinal outcome studies will be able to recommend more definitive exercise dosing guidelines for maintaining and/or improving brain health over a lifetime. Even then, the recommendations will likely be for specific populations, a specific gender, or specific types of physical activity. It will take several years to arrive at the more global health fitness recommendations now common in the cardiovascular literature. There is plenty of work ahead for innovative exercise-focused neuroscientists.

4. Media releases

The biggest blunder that has been occurring with the current brain studies is the pseudo-science reporting in the popular press. When public dollars are funding the research, it is important to get the science results out to the public in a media format that is understandable for the layman. However, the information is often unwittingly misrepresented by the media, resulting in conflicting reports when different modalities/populations are investigated, or worse, the media report leaves the impression that brain researchers are somehow privy to reading someone's mind. In the exercise neuroscience field, media interviews with researchers who are not trained in the exercise sciences or knowledgeable in the exercise design of a study has resulted in less than accurate interpretations of the study's purpose, strengths and/or weaknesses. This can have a dampening effect on future exercise neuroscience studies and may lessen the scientific integrity of the research itself. Thus it is critical that researchers understand the basics of the modality being used – in this case, exercise is the modality.

5. The exercise dose-response

To be comparable across studies and to better determine the most efficacious exercise plan for promoting successful brain aging, researchers and clinicians need to attend to the multi-faceted nature of the exercise prescription, or dosing, components. These components can be manipulated in a variety of ways so as to not only meet the research needs but also ensure that the participants will stick with the program. While not everyone is going to love to exercise, the exercise program should be designed to accommodate one's abilities, interests, and health status. Note that the exercise prescription is individualized not as a function of age or gender per se, but rather, it is individualized as a function of personal interests and health-fitness limitations. For research, the trick is to create a general exercise prescription for an entire group while maintaining an individualistic approach, to ensure the safety of each participant, prevent drop-outs, yet still be efficacious for the research goal. That is the "art" of an exercise prescription.

5.1 Components of an exercise prescription
When exercise is being used as a research tool, neurobiology researchers should consider the FITT + P paradigm (frequency, intensity, time, type, progression) of an exercise prescription

recommended by the American College of Sports Medicine (ACSM, 2009). Precisely identifying each of these components within an exercise neurobiology study makes comparison across studies, replication of results, and advancement of the exercise science of neurobiology much more accurate. Furthermore, it makes providing global recommendations to the public easy. Vaguely described exercise protocols are one of the major pitfalls encountered in the neurobiological literature utilizing exercise as a treatment modality. Often the research outcomes are either un-interpretable or non-generalizable. Manipulation of any one of the five components in the FITT + P paradigm can alter the intervention outcome significantly, and varying more than one component within a study must be done carefully. Ultimately the goal is to determine what type(s) of exercise recommendation(s) will best facilitate brain health maintenance. Reproducibility of the exercise prescription is paramount so that the findings can be applied across various physical activities and different populations.

5.1.1 Frequency ("F") of exercise

How "often" one exercises is a critical component of the exercise dose-response. It depends not only upon the health status of the individual, but also the type (or modality) of exercise. To improve cardiovascular health (or aerobic fitness), metabolic and lipid profiles, and body composition, 3 days per week is the recommended minimum number of times one should exercise (ACSM, 2009). However, if a person is at either extreme of the physical fitness continuum, (i.e., extremely deconditioned/inactive versus highly fit/active), then multiple daily sessions of very short duration (i.e. time) or nearly daily sessions of moderately long sessions may be instituted. Hence, there is a distinct relationship between frequency of exercise and duration of exercise. Simply put, the amount of time (in minutes) one should expend in a given exercise session is partially determined by how frequently one is exercising on a daily or weekly basis. Furthermore, the 3-days-per week minimum recommendation only applies to aerobic conditioning. Strength conditioning should be performed 2-3 days per week with the goal to alternate muscle groups being trained, and flexibility training recommendations is a minimum of 2 days weekly. Fitting all three of these exercise components (aerobics, strength, flexibility) into one exercise session can cause an exercise session to require at least one hour of time. Therefore, it is common to break up the exercise program into "aerobic" training days and "strength/flexibility" training days, resulting in exercising almost daily.

5.1.2 Intensity ("I") of exercise

How "hard" one exercises has many physiological parameters to consider including heart rate response, perception of effort, and workloads on various types of equipment. All of these factors contribute to the "intensity" of the exercise prescription and are manipulated according to the desired outcomes (Nieman, 2010).

5.1.2.1 Heart rate

If aerobic conditioning is desired, then the recommendation is for one to exercise within a ""stimulus zone". This zone is based upon one's health status and a percentage of one's age-predicted maximum heart rate (220 - age). For the average individual, a "moderate" intensity stimulus zone is recommended. As can be seen in *Table 1*, a moderate heart rate stimulus zone would be 64 – 76% of one's maximal predicted heart rate. So if one is 50 years old, the predicted maximal heart would be 170, and the heart rate training stimulus zone would be 109 to 129 bpm.

Intensity	%HRR	%Max HR (bpm)	RPE Range	% 1-RM
Moderate	40-59	64-76	12-14	40-69
Hard /Vigorous	60-84	77-93	14-15	50-69

Source: Modified from: Nieman, D. *Exercise Testing and Prescription, A Health Related Approach.* 7th Edition, New York: McGraw Hill Publishers, 2011, pp 180, Table 6.3, Classification of Physical Activity Intensity

Table 1. Intensity scales equating verbal descriptions to percent heart rate reserve (%HRR), percent heart rate max (%HRmax), rating of perceived exertion (RPE) based on the Borg 6-20 scale, and percent of a one-repetition maximum (%1-RM) strength test.

A slightly more complex, but more accurate way to prescribe aerobic exercise intensity is by using the Karvonen formula, a mathematical formula using percentage of one's heart rate reserve (maximal heart rate – resting heart rate). This requires knowing one's maximal heart rate (or estimating it as shown above), knowing one's resting heart rate (being able to take one's pulse rate at rest) and using the percentages listed in *Table 1*. Because this calculation more closely represents oxygen consumption requirements, the percentages shown in the table are slightly lower than the ones used with the age-predicted heart rate max method just described. Thus, the formula for determining a moderate-intensity heart rate stimulus zone using the Karvonen Method is as follows:

[(Maximal Heart Rate – Resting Heart Rage) * 40%] + Resting Heart Rate

[(Maximal Heart Rate – Resting Heart Rage) * 59%] + Resting Heart Rate

Thus, if our 50-year old person had a resting pulse rate of 75 bpm, using the Karvonen method to determine his exercise stimulus zone, his heart rate training stimulus zone would be 113 to 131 bpm.

5.1.2.2 Perception of effort

Sometimes heart rate responses are modified by medications or the exercise participant simply cannot take his/her pulse rate. In that case, exercise can be prescribed based on one's perception of the exercise intensity. This is called "rating of perceived exertion", or RPE. The most common RPE scale used is Borg's 6-20 scale, which at moderate intensity exercise, correlates well with the heart rate response. For instance if a person rates his level of exertion to be between 12-14, the heart rate is generally within 120-140 beats per minute. It does take about 3 practice sessions for the user to become familiar and comfortable with this scale in order to get the most accurate RPE scores (Borg, 1985). For a more complete understanding of using perceived exertion, an excellent applied book is "*Perceived Exertion for Practioners*" (R.J. Robertson, 2004, Human Kinetics Publishers).

5.1.2.3 Workload

When utilizing equipment for exercise training, the intensity of training will in part be mediated by the workload setting employed. For instance, if a moderate intensity is desired for lifting weights on a machine, a percentage of what a person is able to lift maximally one time (% 1-RM) maybe used. As seen in *Table 1*, to strength train at a moderate intensity, approximately 40-69% of a 1-RM will be recommended. That means, if the maximum weight one is able to lift is 100 pounds, then the training weight stack should be between 40 and 69 pounds (or, 45 kg max = 18 to 31 kg). If using a treadmill, the exerciser would need instructions as to how to set the speed and percent grade; if using a cycle ergometer, the exerciser would need to know how to set the resistance and at what speed to pedal. Sometimes this is determined by an entry exercise test and the settings are based upon a percentage of their max test results; other times it is arbitrarily determined and governed simply by determining a "comfortable" pace in order to attain a desired heart rate or RPE range. Using the latter method will enable the researcher to permit the exerciser to exercise on a greater variety of equipment, thereby helping to reduce exercise boredom and dropping out of a study. However, a word of caution: if the goal of the research is to determine the impact of a certain TYPE of exercise on the brain over a certain period of time, then the researcher must give explicit instructions as to which equipment use is permissible for exercise research participation. Sometimes, giving a research volunteer too many choices can truly confound interpretation of the research results. Thus, while that new exercise club down the road may be convenient and affordable for the study, the researcher must determine how precisely the exercise prescription must be adhered to and consider the consequences if a subject veers off course.

5.1.3 Time ("T"), or duration, of exercise

The first "T" of the FITT + P paradigm is Time. How "long" one exercises, or how much time is required to achieve a desired fitness benefit, depends upon one's health status and/or fitness goals, and as stated above, the   frequency of exercise. If one is very deconditioned, then multiple sessions of brief duration may be recommended. These brief durations may be as little as 5 minutes. It is common for those with a fragile health status or simply deconditioned due to inactivity (but otherwise considered healthy) to be given an intermittent exercise prescription consisting of 5 minutes of physical activity interspersed with an equal amount of rest, with that dose repeated twice more in succession so that an equivalent of 15 minutes can be accrued. As one successfully adapts to the exercise stimulus, the rest sessions will be reduced so that eventually the previously deconditioned person can exercise for 15 continuous minutes. Once a baseline level of aerobic endurance is attained, then strength conditioning can be safely and effectively added to the exercise program. As indicated above, an exercise session focusing only on aerobic conditioning can require 15 to 30+ minutes. A strength conditioning program may also require 30+ minutes if the entire body is to be trained in one session. Flexibility training can be a stand-alone program or be incorporated into the regular exercise program as part of a warm-up and/or cool-down routine. Thus, flexibility training can take as little as 5 minutes or as long as 30 minutes, depending upon the nature of the training.

While any one component of an exercise program may eventually take about 30+ minutes, it is standard to also incorporate a brief 5-10 minute warm–up before entering the "stimulus zone" and a 5-10 minute cool-down after completing the "stimulus zone" work-out. The warm-up is usually a lighter version of the stimulus and is to ensure the body is prepared to be stressed, whereas the cool-down is usually a relaxing set of stretches to enable the body to return to the pre-exercise non-stressed state. Therefore, at least 30 minutes needs to be allotted for the first week of a beginning exercise session (5 minute warm-up, ~20 minute stimulus, 5 minute cool-down), and more time thereafter as one's exercise prescription is upgraded, or progressed through several weeks of a research study.

Another aspect of "time" is the actual timing of the exercise – that is, time of day. While this does not impact the dose-response of exercise per se, it does impact the effectiveness of the exercise plan if the time of day allotted to exercise is not compatible with the exerciser's lifestyle. For instance, if exercise is to take place under supervised conditions at a facility, the hours must be agreeable with the exercise's life – are there times available before or after one's work day, or at lunch? If recruiting a person with child care responsibilities, are there childcare services? Are weekend hours available? Other concerns are parking, commuting time, or easy bus/rail access. Will the research study pay for on-site childcare or parking?

5.1.4 TYPE ("T") of exercise

The other "T" component of the FITT + P paradigm is the TYPE of exercise (or activity) needed to achieve the stated research goals. The exercise prescription type is subdivided into three broad categories: aerobic endurance (or fitness), muscular strength/endurance, and flexibility. Of course each of these broad activity categories has numerous subtypes, thus it is crucial to specifically describe the type of activity one is to engage in. For instance, an aerobic activity is any activity that a person can complete continuously for 15 minutes or more that utilizes a large portion of the body's musculature in a rhythmic fashion. This includes common individual activities such as walking, running, swimming and cycling but it can also include games, sports and various types of dance. Muscular strength/endurance training also has many sub-types. It can consist of the traditional lifting of weights (aka weight training) or it can be termed resistance training or core training and involve not only dumbbells, free weights, or machines, but also medicine balls, resistance bands and tubing, kettle balls and one's own weight (e.g. push-ups, sit-ups). Other types of musculoskeletal training can include balance training, plyometric training, neuromuscular facilitation training, yoga, and tai chi. Flexibility training can involve static, ballistic, or dynamic stretching. Often times, strength and conditioning programs are simply called "stretching and toning", which really provides no concrete idea of the type of training actually provided. Thus, with all these options available to the researcher, creating a reproducible exercise program to investigate a particular health parameter becomes an art form. Obviously it is not possible to investigate every aspect of exercise within one study, so the researcher must narrow his/her focus to a select few options and describe them well-enough for the reader to be able to replicate. Ultimately, with enough well-designed neurobiology exercise studies, general recommendations for cerebral health will be able to be created, similar to those that now exist for cardiovascular health.

5.1.5 Progression ("P") of exercise

There are a variety of ways to "progress" an exercise prescription so that it remains challenging yet doable for the participant and prevents boredom or staleness. The progression of exercise is increased over the ensuing weeks at a percentage that is both safe and effective for that particular individual. The eventual goal is for one to attain a minimum of 30 or more minutes of continuous exercise on most days of the week (Haskell et al., 2007). One rule of thumb has been to increase any given exercise dose by as little as 2% or as much as 30% weekly or every other week. Another practice is to increase the duration of exercise by approximately 5 to 10 minutes every week, which might translate to a 15% increase in time week to week. If there is little room for adding additional time to an exercise session, then an extra day of training can be added on. If neither time nor frequency is an option to increase, then intensity becomes the progression target. When a person's perception of effort decreases along with lower heart rate responses with any given exercise stimulus, it is time to increase the exercise intensity. The goal is to make sure a slight overload is placed upon the physiological systems so that the body can continually respond and successfully adapt to the overload. Unsuccessful adaption to an overload will result in undue fatigue, unnecessary muscle soreness, and if extreme, illness and/or injury.

Perhaps the most important concept to understand is the complex interaction between intensity, frequency and duration of the exercise prescription and how manipulation of any one of these variable impacts the exercise progression and adaption. The way to avoid unsuccessful overloading is to increase only one exercise prescription component in any given exercise session. For example, if the frequency of exercise training is scheduled to be increased from 3 days a week to 4 days a week, then the duration (total time) and intensity of the exercise session should remain the same as the previous training session. If on the other hand, the intensity of exercise needs to be increased, then the duration of the exercise session should either remain the same or be decreased slightly to accommodate for the increased effort required. On the following day, the duration can be returned to its previous level as long as the "new" exercise intensity remains the same. *Figure 1* outlines the basic components of the exercise prescription and can serve as a quick-reference exercise dosing

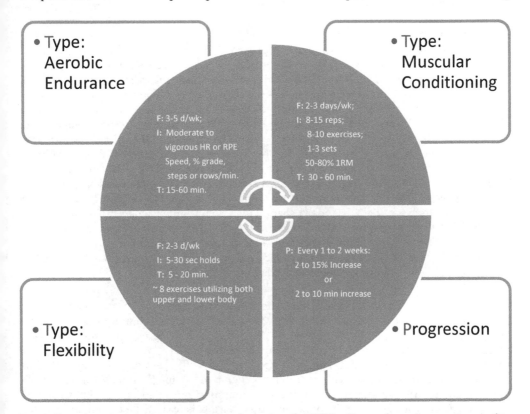

Fig. 1. Exercise prescription components featuring the FITT + P paradigm. Less active, unfit individuals would have exercise dosing at the lower ranges where as more active, higher fit individuals would have exercise dosing at the higher ranges. HR = heart rate; RPE = rating of perceived exertion.

guide. More complete exercise prescription information is available in the ACSM's Guidelines for Exercise Testing and Prescription book (2009), updated every four years. The best advice for researchers using exercise as a research treatment arm, or clinicians using exercise as a therapeutic agent is to make sure one or more ACSM-certified exercise physiologists are a part of your team.

6. Structural neuroimaging and exercise impact

What type of neuroimaging is best when trying to determine how exercise impacts the [aging] brain? That depends on the question(s) one needs to answer. If the goal is to determine the long-term impact of exercise on brain structure, then structural MRIs are appropriate. Structural imaging can track changes over time due to a stimulus such as exercise. Structural imaging can involve gray and white matter volume determination ("quantity"), cerebral white matter integrity ("quality") using diffusion tensor imaging (DTI), or both. It can also involve investigating the cerebral blood vessels utilizing magnetic resonance angiography (MRA).

6.1 Voxel-wise or ROI approach?

The MRI analysis can take a voxel-wise approach if the researchers have no particular hypotheses regarding expected areas of impact, or the MRI analysis can take a regions of interest (ROI) approach if there are research-driven hypothesis regarding expected areas of impact from physiological knowledge. There are pros and cons to both methods. It is argued that the voxel-wise approach is less biased, less time consuming, and therefore less costly. The ROI approach is argued to be driven by scientific knowledge of the physiology, more targeted and less "look-see" exploratory type research. While the ROI approach can be more costly due to the labor-intensive outlining of the specific ROI, and costly if ROI mapping is being done by more than one investigator for reliability purposes, if automated ROI templates are available, the cost and time decrease substantially. Unfortunately, not all ROI have templates. The "con" to template mapping is that a small degree of accuracy is sacrificed due to assuming a "standard shape" for a brain region when in fact there is no true standard shape (Scheibel, 2009). Thanks to the NIH Neuroscience Roadmap Initiative, there are a variety of free resources, including software mapping templates, available on the internet to download. One such site is called *MIDAS* and offers brain images as well as toolkits: http://www.insight-journal.org/midas/gallery/?flash=true

6.2 How long does it take for exercise to alter brain structure?

While rate of decline in brain mass with aging is highly individualized, it is often stated that the "normal" brain gradually decreases in size 10-15% with aging, and this shrinkage becomes particularly evident in octogenarians (Scheibel, 2004). The average rate of brain atrophy is between 0.9 to 1.5% per year after age 52, with the steepest rate of decline occurring in the frontal region with concomitant cognitive decline (Dennis & Cabeza, 2008). While it is not currently known precisely how much time is needed to facilitate structural changes (i.e., improvements) in the brain due to exercise, it is reasonable to hypothesize that relatively short-term structural change may be possible. In two separate studies demonstrating brain plasticity, as little as 1.5 to 3 months of cognitive training resulted in cortical changes in younger populations (Driemeyer et al., 2008; Haier et al., 2009). As for exercise, six months of aerobic exercise using moderate intensity walking 3 days per week for an hour each session not only prevented brain volume atrophy but resulted in brain volume improvement in older adults (Colcombe et al., 2006). Using voxel-based morphology, improvements in brain volume were noted in both the gray and white matter regions associated with executive function, long term memory, and general intelligence (i.e., the prefrontal and temporal cortices). These improvements were cautiously reported in terms of brain atrophy risk reduction in comparison to a stretching/toning control group such that a 16% improvement in aerobic fitness resulted in a 27 to 42% risk reduction of brain atrophy. The greatest risk reduction was in the anterior cingulate cortex. The stretching/toning group experienced a non-significant 5% increase in aerobic fitness but no volumetric information was reported for them. Although it is not known if the 5% improvement in aerobic fitness also resulted in some volumetric improvement, it might be surmised that embarking upon a moderate-intensity aerobic exercise program which produces at least a 1% increase in aerobic fitness may attenuate aging-related brain atrophy. This was one of the first longitudinal outcome studies reporting the impact of aerobic versus musculoskeletal-type exercise on the aging brain.

Currently, little neuroimaging information is available on other modes or durations of exercise training; nor is there information regarding how quickly the human brain structure detrains. But if the brain/cerebrovasculature mirrors the heart/cardiovasculature in exercise adaptations, then like the cardiovascular system, the cerebrovascular system may lose that 11% gain in as little as 3 weeks of no training (Coyle et al., 1984). Thus, the protective effect against brain atrophy may be lost in one short month if one is unable to exercise sufficiently. An intriguing question remains, can cognitive brain training (e.g. suduko, puzzles, playing chess, Wii-games) supplant physical activity during periods of physical inactivity in order to maintain brain structure and function?

6.3 Exercise neuroimaging study shortcomings

Being a pioneer in exercise and aging neuroscience research also means there will likely be design flaws in the research. For instance, in Colcombe et al's study (2006), the age range was wide, 60 to 79 years with a mean age of 66 years. The study age range spanned two decades with three standard aging cohorts: the older end of middle-aged (45-64 years old), the young-old (65-74 years old), and the younger end of old (75-84 years old). No mention was made regarding how many subjects fell within each of these age cohorts, therefore it is not known if these age cohorts responded differently to the exercise programs. With no variance measure or age range provided *per group* on any variable, it is difficult to assume the study did not have a few inadvertent biases. A potential younger-age bias may have pre-existed in the aerobic treatment group (the treatment group was on average 1.4 years younger). The stretching/toning control group had a slightly higher percentage of females (4% more), creating a potential gender bias. Further, the actual pre-aerobic fitness distribution per grouping was unclear. Although the mean aerobic fitness (VO_2) values were not significantly different between groups (~ 23 ml/kg/min), the pre-intervention VO_2 values ranged from 12.9 to 49.9 ml/kg/min. Thus there were some older individuals with pre-intervention VO_2 values who would be considered highly fit and therefore have less room for improvement from any type of intervention. It is not known if an attempt was made to balance the placement of these higher-fit individuals into the two groups since the methods claim group assignment was totally randomized. Furthermore, it was reported that the aerobic group was previously sedentary, however older adults with VO_2's exceeding 40 ml/kg/min are not likely habitually sedentary. Individually, the between group differences highlighted here are small and were reported to be non-significant, but considered collectively, these small biases could contribute to confounding the interpretation of the results.

Sociological studies have shown that women outlive men by 4 to 10 years, thereby partially explaining why there are usually more women in research studies involving older adults. Although women tend to live about a decade longer than men, they also experience an accelerated pace of physiological decline between their seventh and eighth decade of life. Older men tend to weigh more, be more physically active and have a higher degree of aerobic fitness than older women of the same age (Spriduso et al. 2005) and women's brain volumes are smaller than men (Allen et al., 2003). Thus care must be taken when studying variables with inherent age or gender differences. Colcombe et al. (2006) made no mention of controlling for age or gender in the statistical analyses of their data in order to determine if improvements attributed to aerobic fitness change was independent of age or gender influences. It is well known that both age and gender can impact brain volumes and cognition independently (Madden et al, 2009). Failure to control for these variables can lead to potentially erroneous conclusions. For example, Marks et al. (2010) initially noted moderate positive relationships in the anterior cingulum segment between cerebral white matter integrity and aerobic fitness as measured by diffusion tensor imaging (DTI). However, upon controlling for both age and gender, only the middle and posterior cingulum segments remained significantly related to aerobic fitness. Similarly, this pattern of reduced significance was repeated in a voxel-wise brain analysis on the same data (Liu et al. 2009). Thus it is critical to control for factors that are known to impact the brain and/or aerobic fitness parameters. Lastly, neither the exercise test protocol nor the "stretching and toning" prescription was ever fully described by Colcombe et al. (2006). This lack of information makes it difficult to determine the validity of the aerobic fitness and strength training outcomes, and it is even more difficult to impart health recommendations with confidence. Hence the encouraging conclusions regarding aerobic fitness and brain improvement from this study by Colcombe et al. (2006) must be viewed with cautious optimism. There are currently a few new NIH-funded exercise trials involving both healthy and diseased older adults in progress (http://projectreporter.nih.gov/reporter.cfm), with intervention timelines and exercise protocols seemingly mirroring Colcombe et al. 's initial study (2006) . Hopefully, these newer studies will not only control for potential confounding variables but also provide sufficient exercise testing and training details to render their studies replicable.

6.4 Magnetic resonance angiography and exercise impact

Magnetic resonance angiography (MRA) in conjunction with DTI is helpful in determining the status of one's cerebral blood vessels. Using a process known as arterial spin labeling (ASL), the quality and quantity of the cerebral blood flow can be determined with or without perfusion. It is believed that the progressive reduction in cerebral blood flow attributed to the aging process may be caused by a reduced metabolic demand due to a reduction in neurotransmitter synthesis (Orlandi & Murri, 1996) and/or underlying microvascular disease (Bullitt et al., 2010). The consequential neural atrophy results in smaller cerebral arteries, increased intracranial resistance and slower arteriole vasomotor reactivity (Orlandi & Murri, 1996). Even though studies suggested aging may be associated with smaller cerebral vessels, Bullitt et al. (2010) reported that vessel diameter reductions may be compensated for by an increase in vessel number and that both larger and smaller vessels were impacted. In a sub-study comparing active versus inactive older adults, Bullitt et al. (2009) reported significantly lower vessel tortuosity along with a higher number of smaller vessels. In a separate conference paper, although cerebral blood flow velocity did not change, Rahman et al. (2008) reported less variance in the cerebral blood flow velocity in those with higher physical activity levels. To examine both the cerebral vasculature as well as cerebral blood flow, arterial-spin labeling (ASL) would be required. For either the blood oxygen level-dependent effect (BOLD) or ASL methods, intravenously (IV) injected contrast agents will produce more distinct images. However decent (but not great) images can be obtained without the IV injections. Not using invasive procedures is certainly more appealing to the volunteer subject and helps to contain the imaging costs as well.

7. Functional neuroimaging and exercise

If one is interested in determining which regions of the brain are being activated /oxygenated during an exercise or cognitve task, a functional MRI (fMRI) using the BOLD response would be needed. For exercise studies, the obvious hurdle to overcome is movement as most movement causes disruption in the scanning process and poor images are created. Whereas cognitive psychology has forged numerous research pathways using fMRI with BOLD contrasts to determine regions of activation in the brain during various cognitive tasks, this has not been the case with exercise training interventions. Clearly there is a need for this type of research if one desires to investigate changes in cerebral blood flow or neural hormonal factors due to an exercise stimulus from either an acute exercise bout or in response to a chronic adaptation. The stumbling block to overcome is the exercise test itself. Most exercise studies use upright testing protocols on equipment that are large and bulky with both metal and electronic parts. All of this precludes testing within the scanning room due to the magnetic field. Furthermore, by the time the subject could be transferred from the exercise apparatus to the scanning bed, critical time would be lost such that the exercise impact on the cerebrovascular system would likely be missed in all but the most deconditioned subjects.

7.1 MRI-friendly leg cycle ergometer

Therefore, up to this point, the more feasible methodology for cerebral blood flow investigations with exercise have been with using transcranial dopplers (TCD) and/or electroencephalography (EEG). Although these methods also have difficulty with accurate measures during movement, they are in comparison, lower in cost and easier to administer than an fMRI study. However, for approximately $75,000 (US$), the Lode MRI-compatible recumbent leg cycle ergometry system can now be purchased from ELECTRAMED Corporation, located in Flint, Michigan, http://www.electramed.com/MRI%20ERGOMETER %20CARDIOLOGY%20_Details.htm. This would enable the researcher to conduct exercise tests while the subject remains in the MRI unit. Also available are MRI-compatible electrocardiography and blood pressure measurement units, thereby solving the equipment issue. Unfortunately, this particular equipment model is only compatible with a 1.5 T MRI scanner and only with select manufacturers. Given that most research is now being done on 3.0 T or 4.0 T scanners, this ergometer may not be useable for many research protocols. The final issue left to resolve is an acceptable exercise protocol that would be taxing enough yet involve minimal movement from the torso up during scanning sequences. One potential resolution would be to develop an intermittent exercise test protocol so that exercise bouts would take place during the imaging sequence changes, akin to an event-related design. Since stimuli in an event-related design are presented as isolated events of short duration, a brief cycling set that progressed in intensity with each event presentation could be incorporated (Carter and Sheih, 2010). Obviously, much pilot work would need to be done to determine the exact power outputs required to elicit measureable BOLD signals.

7.2 Exercise mental imagery

If actual physical exercise testing is not possible, there is still one other avenue to determine cerebral activation during an exercise task: mental imagery. For example, a sport psychology study investigated motor imagery of the golf swing to determine brain region activation. Using the sensori-motor homunculus map as a guide, Ross et al. (2003) compared the amount of fMRI BOLD response in brain regions related to the golf swing between novice versus expert golfers. It was determined that the greater the golf handicap, the greater the region of activation (greater than 2%) in specific somatatropic regions of interest relevant to golf. The powerpoint presentation can be downloaded from the internet with a search engine. A very recent BOLD fMRI study (Cremers et al., 2011) investigated mental imagery consisting of subjects envisioning themselves either walking, standing, or lying down (block design). Their imagined walking (speed = 2.3 ± 0.4 m/s) was associated with activation in the right dorsolateral prefrontal cortex, posterior parietal lobule, and the left cerebellar hemisphere. Therefore, it might be interesting to conduct an imagery intervention study to determine the acute response to an imagined exercise stress test as well as an imagined chronic response to a long-term exercise intervention. Studies of this nature have not yet been reported.

8. Testing pearls and pitfalls

Neuroimaging studies are expensive. Exercise testing and training are expensive. Recruitment drop-outs are expensive. And botched tests are expensive. They are expensive in terms of time, money and patience. Neuroimaging and exercise testing aged individuals bring a unique set of challenges to intervention research. There are the standard safety issues to consider when using a neuroimaging technique or conducting a physical exercise test; but the less obvious issues of comfort and trust sometimes slip by unasked, until it is too late and the subject has dropped out of the study. Therefore, when screening an older individual for an imaging and/or an exercise study, the following question must be asked: can the volunteer complete the testing protocol accurately and in relative comfort? The researcher must ascertain that the older volunteer can hear, see, follow directions, and adhere to the instructions. Volunteers must be able to complete enough of the exercise protocol to get valid physiological baseline data and/or remain motionless and pain free in the MRI scanner anywhere from 15 to 120 minutes. The brief breaks afforded between imaging sequences when a subject is free to move slightly may be insufficient. Arthritis, nasal-sinus drainage, and circulatory issues have thwarted many research MRI scans. For a first-time MRI scan, volunteers may back out at the last minute due to unanticipated fright (hence a simulator is an invaluable resource) or the irrational worry that the MRI will read their minds (thanks to outlandish media stories). Thus, the researcher must design protocols with both the science and the targeted subject population in mind.

8.1 Exercise testing versus physical activity recalls

Actual measurement of aerobic fitness, as opposed to estimating it in some fashion, is usually preferable. There are a variety of reference books available detailing exercise protocols for various health and fitness statuses. The researcher who wants to include exercise in the research design should obtain the ACSM Guidelines for Exercise Testing and Training (2009). A good textbook is Nieman's (2010) exercise prescription textbook used for training undergraduates in exercise science. However, there are times when it is inconvenient, illogical, or cost-prohibitive to conduct a fitness test. For those times when actual exercise testing is ruled out, there is a rather good non-exercise aerobic fitness estimation equation that is quite easy to use, providing one is trained in obtaining a valid physical activity recall. While it can be difficult to get accurate physical activity recalls beyond a few weeks, a seasoned investigator in physical activity recall questionnaires can elicit excellent responses, even recalls spanning several years.

One physical activity recall formula for estimating aerobic fitness has been in the literature since 1990. It was gathering dust until recently when we used it for a retrospective analysis exploring the role aerobic fitness might have on cerebral white matter integrity on both younger and older adults (Marks et al., 2007). Ever since that publication, we have been getting inquiries about the formula and how to use it. The formula was developed and tested at the Cooper Aerobic Institute in Texas on over 2,000 U.S. Air Force personnel ranging in age from 18 to 70 years. The subject population included males and females, fit and unfit, healthy and unhealthy. The estimated aerobic fitness value (VO_2) has a standard error of about 5 ml/kg/min. This formula is very good for cross-sectional, population-based studies when the purpose is to simply categorize one's fitness level. However, the error range is a bit too high and the fitness categorizing a bit too vague for pre-post research designs where VO_2 change is a critical factor. For that, VO_2 does need to actually be measured. Although the formula tends to underestimate the highly fit and over-estimate the very low fit, all subjects are still able to be categorized accurately into a fitness level (e.g., low fit, average fit, high fit). The estimation formula and its accompanying physical activity rating scale (PARS) are contained in *Table 2* and *Table 3* below:

VO_2 max ≈ 56.363 – (0.381 * age) + (1.951 * PARS) – (0.754 * BMI) + (gender * 10.987)

where: *Gender*: 0 = women; 1 = men

BMI = body mass index = weight (kg) / (height in meters^2)

PARS = physical activity rating scale from 0 to 7 (see Table 3)

Table 2. Estimated Aerobic Fitness (VO_2 max) (Jackson et al., 1990).

9. Limitations and suggestions

The good news is, lines of inquiry utilizing neuroimaging are still rather novel and as such, there is much to study. The bad news is, these lines of inquiry utilizing neuroimaging are still rather novel and there is much to learn, so omissions and/or mistakes in research design are to be expected. Investigating how exercise impacts the brain is akin to the first studies investigating how exercise impacted the heart and its related vasculature several decades ago.

A limitation in several structural imaging studies (e.g., Marks et al. 2010; Bullitt et al. 2009; Colcombe et al., 2006) was lack of cognitive function testing – it is unknown if the improved brain structures found in the more active subjects would have translated into better cognitive function. Adding cognitive testing with magnetic resonance imaging (MRI) may help detect subtle changes that the standard cognitive test batteries if used alone, cannot. If the MRI is able to detect changes, independent of the cognitive tests, a therapeutic program could be implemented at an earlier stage of decline and perhaps be more effective in reducing further impairment.

Directions: Query the participant regarding his/her extent of physical activity using the activity descriptors below as well as established metabolic tables for physical activity.

A. No regular participation in programmed recreational sport or physical activity:
0 = avoid walking or exertion (always use elevator, drive whenever possible instead of walking.)
1 = pleasure slow walking, routinely use stairs, occasionally heavy breathing or perspiration

B. Regular participation modest/moderate physical activity (e.g. golf, horseback riding, calisthenics, gymnastics, table tennis, bowling, weight lifting, yard work etc):
2 = 10 to 60 minutes per week
3 = over one hour per week

C. Regular participation in heavy physical exercise (e.g. jogging, running, swimming, cycling, rowing, skipping rope, running in place, tennis, basketball, or handball etc.):
4 = run less than 1 mile per week or spend less than 30 minutes per week in comparable heavy physical activity
5 = run 1 to 5 miles per week or spend 30 to 60 minutes per week in comparable heavy physical activity
6 = run 5 to 10 miles per week or spend 1 to 3 hours per week in comparable heavy physical activity
7 = run over 10 miles per week or spend over 3 hours per week in comparable heavy physical activity

Table 3. Physical Activity Rating Scale (PARS; Baumgartner and Jackson, 1995).

There are also scanner issues to deal with when a study design goes from a single acute scan to repeated scans over several months or years. Your scanner must be intra-reliable (i.e, a measure today will yield relatively the same results tomorrow). It is well known among neuroimaging technicians that scanners "drift" over time, therefore it is important to keep track of the drift so you can be sure changes that are seen months from the initial scan are corrected for the drift. Along these same lines, in order to get larger sample sizes, multiple sites may be needed. Therefore all the scanners used must be determined to be inter-reliable. This is generally accomplished with phantom testing.

It is equally important to account for individual brain plasticity - the investigator must understand the normal brain changes over time independent of any treatment so that intervention changes seen can be distinguished from random occurrence or normal aging.

Lastly, dehydration is an issue that only recently has begun to be accounted for in neuroimaging research studies. Care must be taken to ensure the research volunteers are euhydrated, otherwise, the question that may arise when a brain volume increase is reported: Is the increase in brain volume "true"? Or is it due to dehydration known to plague not only the elderly but also exercisers who exercise in a hot environment and may not have hydrated sufficiently? A simple way to account for hydration status is to obtain a urine sample and test it for urine specific gravity using either a dip stick (aka chem. strip) or a small handheld refractometer. A non-smelly light straw-colored urine would suggest the person was adequately hydrated. If a more precise objective measure is needed, the urine specific gravity reading should be between 1.010 to 1.020 (Armstrong et al., 1998).

10. Conclusions

Aerobic fitness not only facilitates improved oxygen delivery and utilization in the cardio-cerebral vascular systems, improved oxidative capacity has been shown to up-regulate expression of important neuronal growth factors such as insulin-like growth factor I (IGF-I), brain-derived neurotrophic factor (BDNF) and related protein precursors in animal models (Ding et al., 2006; van Praag et al., 2005). Furthermore, aerobic fitness may mediate improved cerebral white matter integrity via the intricate adaptations that take place on the neural-humoral level during exercise (Marks et al., 2010). Therefore, exercise outcome studies trials need to include not only structural imaging detailed in this paper, but also hormonal measurements and perfusion imaging.

In summary, the research questions that remain to be answered are: What is a sufficient exercise dose for the brain? How much, or how little, exercise is really needed to maintain brain structure and cognitive function? Will any type of physical activity do? Will the resultant health recommendations for the brain be complementary to the current guidelines for cardiovascular health?

To move the future of brain training research forward, we must continue to revisit the past ground-breaking cardiovascular research studies and modify them for the brain. Ancient physicians and philosophers like Hippocrates and Cicero espoused the benefits of exercising both the body and the mind, and here we are, 2,000 years later, scientifically documenting the neurobiological benefits of exercise. Several investigators have been using a few standard cardiovascular disease risk reduction guidelines with success in maintaining brain volume in older adults, but so many more exercise options remain to be explored. Hopefully it will not take another 50 years to firmly establish exercise guidelines for maintaining and enhancing brain health with exercise.

11. Acknowledgment

The University of North Carolina at Chapel Hill's Libraries provided support for open access publication.

12. References

Allen, J.S., Damasio, H., Grabowskia, T.J., Brussa, J. and Zhang, W. (2003). Sexual dimorphism and asymmetries in the gray–white composition of the human cerebrum, *NeuroImage*, 18:880-894

American College of Sports Medicine. (2009). *ACSM's Guidelines for Exercise Testing and Prescription*, 8th Edition, New York: Lippincott, Williams and Wilkins

American College of Sports Medicine. (1990). The recommended quantity and quality of exercise for developing and maintaining cardiorespiratory and muscular fitness in healthy adults. *Med Sci Sports Exerc*, 22:265-274

Armstrong, L.E., Soto, J.A., Hacker, F.T., Casa, D.J., Kavouras, S.A., Maresh, C.M. (1998). Urinary indices during dehydration, exercise, and rehydration. *Int. J. Sport Nutr.* 8: 345-355

Borg GAV. (1985). *An introduction to Borg's RPE Scale*. Ithaca, NY:Movement Publications.

Baumgartner, T.A. & Jackson, A.S. (1995). *Measurement for Evaluation in Physical Education and Exercise Science*, (p. 289) Brown & Benchmark Publ., Madison:WI

Bullitt E, Zeng D, Ghosh A, Aylward SR, E, Lin W, Marks BL, Smith K. (2010). The effects of healthy aging on intracranial blood vessels visualized by magnetic resonance angiography. *Neurobiology of Aging*, 31:290-300

Bullitt E, FN Rahman, JK Smith, E Kim, D Zeng, Katz LM, Marks, BL. (2009). The effect of exercise on the cerebral vasculature of healthy aged subjects as visualized by magnetic resonance angiography. *Am J Neuroradiol*, 30:1857-1863

Burns JM, Cronk BB, Anderson HS et al. (2008). Cardiorespiratory fitness and brain atrophy in early Alzheimer's disease. *Neurology*, 71:210-216

Caspersen CJ Powell KE, Christenson GM. (1985). Physical activity, exercise, and physical fitness: Definitions and distinctions for health-related research. *Public Health Reports*, 100:120-131

Colcombe SJ, Kramer AF. (2003). Fitness effects on the cognitive function of older adults: a meta-analytic study. *Psychol Sci*, 14:125-130

Colcombe SJ, Erickson KI, Scalf PE et al. (2006). Aerobic exercise training increases brain volume in aging humans. *J Gerontol-A Biol Sci Med Sci*, 61:1166-70

Cotman CW, Berchtold C, Christie L. (2007). Exercise builds brain health: key roles of growth factor cascades and inflammation. *Trends in Neuroscience*, 39:464-472

Coyle EF, Martin WH, Sinacore DR, Joyner MJ, Hagberg IM, Holloszy JO. (1984). Time course of loss of adapatations after stopping prolonged intense endurance training. *J Applied Physiology: Respiratory, Environmental and Exercise Physiology*, 57:1857-64

Crémers J, Dessoullières A, Garraux G (2011). Hemispheric specialization during mental imagery of brisk walking. *Hum Brain Mapp*, Mar 21. doi: 10.1002/hbm.21255. [Epub ahead of print] Last Accessed April 25, 2011

Cronk BB, Johnson DK, Burns JM. (2009). Body mass index and cognitive decline in mild cognitive impairment. *Alz Dis Assoc Dis.*, Epub Ahead of Print: 2009 June 30. PMED:19571736

Dennis NA & Cabeza R (2008). Neuroimaging of Healthy Cognitive Aging. In: *The Handbook of Aging and Cognition, 3rd Ed.* Ed: FIM Craik & TA Salthouse, pp. 1-54, Psychology Press, ISBN-13:978-0-8058-5990-4, New York

Ding, Q, Vaynman S, Akhavan M et al. (2006). Insulin-like growth factor I interfaces with brain-derived neurotrophic factor-mediated synaptic plasticity to modulate aspects of exercise-induced cognitive function. *Neuroscience*, 140:823-833

Driemeyer J, Boyke J, Gaser C, Buchel C, May A. Changes in gray matter induced learning-revisted. *PLoS ONE*, July 2008 Volume 3, Issue 7, e2669, www.plosone.org

Erickson KI, Prakash RS, Voss MW, Chaddock L, Hu L, Morris KS, White SM, Wójcicki TR, McAuley E, Kramer AF. (2009). Aerobic fitness is associated with hippocampal volume in elderly humans. *Hippocampus*, 19:1030-1039 doi:10.1002/hipo.20547 [published Online First: 2 January 2009]

Etnier JL, Nowell PM, Landers DM et al. (2006). A meta regression to examine the relationship between aerobic fitness and cognitive performance. *Brain Research Reviews*, 52:119-130

Ferris LT, William JS, Shen CL. (2007). The effect of acute exercise on serum brain-derived neurotrophic factor levels and cognition. *Med Sci Sports Exerc*, 39:728-734

Gunstad JP, Cohen RA,Tate DF, et al. (2008). Relationship between body mass index and brain volume in healthy adults. *Int J Neurosci*, 119:1582-1593

Gustafson D, Lissner, L, Bengtsson, C et al. (2004). A 24-year follow-up of body mass index and cerebral atrophy. *Neurology*, 63:1876-1881

Haier RJ, Karama S, Leyba L, Jung RE. MRI assessment of cortical thickness and functional activity changes in adolescent girls following three months of practice on a visual-spatial task. *BMC Research Notes*, 2009, 2:174 doi:10.1186/1756-0500-2-174. Published 1 September 2009

Haskell WL, Lee IM, Pate RR, et al. (2007). Physical activity and public health: updated recommendation from the American College of Sports Medicine and the American Heart Association. *Med Sci Sports Exerc.* 39:1423-34

Heyn P, Abreu BC, Ottenbacher KJ. (2004). The effects of exercise training on elderly persons with cognitive impairment and dementia: a meta analysis. *Arch Phys Med Rehabil*, 85:1694-1700

Jackson AS, Blair SN, Mahar MT, et al.(1990). Prediction of functional aerobic capacity without exercise testing. *Med Sci Sports Exerc*, 22:863-870

Kharti P, Blumenthal JA, Babyak MA, et al. (2001). Effects of exercise training on cognitive functioning among depressed older men and women. *J Aging and Physical Activity*, 9:43-57

Leasure JL, Jones M. (2008). Forced and voluntary exercise differentially affect brain and behavior. *Neuroscience*, 56:456-465

Liu Z, Zhu H, Marks, BL, Katz LM, Goodlett CB, Gerig G, Styner M. (2009). Voxel-wise group analysis of DTI. *IEEE International Symposium on Biomedial Imaging* (June 28-July 1, 2009, Boston, MA) Proceedings of the 6th IEEE International Symposium on Biomedical Imaging: From Nano to Macro, NA-MIC, June 2009; 807-810

Lommatzsch M, Zingler D, Schuhbaeck K, et al. (2005). The impact of age, weight and gender on BDNF levels in human platelets and plasma. *Neurobiology of Aging*, 26:115-23

Madden DJ, Bennett HJ, Song AW. (2009). Cerebral white matter integrity and cognitive aging: contributions from diffusion tensor imaging. Neuropsychol Rev. Epub Ahead of Print: 25 August 2009. doi 10.1007/s11065-009-9113-2

Marks BL, Katz LM, Styner M, Smith JK. (2010). Aerobic Fitness and Obesity: Relationship to Cerebral White Matter Integrity in the Brain of Active and Sedentary Older Adults. *British Journal of Sports Medicine*, online first, doi:10.1136/bjsm.2009.068114

Marks BL, Madden DJ, Bucur B, et al. (2007). Role of aerobic fitness and aging on cerebral white matter integrity. *Annals NY Acad Sci*, 1097:171-174

Marks, BL, Katz, LM, Nunley, DC, Neelon, V, Daniel, P. (2000). Cerebral blood flow and cognitive function is maintained in aerobically active older adults. *Circulation*, Suppl, 102(18): 4198

Meriam Webster Free Dictionary, http://www.merriam-webster.com/dictionary/exercise, last accessed April 23, 2011

Nieman, D. (2011). *Exercise Testing and Prescription, A Health Related Approach.* 7th Edition, New York:McGraw Hill

Orlandi G, Murri L. (1996). Transcranial doppler assessment of cerebral flow velocity at rest and during voluntary movements in young and elderly subjects. *Internat J Neurosci*, 84(1-4):45-53

Rahman, F, Smith K, Bullitt E, Marks B. (2008). Relationships between exercise and cerebral blood flow in older adults. American Society of Neuroradiology Conference, New Orleans, May 31 – June 5. Abstract ID: 6009535

Raji CA, Ho AJ, Parikshak NN, Becker JT, Lopez OL, Kuller LH, Hua X, Leow AD, Toga AW, Thompsom PM. (2009). Brain structure and obesity. *Human Brain Mapp*, Published Online First: 6 August 2009; doi: 10.1002/hbm.20870

Ross JS, Tkach J, Ruggieri PM, Lieber M, Lapresto E. (2003). The Mind's Eye: Functional MR imaging evaluation of golf motor imagery. *American Journal of Neuroradiology*, 24:1036-1044

Scheibel AB. (2009). Aging of the Brain, In: *Handbook of the Neuroscience of Aging, Ed: PR Hoff & CV Mobbs*, pp. 5-9, Academic Press, ISBN: 978-0-12-374898-0, New York:NY

Soreca I, Rosana C, Jennings R, et al. (2009). Gain in adiposity across 15 years is associated with reduced gray matter volume in healthy women. *Psychosom Med*, 71:485-490

Spirduso WW, Francis KL, MacRae PG. (2005). *Physical Dimensions of Aging*, 2nd Edition. Human Kinetics, Champaigne:IL

Stebbins GT, Murphy CM (2009). Diffusion tensor imaging in Alzheimer's disease and mild cognitive impairment. *Behav Neurol*, 21(1):39-49

US Department of Health and Human Services (USDHHS). 2008 Physical Activity Guideline for Americans. ODPHP Pub. No. U0036, October 2008
www.health.gov/paguidleines last accessed April 23, 2011

US Department of Health and Human Services (USDHHS). National Institutes of Health Research Portfolio Online Reporting Tools (RePORT)
http://projectreporter.nih.gov/reporter.cfm) Last accessed April 25, 2011

Ward M, Carlsson CM, Trivedi MA, Sager MA, Johnson SC. (2005). The effect of body mass index on global brain volume in middle-aged adults: a cross-sectional study. *BMC Neurol*, 5:23 doi:10.1186/1471-2377-5-23. [Published Online 2005 December 2]

Vachet C, Bullitt E, Katz L, Marks B, Davis B, Styner M. (2009). UNC Elderly Brain Atlas,
http://www.insight-journal.org/midas/item/view/2330 and
http://www.insight-journal.org/midas/gallery
In collection MIDAS/National Alliance for Medical Image Computing (NAMIC)/ NAMIC: Public Data Repository; NIH Neuroscience Roadmap Initiative

van Praag H, Christie BR, Sejnowski TJ, Gage FH. (1999). Running enhances neurogenesis, learning, and long-term potentiation in mice. *Proc Natl Acad Sci*, 96:13427-13431

Permissions

The contributors of this book come from diverse backgrounds, making this book a truly international effort. This book will bring forth new frontiers with its revolutionizing research information and detailed analysis of the nascent developments around the world.

We would like to thank Dr. Peter Bright, for lending his expertise to make the book truly unique. He has played a crucial role in the development of this book. Without his invaluable contribution this book wouldn't have been possible. He has made vital efforts to compile up to date information on the varied aspects of this subject to make this book a valuable addition to the collection of many professionals and students.

This book was conceptualized with the vision of imparting up-to-date information and advanced data in this field. To ensure the same, a matchless editorial board was set up. Every individual on the board went through rigorous rounds of assessment to prove their worth. After which they invested a large part of their time researching and compiling the most relevant data for our readers. Conferences and sessions were held from time to time between the editorial board and the contributing authors to present the data in the most comprehensible form. The editorial team has worked tirelessly to provide valuable and valid information to help people across the globe.

Every chapter published in this book has been scrutinized by our experts. Their significance has been extensively debated. The topics covered herein carry significant findings which will fuel the growth of the discipline. They may even be implemented as practical applications or may be referred to as a beginning point for another development. Chapters in this book were first published by InTech; hereby published with permission under the Creative Commons Attribution License or equivalent.

The editorial board has been involved in producing this book since its inception. They have spent rigorous hours researching and exploring the diverse topics which have resulted in the successful publishing of this book. They have passed on their knowledge of decades through this book. To expedite this challenging task, the publisher supported the team at every step. A small team of assistant editors was also appointed to further simplify the editing procedure and attain best results for the readers.

Our editorial team has been hand-picked from every corner of the world. Their multi-ethnicity adds dynamic inputs to the discussions which result in innovative outcomes. These outcomes are then further discussed with the researchers and contributors who give their valuable feedback and opinion regarding the same. The feedback is then collaborated with the researches and they are edited in a comprehensive manner to aid the understanding of the subject.

Apart from the editorial board, the designing team has also invested a significant amount of their time in understanding the subject and creating the most relevant covers. They scrutinized every image to scout for the most suitable representation of the subject and create an appropriate cover for the book.

The publishing team has been involved in this book since its early stages. They were actively engaged in every process, be it collecting the data, connecting with the contributors or procuring relevant information. The team has been an ardent support to the editorial, designing and production team. Their endless efforts to recruit the best for this project, has resulted in the accomplishment of this book. They are a veteran in the field of academics and their pool of knowledge is as vast as their experience in printing. Their expertise and guidance has proved useful at every step. Their uncompromising quality standards have made this book an exceptional effort. Their encouragement from time to time has been an inspiration for everyone.

The publisher and the editorial board hope that this book will prove to be a valuable piece of knowledge for researchers, students, practitioners and scholars across the globe.

List of Contributors

Lazaros C. Triarhou
University of Macedonia, Thessaloniki, Greece

James Danckert
Dept of Psychology, University of Waterloo, Canada

Seyed M. Mirsattarri
Depts of CNS, Med Biophys, Med Imaging, & Psychology, University of Western Ontario, Canada

Manuel Martín-Loeches and Pilar Casado
Center UCM-ISCIII for Human Evolution and Behavior, UCM-ISCIII, Madrid, Spain

Fabrizio Esposito
Neurological Institute for Diagnosis and Care "Hermitage Capodimonte", Italy
Department of Neuroscience, University of Naples "Federico II", Italy
Department of Cognitive Neuroscience, Maastricht University, The Nethelands

Gioacchino Tedeschi
Department of Neurological Sciences, Second University of Naples, Italy
Neurological Institute for Diagnosis and Care "Hermitage Capodimonte", Italy

Satoru Yokoyama
Tohoku University, Japan

Joshua Goh
National Institute on Aging, Baltimore, MD, USA

Chih-Mao Huang
University of Illinois, Urbana-Champaign, IL USA

Nobuhisa Kanahara, Eiji Shimizu, Yoshimoto Sekine and Masaomi Iyo
Chiba University, Japan

Roumen Kirov and
Institute of Neurobiology, Bulgarian Academy of Sciences, Bulgaria

Serge Brand
Depression Research Unit, Psychiatric Hospital of the University of Basel, Switzerland

Silvia Marino, Rosella Ciurleo, Annalisa Baglieri, Francesco Corallo, Rosaria De Luca, Simona De Salvo, Silvia Guerrera, Francesca Timpano, Placido Bramanti and Nicola De Stefano
IRCCS Centro Neurolesi "Bonino-Pulejo", Messina, Dept. of Neurology, Neurosurgery & Behavioral Sciences, University of Siena, Siena, Italy

Trevor Archer
Department of Psychology, University of Gothenburg, Gothenburg, Sweden

Peter Bright
Department of Psychology, Anglia Ruskin University, East Road, Cambridge, UK

Bonita L. Marks and Laurence M. Katz
University of North Carolina at Chapel Hill, USA

9 781632 411822

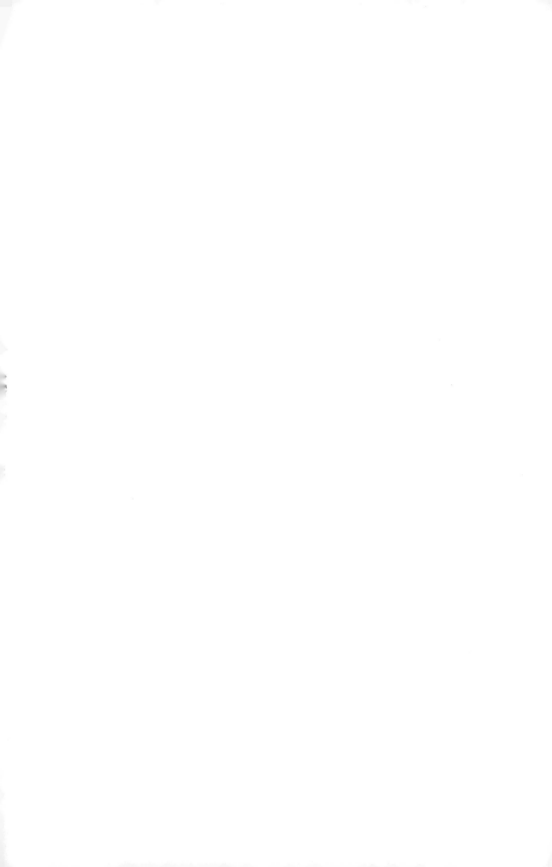